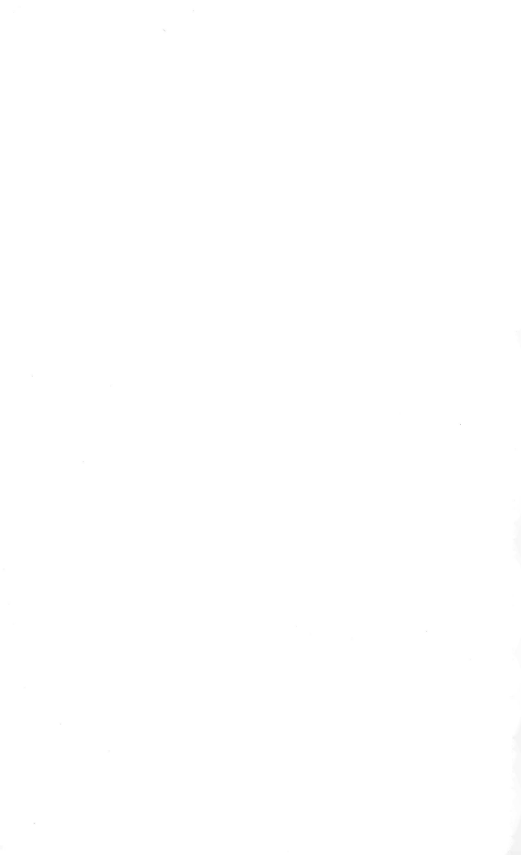

Disease and Discovery

Disease and Discovery

A History of the
Johns Hopkins School
of Hygiene and Public Health,
1916–1939

Elizabeth Fee

Johns Hopkins University Press
Baltimore

Johns Hopkins University Press
2715 North Charles Street
Baltimore, Maryland 21218
www.press.jhu.edu

Library of Congress Cataloging-in-Publication Data for the 1987 edition

Fee, Elizabeth.
Disease and discovery.

Bibliography: p.
Includes index.
1. Johns Hopkins University. School of Hygiene and Public Health—
History   2. Public health—Study and teaching—United States—
History.   3. Public health—Research—United States—History.   I. Title.
[DNLM: 1. Johns Hopkins University. School of Hygiene and Public
Health.   2. Schools, Public Health—history—Maryland. WA 19 F295d]
RA440.7.U62M34   1987   610'.7'1175271   86-46277
ISBN 0-8018-3460-0 (alk. paper)

ISBN-13 978-1-4214-2110-0
ISBN-10 1-4214-2110-0

Special discounts are available for bulk purchases of this book. For more information, please contact Special Sales at 410-516-6936 or specialsales@press.jhu.edu.

Johns Hopkins University Press uses environmentally friendly book materials, including recycled text paper that is composed of at least 30 percent post-consumer waste, whenever possible.

To my father

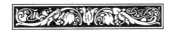

Contents

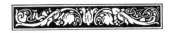

List of Illustrations

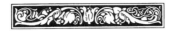

Preface

I began to examine the history of the School of Hygiene and Public Health because I wanted to understand the institution in which I was working. I also wanted to convince students of public health that history, even if neither scientific nor statistical, could give them important insights into the nature of their field and provide a medium for critical reflection on their own work and purposes of study. Over the several years of research and writing leading to the production of this book, I have had strong support from Dean D. A. Henderson, the late Abraham Lilienfeld, and the other members of the School of Hygiene faculty. The members of the school history committee—D. A. Henderson, Abraham Lilienfeld, Ernest Stebbins, Lloyd Stevenson, Genevieve Miller, Roger Herriott, and Jacqueline Corn—were particularly helpful in encouraging the project. The chapters on the history of the School of Hygiene in Thomas B. Turner's *Heritage of Excellence* (Baltimore: Johns Hopkins University Press, 1974) provided the starting point for my research.

I am grateful to Karen Davis, Barbara Starfield, and the faculty and students of the Division of Health Policy for providing a supportive intellectual and academic environment in which to work. They have encouraged a diversity of approaches to understanding the critical health issues of our time and cheerfully assented to the proposition that historical studies could make important contributions to the research and teaching program in health policy. Vicente Navarro has been especially helpful as a friend and colleague in challenging me to think more carefully about the politics of public health.

Many individuals have been generous with their time in sharing with me their knowledge of different aspects of the history of the school and its development. I am especially grateful to Margaret Merrell, Anne Clark Rodman, Susan Frost Parrish, Abel Wolman, Anna Baetjer, Roger Herriott, Morton Kramer, Paul Lemkau, Ernestine McCollum,

Agatha Rider, Lloyd Rozeboom, Lydia Arden, Philip Sartwell, Huntington Williams, Gerald Winfield, Carl Taylor, Arthur Bushel, Edward Kupka, Marie Koch, George Comstock, Ernest Stebbins, Noel Rose, and Gert Brieger for their assistance. Members of the alumni will forgive me if I do not mention individually the many people who have shared their memories of the school in its earlier days; some of their contributions are noted in the references, and all were helpful in expanding my understanding of the history of the school as lived experience.

Many librarians and archivists have been helpful in researching the written records of the school. I would especially like to thank A. McGehee Harvey, Nancy McCall, and Gerard Shorb, of the Alan Mason Chesney Medical Archives, the Johns Hopkins Medical Institutions; Julia Morgan, of the Hamburger Archives, the Johns Hopkins University, Baltimore, Maryland; and Tom Rosenbaum, of the Rockefeller Archive Center at Pocantico Hills, Tarrytown, New York. Susan Frost Parrish and Anne Clark Rodman were generous in sharing their private collections of papers, photographs, and other unpublished documents.

I would like to thank the Rockefeller Archive Center of the Rockefeller University for a research grant that enabled me to spend several happy and productive weeks at the Rockefeller Archive Center examining their splendid collection of historical documents. A research grant from the Program in Ethics and Values in Science and Technology of the National Science Foundation and the National Endowment for the Humanities, though not directly supporting this project, enabled me to work with a rich source of ideas and information about the history of public health and the issues of professional public health education.

My students at the School of Hygiene have provided an attentive, encouraging, and critical audience for many parts of this study. Greg Silsbee cheerfully combed through voluminous administrative records during the early stages of this project; in the later stages, Ruth Finkelstein has been a delightful friend and a most thoughtful and creative editor during the process of manuscript revision. Ann Pritchard-Smith has lived with this project from the beginning and has been an invaluable assistant in all stages of my work. I would also like to thank Gert Brieger, Daniel Todes, Noel Rose, Abel Wolman, Thomas B. Turner, Vicente Navarro, and Roger Herriott for their helpful suggestions on drafts of the manuscript, and Wendy Harris, of the Johns Hopkins University Press, for her gentle and patient editorial direction.

Disease and Discovery

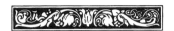

Introduction

his book tells the story of the founding, organization, and early development of the Johns Hopkins School of Hygiene and Public Health. As the first independent, degree-granting institution for research and training in public health, the School of Hygiene was crucial to the process of professionalization of public health in the United States. As a leading research center, it helped shape the form and content of public health by developing new scientific knowledge, generating organized research, and training highly educated personnel to put this knowledge into practice. As a center for training international public health officers, it influenced the development of public health activities around the world. The first and largest of a series of national and international schools of public health funded by the Rockefeller Foundation, the Hopkins school would be the model for those that followed. It was empowered to define the meaning of a "good scientific education" for public health professionals.

In the late nineteenth century, public health was institutionalized in city and state health departments, but few public health officers had any specialized training in the field. They were usually given paid part-time positions through political patronage; they could be promoted or removed from office on the basis of their political alliances and personal friendships. Some of these political appointees were remarkably dedicated and effective; others attempted and achieved little. Any knowledge they might have of public health principles was fortuitous, the result of independent study and practical experience. A few of the better medical schools offered courses in public health or preventive medicine but there was neither standardized training nor were there any recognized credentials necessary to practice public health. Most public health officers had medical degrees, but some were engineers and others were lawyers, chemists, or biologists. Indeed, there was little agreement

1

about the kinds of knowledge necessary or desirable for public health practice.

In that preprofessional period, public health was still largely the province of amateurs and gentlemen; voluntary groups dedicated to a wide variety of social and health reforms often goaded reluctant officials into activity. Thus, the reform commitments of the voluntary groups and the political interests of appointed officials shaped public health activities more directly than did scientific knowledge. Scientific theory might be used as a debating weapon by either side in a struggle, but it was hardly an essential factor. Most important were the political and economic interests of those involved and the energy and enthusiasm with which they defended those interests.

Since that time, a complex and problematic relationship between medicine and public health has structured the history of the professionalization of public health. Medicine and public health are intimately related, often overlapping, and yet they also have contradictory interests. Public health is oriented toward the analysis of the determinants of health and disease on a population basis, while medicine is oriented toward individual patients. Public health professionals are usually dependent on government-funded salaried positions, while physicians—at least in the past—have been independent professionals and entrepreneurs involved in private practice. The economic organization of the two fields has been as different as their methods and perspectives, despite the fact that both deal with the basic problems of human health and disease.

Public health and medicine do not stand in a relationship of equality. Whatever opinion one may hold of their relative social importance and moral legitimacy, there can be little doubt that clinical medicine is the more wealthy and powerful of the two. Where the two enterprises directly compete for resources, medicine usually has the advantage. As the weaker partner in an uneasy marriage, public health strives for autonomy and independence from medicine, while at the same time desiring the stronger partner's status and protection. The two are irrevocably linked, unable either to merge or become completely independent. The tension between them can be the source of problems, confusions, and also creativity: for public health, this tension structures the fundamental unresolved issues of the profession.

A second complex and problematic question for public health is the relationship between technical knowledge and politics. When public health developed as a profession during the progressive era of American politics, its leaders intended a dual commitment to scientific knowledge and social reform. The scientific disciplines constituting public health would be used to improve health conditions, solve practical problems, and shield public health professionals from direct political interference. The mantle of scientific legitimacy could protect against the interference of local political groups whose interests might be challenged; the commitment to social reform on a scientific basis would provide a safer alternative to the revolutionary ideas of the socialists. On the other hand, public health professionals could not be completely independent of politics if they wished to be effective: the planning, organization, and implementation of public health programs required political skills and sensitivity, and, furthermore, their success was largely dependent on larger social, political, and economic currents. The boundaries of public health were fluid: the contours of the field changed over time with the perception of new health and social problems and with political, economic, and ideological shifts within the government and the nation.

The process of defining and redefining public health in the early twentieth century is the central and continuing theme of this book. As in other professions, the organization of research and training helped define the content and practice of the field; as public health became both scientific and professional, its boundaries were drawn by specific modes of attaining knowledge. Scientific training and new credentials allowed public health professionals to distance themselves from the volunteers and amateurs; it also gave them a claim to more secure positions, less political interference, and better pay. It provided a set of methods for producing new knowledge and, often, a preference for the rarefied atmosphere of the laboratory over the dust of city streets.

The creation of public health as a profession—however incomplete the process—was part of a deliberate plan and strategy. We can now look back at specific decisions taken and, with the benefit of hindsight, evaluate their results. In 1914, a small number of public health leaders, meeting by invitation of the General Education Board of the Rockefeller Foundation, identified the need to create formal institutions to train public health personnel; they sketched the broad outlines of the public health education of the future. William Henry Welch and Wickliffe Rose refined these ideas, each inserting his own favored emphasis, in their famous report of 1915. Welch then worked out the implementation of these ideas in a series of negotiations between the Johns Hopkins University and representatives of the Rockefeller Foundation; the men selected for the first professorships in the new school would bring their own interests to working out the details of the plan.

The public health leaders and foundation representatives involved in planning the future of public health education set themselves three main tasks: to remove public health from direct political control, to define the necessary knowledge base for public health practice, and to outline the educational system needed to train a new profession. They were successful in each of these tasks. After the advent of formal professional education, legal restrictions and public expectations would compel city and state health departments to appoint new personnel on the basis of their training and qualifications rather than solely on political influence or personal friendships. The independence of public health from politics could at best be relative, since public health must always be practiced within the context of politics; professional education did, however, give public health officials partial protection from sabotage by slighted local interests. The political struggles of public health were now played out on the national and international stage, rather than the local one.

The second task in planning public health education, to define the necessary knowledge base for public health practice, meant deciding the specific disciplines and skills required. In the early years of the twentieth century, few physicians had any knowledge of bacteriology or sanitary engineering, much less of occupational or environmental health, epidemiology or statistics. After the establishment of schools of public health, public health officials could be expected to have at least some knowledge of these areas, and to be aware of the range of techniques available for public health investigations. The question of what level of skills and training should be required was not a matter of one simple solution, but of ongoing negotiation involving continuous confrontations between intellectual ideals and social reality.

Public health reformers were committed to the idea that public health activities should be planned along scientific lines by a scientifically trained elite, and not left either to the good intentions of amateurs or to changing political pressures and special interests. Public health, they thought, was too important to be left to chance. Social, political, and economic benefits would follow from a new, scientific public health. Trained public health professionals would solve the worst social and health problems of industrial cities, raise the health status of agricultural laborers, mitigate extremes of wealth and poverty, raise levels of productivity and efficiency, and conserve human resources, the source of national wealth. When the federal government was slow to act, the great foundations, and especially the Rockefeller Foundation, took the lead in organizing public health programs and professional public health education.

The men who guided the foundations had an elite vision of social reform. They believed that social improvements could best be implemented by starting at the top; their philosophy was to "make the peaks higher." The reform of medical education, for example, proceeded by funding the strongest institutions while using them as the standard by which to evaluate all others, rather than by trying to help weaker institutions reach an acceptable level of performance. In public health, this philosophy meant creating specialized institutions to provide advanced training for those already highly qualified, rather than providing educational resources for those whose previous training and skills were deficient. They believed that the best way to raise the general standard of public health programs was to provide the best possible education to their leaders.

Who should be the future leaders of public health? What should be the relationship of public health to the medical profession? At the time, there were several possibilities for organizing public health education. One option was to regard public health as a unique amalgam of the biomedical, engineering, and social sciences, requiring administrative talents and political skills, but not specifying any one background as preferred. As an alternative, some suggested public health be regarded as a combination of sanitary engineering and bacteriology, so that engineers and physicians would each bring specific qualifications to the field. A third viewpoint regarded public health as mainly a problem of social reform and social organization, drawing on a range of technical skills as appropriate, but not enveloping the field in any one scientific discipline. Finally, public health could be regarded as a specialized branch of medicine, drawing on physicians' knowledge of disease processes, diagnosis, and therapy. Physicians claimed to make a special contribution to public health, but so did other groups, including chemists, nurses, engineers, lawyers, bacteriologists, and statisticians. How should these rival claims be adjudicated and combined into a single profession?

The question of the relationship of public health to other disciplines and professional groups was simultaneously the question of the content and methods of the newly defined field. Should public health deal mainly with "pathological hygiene"—the study of specific diseases—or with "physiological hygiene"—the study of the general conditions promoting human health? Should public health identify closely with bacteriology and the successes of the germ theory of disease, or should it seek a broader definition, trying to understand the influence of social, economic, and environmental conditions on the health of individuals? These questions were related to others. Should human health and disease be studied in the laboratory or in houses, factories, and fields? Should an investigator begin with the biological study of infectious organisms or with the living conditions and habits of their human hosts?

What was the proper relationship between laboratory and "field" studies? Should the human experience of health and disease pose the questions to be studied in the laboratory or was the social experience of disease only relevant to test conclusions developed by laboratory research? Were the social sciences of fundamental importance to understanding the definition, patterns, and distribution of health and disease, or were they more of an afterthought qualifying the serious business of biological research? If public health constituted the study of disease in society, how much attention should be devoted to disease and how much to society?

The tensions between public health and medicine and between the social and biological approaches to health were fundamental in the design of public health education. A series of other related, but not identical tensions also structured the debates about public health education. The first was the debate about the relative importance of advanced education for the few versus minimal training for the majority of practitioners. These issues mirrored similar questions being raised in other professions, such as the debate whether engineers would be better trained on the shop floor or in the academy. Those advocating the position that training efforts should be directed at practicing public health officers wanted short courses, correspondence courses, and extension courses rather than lengthy full-time degree programs, so that people already working in the field would have access to some specialized education.

The second issue, related to the first, was whether educational programs should concentrate on research and research methods—the means of developing new knowledge—or on the more practical skills needed in running a health department, planning an immunization campaign, or establishing a new clinic. Those advocating a research-oriented education argued that the demands of practice were constantly changing so that education in specific methods would soon be outdated; research training provided the basic scientific principles to deal with a wide range of specific problems. Those arguing for more practically oriented programs maintained that scientific research, however valuable, was not the main need of health departments: more important were organizational and administrative skills. Practical training advocates felt that the most urgent task was to implement existing public health knowledge rather than to devote resources to research.

The proponents of practical, administrative training cited the English model of public health education; several British universities offered a year-long program oriented toward practical and administrative skills in public health. Those advocating the research-oriented model of education referred to the German institutes of hygiene as their model. These specialized institutes, attached to several German universities, were devoted to research rather than practical public health training. In the debates about the orientation of public health education in America, the term "public health" referred to the English administrative model, while "hygiene" implied the German orientation to research.

A third related issue in public health education was the relative importance placed on providing mass education to the general public. Most agreed in principle that public education in the broadest sense was important in improving the public's health, but they differed in their emphasis on popular education. Those oriented toward specialized education and research tended to give a lower priority to popular health education than the advocates of practical training programs. These issues were not, however, synonymous, and some laboratory researchers were ardent proponents of popular education.

These major themes recur frequently in the history of public health education; they are never completely settled, but are continuously debated and negotiated. This book is intended to contribute to contemporary discussions of these and similar questions by placing them in their historical context and introducing some of the men and women who framed early, influential answers.

The first chapter sketches the last nineteenth-century movement toward the professionalization of public health, thus providing the immediate context for the decision to establish specialized schools for public health education. The second chapter focuses on the process of planning for the first schools of public health and the consequent competition among leading universities for the endowment funds offered by the Rockefeller Foundation. The third discusses the process of negotiation between William Henry Welch and representatives of the International Health Board over the structure and purpose of the new school at the Johns Hopkins University, the selection of faculty and students, and the organization of the curriculum. The fourth and fifth chapters outline the early development of the scientific disciplines and departments within the school; following the first curriculum plan, these are organized into physiological hygiene and pathological hygiene. The problems faced during the depression and the new directions taken in adapting to a changed social environment are the subjects of the sixth chapter. The seventh examines new moves into community-based applied research including the establishment of the Eastern Health District in Baltimore for population-based studies and field training. The final chapter shows how the model of education established at Hopkins was extended in the creation of other national and international schools of public health. Here are raised again some of the basic questions and themes of public health education in the early decades of the twentieth century. These themes have shaped and in turn have been reshaped by more recent experience in the field of public health.

This volume ends in 1939. In the history of public health education, World War II marks a watershed between the first period when the schools of public health were established, largely on the basis of private funding, and the period after the war when the stimulus of federal grant support dramatically expanded research and training efforts. The content and focus of public health in the postwar period extended into many new areas, including medical care organization, occupational and environmental health, the epidemiology of chronic diseases, international health, and population planning programs. These later developments will be the subject of a subsequent volume; here, I am concerned with the intellectual and organizational issues of professional public health education in the earlier decades of this century, as reflected in the Hopkins experience.

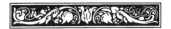

Toward a New Profession of Public Health

n the United States, before the twentieth century, there were few formal requirements for public health positions, no established career structures, no job security for health officials, and no formalized ways of producing new knowledge. Public health positions were usually part-time appointments at nominal salary; those who devoted much effort to public health typically did so on a voluntary basis. Until the mid–nineteenth century, public health, like other governmental functions, was usually the responsibility of the social elite. The public health officer was expected to be a "statesman" acting in the public interest, not a "politician" answering to a class constituency; men of independent property and wealth were believed to be independent of special interests and therefore capable of disinterested judgment. (Only in places with large immigrant populations, like New York City, did machine politicians confront this traditional view with an alternative, organized base of local control.)

Charles Rosenberg has eloquently described an earlier conception of both poverty and disease as consequences of moral failure at the individual and social level.[1] Disease attacked the dirty, the improvident, the intemperate, the ignorant; the clean, the pious, and the virtuous tended to escape. Until the mid-nineteenth century, epidemic diseases were thus seen as the consequence of a failure to obey the laws of nature and of God: they were the indicators of social and moral dissolution. As cleanliness was linked to Godliness, virtue was an essential qualification for managing the state; the conscientious, the respectable, the educated, and the affluent were naturally qualified for public office. Physicians were frequently chosen as public health officers, but lawyers or gentlemen of independent means could also be appointed.

Public health programs, when organized at all, were organized locally. As Robert Wiebe has argued, the United States in the early nineteenth century was a society of "island communities" with considerable economic and political autonomy.[2] The first public health organizations were those of the rapidly growing port cities of the eastern seaboard in the late eighteenth century. Here, the American Republic intersected with the world of international trade. Local authorities tried to protect the population from the threat of potentially catastrophic epidemic diseases, such as the yellow fever epidemic that crippled Philadelphia in 1793, while they also tried to maintain the conditions for successful economic activity.[3]

Public health in this period was largely a police function. Traditionally, port cities had dealt with epidemics by means of quarantine regulations, keeping ships suspected of carrying disease in harbor for up to forty days. However, quarantine regulations clearly interfered with shipping, and were energetically opposed by those whose economic interests were tied to trade.[4] Opponents of quarantine argued that diseases were internally generated by the filthy conditions of the docks, streets, and alleys that provided an ideal environment for "putrefactive fermentation." City health departments attempted to regulate the worst offenders: graveyards, tallow chandleries, tanneries, sugar boilers, skin dressers, dyers, glue boilers, and slaughterhouses; to clean the privies and alleys; and to remove dead animals and decaying vegetable matter from the streets and public spaces.[5]

The causes of disease were much disputed by those who believed that diseases were brought in from overseas, and thus should be fought by quarantine regulations, and those who believed that diseases were internally generated and should therefore be fought by cleaning up the cities. Evidence was marshaled to support both sides of the debate. Health regulations, however, were written and revised more in response to political pressures than to shifts in scientific thinking. Quarantine regulations were alternately relaxed in response to pressure from merchants and strengthened under the immediate threat of epidemics.

Periodically, the dread of yellow fever, plague, and cholera galvanized city authorities into action. The more common endemic diseases with less spectacular lethal capacities—typhoid fever, typhus, smallpox, measles, diphtheria, influenza, tuberculosis, and malaria— were met with a stolid indifference born of familiarity and a sense of helplessness. For these diseases, little was done beyond attempts to maintain general cleanliness, backed up by prayer, fasting, and exhortations to virtue.[6]

The Civil War enforced a national consciousness of epidemic disease:

two-thirds of the 360,000 Union soldiers who died were killed by infectious diseases rather than by enemy bullets.[7] The ravages of dysentery, spread by inadequate or nonexistent sanitary facilities, were appalling. The United States Sanitary Commission, a voluntary organization inspired by Florence Nightingale's work in the Crimean War, promoted the health of the Union Army by inspecting army camps, distributing educational materials, and providing nursing care and supplies for the wounded.

By 1860, public health activities were just beginning to move beyond the confines of local city politics. Between 1857 and 1860, quarantine and sanitary conventions were held in Philadelphia, Baltimore, New York, and Boston.[8] The first state board of health, largely a paper organization, had been created in Louisiana in 1855. In the 1870s and 1880s, however, most of the states created their own boards of health. The first working state health board was formed in Massachusetts in 1869, followed by California (1870), the District of Columbia (1871), Virginia and Minnesota (1872), Maryland (1874), and Alabama (1875).[9] The impact of these state boards of health should not, however, be overemphasized; by 1900, only three states (Massachusetts, Rhode Island, and Florida) spent more than two cents per capita for public health services.[10]

As state boards of health were organizing, public health reformers also urged the formation of a national health board. In 1879, a disastrous yellow fever epidemic, sweeping up the Mississippi Valley from New Orleans, prompted the United States Congress to create a National Board of Health consisting of seven physicians and one representative each from the Army, the Navy, the Marine Hospital Service, and the Department of Justice. Responsible for formulating quarantine regulations among the states, the National Board of Health soon became embroiled in fierce battles over states' rights. In 1883, it was disbanded, and quarantine powers reverted to the Marine Hospital Service. Gradually, the Marine Hospital Service expanded its public health activities into public health research. In 1887, it set aside a single room as a "hygienic laboratory," which was gradually expanded into an important center for investigation of the infectious diseases.[11]

After the Civil War, northern industrialists had begun the process of transforming the country into a single national market. Agricultural and industrial mechanization irrevocably altered the traditional patterns of production and consumption; railroad companies competed to cross the country with railroad lines; small companies merged and collapsed into large corporations. Between 1860 and 1894, the value of manufactured goods multiplied by five. The United States was moving into first place as the most powerful industrial country in the world, bypassing England, Germany, and France.

The belief that epidemic diseases posed only occasional threats to an otherwise healthy social order was shaken by the industrial transformation of the late nineteenth century. The burgeoning social problems of the industrial cities could not be ignored: the overwhelming influx of immigrants crowded into narrow alleys and tenement housing, the terrifying death and disease rates of working-class slums, the total inadequacy of water supplies and sewage systems for the rapidly growing population, the spread of endemic and epidemic diseases from the slums to the homes of the wealthy, the escalating squalor and violence of the streets. Almost all families lost children to diphtheria, smallpox, or other infectious diseases. Poverty and disease could no longer be treated simply as individual failings.

The early efforts of city health department officials to deal with health problems represented some attempt to mitigate the worst effects of unplanned and unregulated growth: a kind of rearguard action against the filth and congestion created by anarchic economic and urban development.[12] As cities grew in size, as the flow of immigrants con-

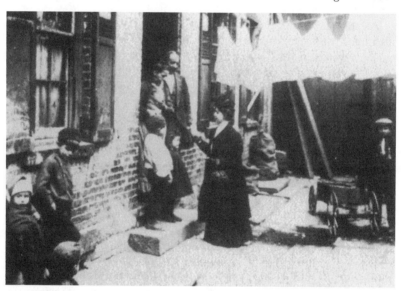

Figure 1. A public health nurse greeting her clients at the door of a tenement building in New York City, 1895. (Courtesy of the New York City Department of Health. Photo reproduced from the Slide Archive of Historical Medical Photographs, Health Sciences Library, State University of New York at Stony Brook.)

tinued, and as public health problems became ever more obvious, pressures mounted for more effective responses to the problems. New York, the largest city, and the one with some of the worst health conditions, produced some of the most active and progressive public health leaders; Boston and Providence were also noted for their public health programs; Baltimore and Philadelphia trailed far behind.[13]

Industrialization had meant new sources of affluence as well as of misery. America no longer fit its self-image of a country of independent farmers and craftsmen; like the European countries, it displayed extremes of wealth and privilege, social misery and deprivation. Labor and social unrest pushed awareness of the need for social and health reforms. The great railroad strike of 1877, the assassination of President Garfield in 1881, the Haymarket bombing of 1886, the Homestead strike of 1892, and the Pullman strike of 1894 were just a few of the reminders that all was not well with the Republic. The Noble Order of the Knights of Labor—dedicated to such measures as an income tax, an eight-hour day, social insurance, labor exchanges for the unemployed, the abolition of child labor, workmen's compensation, and public ownership of railroads and utilities—grew from a membership of 11 to over 700,000 within a few years. Massive strikes for better wages and working conditions revealed deep class divisions and seemed to threaten social stability. At the same time, the development of democratic machine politics challenged the dominance of the political and social elite, permitting some labor leaders to establish local bases of influence and power. The perceived social anarchy of the large industrial cities mocked the pretensions to social control of the traditional forces of church and state, and highlighted the need for more activist responses to the many problems.

An increasing number of reform groups devoted themselves to social issues and improvements of every variety. Health reformers, physicians, and engineers urged improved sanitary conditions in the industrial cities. Medical men were prominent in reform organizations, but they were not alone.[14] Barbara Rosenkrantz contrasted public health in the late nineteenth century with the internecine battles within general medicine: "The field of public hygiene exemplified a happy marriage of engineers, physicians, and public spirited citizens providing a model of complementary comportment under the banner of sanitary science."[15] The most formally organized and professional body, the American Public Health Association, was founded in 1872, and included scientists, municipal officials, physicians, engineers, and the occasional architect and lawyer.[16]

Middle- and upper-class women, seizing an opportunity to escape from the narrow binds of domestic responsibilities, joined in campaigns from improved housing, for the abolition of child labor, for maternal and child health, and for temperance; they were active in the settlement house movement, trade union organizing, the suffrage movement, and municipal sanitary reform. The last, as "municipal housekeeping," was viewed as particularly suitable for women, a natural extension of women's training and experience to become the housekeepers of the world.[17] These voluntary movements, organized to support specific issues, provided the organizational framework for many public health reforms. By the early years of the twentieth century, many voluntary health organizations were established and active.[18]

The progressive reform groups in the public health movement advocated immediate change tempered by scientific knowledge and humanitarian concern. Sharing the revolutionaries' perception of the plight of the poor and the injustices of the system, they counseled less radical solutions.[19] They urged public health reforms on political, economic, humanitarian, and scientific grounds. Politically, public health reform offered a middle ground between the cutthroat principles of entrepreneurial capitalism and the revolutionary ideas of the socialists, anarchists, and utopian visionaries. As William H. Welch expressed it to the Charity Organization Society, sanitary improvement offered the best way of improving the lot of the poor, short of the radical restructuring of society.[20]

The progressive reformers argued in economic terms that public health should be viewed as a paying investment, giving higher returns than the stock market. In Germany, Max von Pettenkofer had first calculated the financial returns on public health "investments" to prove the value of sanitary reform in reducing deaths from typhoid, and his argument was repeated many times by American public health leaders.[21] As Welch explained, "Merely from a mercenary and commercial point of view it is for the interest of the community to take care of the health of the poor. Philanthropy assumes a totally different aspect in the eyes of the world when it is able to demonstrate that it pays to keep people healthy."[22]

Whether progressives stressed the humanitarian need for reform or the business efficiency of improving public health, they emphasized the need for more scientific knowledge and training for those responsible for public health activities. They argued that public health should be a profession with appropriate training and income.

We hope that every local unit of government will have its health officer and that the iceman and the undertaker will not be considered suitable candidates, but that every health officer will be trained for his work. We

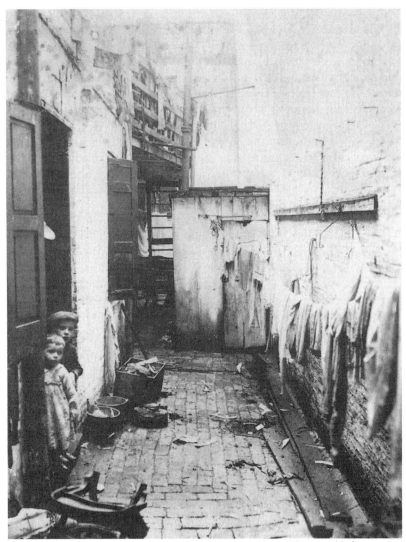

Figure 2. Children in an enclosed courtyard in the tenement district of Baltimore, Maryland, 1910. Recent European immigrants and black rural migrants were exposed to the most unsanitary and dilapidated housing in the tenements and alleys. (Courtesy of the State Historical Society of Wisconsin.)

hope that he will receive a reasonable reward for his services, and that the pay for saving a child's life with antitoxin will at least equal that received by a plumber for mending a leaky pipe; and that for managing a yellow fever outbreak a man may receive as much per week as a catcher on a baseball nine.[23]

Toward a New Profession of Public Health / 15

The demand for centralized planning and business efficiency required scientific knowledge rather than the undisciplined enthusiasms of voluntary groups.[24] Public health decisions should be made by an analysis of costs and benefits "as an up-to-date manufacturer would count the cost of a new process." The health officer, like the merchant, should learn "which line of work yields the most for the sum expended."[25]

Existing health departments were dominated more by patronage and political considerations than by concern for economic or administrative efficiency. Progressives regretted "the evil of politics" and wanted to increase the pay and minimum qualifications for health officers to attract personnel on the basis of skill rather than influence. The attempt to insulate boards of health from local political control was part of a broader movement to make all forms of public administration more "rational" and "efficient" by reducing the influence of political bosses and by promoting a new group of professional administrators.[26] The reformers wanted a well-trained professional elite to make social improvements along scientific lines. It seemed only a matter of selecting the right people and giving them the best possible training for the job. As William Sedgwick argued:

If, as I believe, we are in fact moving irresistibly towards a bureaucracy, while clinging to the ideals of a democracy, we shall do well to pause and inquire what kind of bureaucracy we are building up about ourselves. . . . Scientists and technicians alike . . . must be employed and paid by the people, to rule over them as well as to guide and to guard them, to constitute a kind of official class, a kind of bureaucracy constituted for themselves by the people themselves. . . . What kind of scientists and technicians shall we have in our public service? . . . I honestly believe that upon our ability to solve, and solve wisely, these fundamental problems of our American life will depend in large measure our comfort and success as a people in the 20th century.[27]

Public health was quickly becoming a national and even international issue. Although the United States Congress was reluctant to enact federal health legislation, pressures mounted for the United States to attend to public health abroad. As American businessmen were seeking enlarged foreign markets, a vocal group of intellectuals and politicians argued for an assertive foreign policy. The United States began to challenge European dominance in the Far East and Latin America, seeking trade and political influence more than territory, but taking territory where it could. National defense goals included broadening control of trade routes, building a Central American canal, and establishing strategic bases in the Caribbean and Western Pacific.

In 1898, the United States entered the Spanish-American War, expanded the army from 25,000 to 250,000 men, and sent troops to Cuba. That war showed that the United States could not afford military adventures overseas unless it paid more attention to sanitation and public health: 968 men died in battle, but 5,438 died of infectious diseases.[28] Nonetheless, the United States defeated Spain, and installed an army of occupation in Cuba. When yellow fever threatened the troops in 1900, the response was efficient and effective. An army commission under Walter Reed was sent to Cuba to study the disease and, in a dramatic series of human experiments, confirmed the hypothesis that it was spread by mosquitoes; Surgeon Major William Gorgas then eliminated yellow fever from Havana.[29]

This experience confirmed the importance of public health for successful United States activities overseas. Earlier efforts to dig the Panama Canal had been attended by enormous mortality rates from disease.[30] But, in 1904, Gorgas, now promoted to general, took control of a campaign against the malaria and yellow fever threatening canal, operations. He was finally able to persuade the Canal Commission to institute an intensive campaign against mosquitoes. In one of the great triumphs of practical public health, yellow fever and malaria were brought under control and the canal successfully completed in 1914.

Industrialists brought some of the lessons of Cuba and the Panama Canal home to the southern United States. The South at that time resembled an underdeveloped country within the United States, characterized by poor economic and social conditions. The northern industrialists were already investing heavily in southern education as well as in cotton mills and railroads; John D. Rockefeller had created the General Education Board to support "the general organization of rural communities for economic, social, and educational purposes."[31] Charles Wardell Stiles managed to convince the secretary of the General Education Board that the real cause of misery and lack of productivity in the South was hookworm, the "germ of laziness." In 1909, Rockefeller agreed to provide $1 million dollars to create the Rockefeller Sanitary Commission for the Eradication of Hookworm Disease, with Wickliffe Rose as director.[32] This grant was to be the first installment in Rockefeller's massive national and international investment in public health.

Rose went beyond the task of attempting to control a single disease and worked to establish an effective and permanent public health organization in the southern states.[33] At the end of five years' intensive effort, the campaign had failed to eradicate hookworm, but had greatly expanded the role of public health agencies. Between 1910 and 1914, the combined total of county appropriations for public health work

increased from $240 to $110,000.[34] In 1914, the organizational experience gained in the southern states enabled the Rockefeller Foundation
to extend the hookworm control program to the Caribbean, Central
America, and Latin America.

Meanwhile, in Washington, the Committee of One Hundred on
National Health, composed of such notables as Jane Addams, Andrew
Carnegie, William H. Welch, and Booker T. Washington, campaigned
for the federal regulation of public health.[35] Its president, the economist
Irving Fisher, argued that a public health service would be good policy
and good economics in conserving "national vitality."[36] The federal
government made its first real commitment to public health in 1912,
when it expanded the responsibilities of the Public Health Service,
empowering it to investigate the causes and spread of diseases and the
pollution and sanitation of navigable streams and lakes.[37] By 1915, the
Public Health Service, the United States Army, and the Rockefeller
Foundation were the major agencies involved in public health activities, supplemented on a local level by a network of city and state
health departments.

These developments had led to an increasing demand for public
health researchers and workers for the new programs on local, state, and
national levels. Those promoting such programs became increasingly
critical of the lack of properly trained personnel in public health;
part-time public health officers were simply not adequate to staff the
ambitious new projects. Public health reformers agreed on the need for
full-time practitioners, especially trained for the job. In 1913, the New
York State legislature passed a law requiring public health officers to
have specialized training. Where were such people to be found, and
what training should they receive?

Public health had been defined in terms of its aims and goals—to
reduce disease and maintain the health of the population—rather than
by any specific methodology or body of knowledge. Many different
disciplines contributed to effective public health work: physicians
diagnosed contagious diseases; sanitary engineers built water and sewage
systems; epidemiologists traced the sources of disease outbreaks and
their modes of transmission; vital statisticians provided quantitative
measures of births and deaths; lawyers wrote sanitary codes and regulations; public health nurses provided care and advice to the sick in their
homes; sanitary inspectors visited factories and markets to enforce
compliance with public health ordinances; and administrators tried to
organize everyone within the limits of health department budgets.

Public health leaders wanted public health training to embody a
specific field of scientific knowledge. Public health practice required a

diverse set of disciplines and skills: economics, sociology, psychology, politics, law, statistics, and engineering, as well as the biological and clinical sciences. In the period immediately following the brilliant experimental work of Pasteur, Koch, and the German bacteriologists, however, the bacteriological laboratory became the primary symbol of a new, scientific public health.

The clarity and simplicity of bacteriological methods and discoveries gave bacteriology tremendous cultural importance: the agents of particular diseases had been made visible under the microscope. The identification of specific bacteria had cut through the misty miasmas of disease and had defined the enemy in unmistakable terms. Bacteriology thus became an ideological marker, sharply differentiating the "old" public health, the province of untrained amateurs, from the "new" public health, which belonged to scientifically trained professionals.

Young Americans who had studied in Germany brought back new knowledge of laboratory methods in bacteriology and started to teach others: William Henry Welch and T. Mitchell Prudden in New York, George Sternberg in Washington, and A. C. Abbott in Philadelphia were among the first to introduce the new laboratory methods to the United States. These young scientists were convinced that other physicians spent too much time squabbling over medical ethics and politics, while they exemplified commitment to the purer values of laboratory research. The laboratory ideal rapidly influenced leading progressives in public health. By the 1880s, Charles Chapin had established a public health laboratory in Providence, Rhode Island; Victor C. Vaughan had created a state hygienic laboratory in Michigan; William Sedgwick had used bacteriology to study water supply and sewage disposal at the Lawrence Experiment Station in Massachusetts.[38] Sedgwick demonstrated the transmission of typhoid fever by polluted water supplies and developed quantitative methods for measuring the presence of bacteria in the air, water, and milk. Describing the impact of bacteriological discoveries, he said: "Before 1880 we knew nothing; after 1890 we knew it all; it was a glorious ten years."[39]

The powerful new methods of identifying diseases through the microscope drew attention away from the larger and more diffuse problems of water supplies, street cleaning, housing reform, and the living conditions of the poor. The approach of locating, identifying, and isolating bacteria and their human hosts was a more elegant and efficient way of dealing with disease than worrying about environmental reform. The public health laboratory demonstrated the scientific and diagnostic power of the new public health. By focusing on the diagnosis of infectious diseases, however, it narrowed the distance between medicine and public health, and brought public health into potential conflict with private medical practice. The use of bacteriological laboratory techniques also emphasized the importance of scientific training. Bacteriology thus narrowed the focus of public health, distinguished it from more general social and sanitary reform efforts, and reinforced the importance of scientific knowledge.

The new epidemiology, like the new bacteriology, was firmly oriented to the control of specific diseases. Charles Chapin, the superintendent of health of Providence, Rhode Island, was one of the leading proponents of the new epidemiology. Chapin had published a comprehensive text on municipal sanitation in 1901,[40] but soon concluded that much of the effort devoted to cleaning up the cities was wasted; instead, public health officers should concentrate on controlling specific routes of infection. In 1910, Chapin published a new text, *The Sources and Modes of Infection*, which became a gospel of infectious disease control.[41]

Hibbert Winslow Hill, director of the Division of Epidemiology of the Minnesota Board of Health, popularized Chapin's work in a lively series of articles first printed in 1,100 newspapers across the United States, and later published as a book, *The New Public Health*.[42] Hill likened the epidemiologist to a hunter trying to find a sheep-killing wolf. The old-fashioned amateur hunter covered the mountains with his assistants, and told them to follow all wolf trails until they found the one that led to the slaughtered sheep. The new, professional hunter, however, took a different approach: "Instead of finding in the mountains and following inward from them, say, 500 different wolf trails, 499 of which must necessarily be wrong, the experienced hunter goes directly to the slaughtered sheep, finding there and following outward thence the only right trail . . . the one trail that is necessarily and inevitably the trail of the one actually guilty wolf."[43] The new epidemiologist started with the "slaughtered sheep," the sick patient. From there, he traced back the single trail to the source of disease. All other unrelated environmental trails—decaying milk, flies in the marketplace, outdoor privies—were irrelevant.

Hill urged his readers to adopt the scientific concept of specific diseases instead of the popular notion of good or poor health. Disease, he suggested, should be conceptualized as a bullet entering the body from outside: clearly, a bullet would travel at the same speed through a healthy body as through a sick one. Only one thing mattered—physical contact with an infectious organism.

Hill explained that modern scientific methods were more efficient than old-fashioned approaches to social reform. To control tuberculosis, for example, it was not necessary to improve the living conditions of the one hundred million people in the United States, only to prevent the 200,000 active tuberculosis cases from infecting others. He contrasted the expense and difficulty of trying to secure good food, decent housing, and safe working conditions for the entire population with "the expense of supervision of two hundred thousand people *merely to the extent of confining their infective discharges*. . . . Need any more be said to indicate the superiority of the new principles, as practical business propositions, over the old?"[44] The vital statistician, Hill said, would be the future scientific manager of public health expenditures: "Much abused, laughed at, neglected, he is, or will be, like the cost-of-production scientific manager of modern business, 'the most indispensable man on the staff' . . . a man who knows costs in each department in proportion to production, and where to cut cost, increase production, save time, unnecessary work, and waste in general."[45]

The dominance of the disease-oriented approach to public health was evident in the first handbook for practicing public health officers, *Manual for Health Officers*, published in 1915 by J. Scott MacNutt, and echoing the views of Chapin and Hill.[46] MacNutt devoted approximately half of his six-hundred page handbook to the contagious diseases, four pages to industrial hygiene, and gave only passing notice to housing, water supplies, public education, and environmental health.

Although the narrow bacteriological view was dominant, there were several alternate, competing models for public health research and practice. Public health was not yet characterized by a single paradigm, but by a diversity of views and approaches. Compare, for example, Hill's narrow focus with the broad and expansive gaze of Charles-Edward A. Winslow:

Public health is the science and art of preventing disease, prolonging life, and promoting physical health and efficiency through organized community efforts for the sanitation of the environment, the control of community infections, the education of the individual in principles of personal hygiene, the organization of medical and nursing service for the early diagnosis and preventive treatment of disease, and the development of the social machinery which will ensure to every individual in the community a standard of living adequate for the maintenance of health.[47]

Winslow's was not the only alternative view. In the same year that Hill published his book on the new public health, Alice Hamilton in Illinois conducted a survey of industrial lead poisoning and established the fact that white lead was slowly killing thousands of American workers.[48] Hamilton's method was not that of following the single trail to the guilty wolf, but of following hundreds of trails to find the many guilty wolves in pottery glazing, bathtub enameling, cut glass polishing, cigar wrapping, can sealing, and dozens of other industrial processes. Unaided by legislation, Hamilton argued, persuaded, shamed, and flattered individual employers into improving working conditions. Almost single-handedly, she created the foundations of industrial hygiene in America.

Joseph Goldberger's epidemiological studies of pellagra for the Public Health Service offer an example of yet another approach to public health. In 1914, Goldberger announced that pellagra was due to dietary deficiencies and not to some unknown microorganism; he and his colleagues had cured endemic pellagra in a Mississippi orphanage by feeding the children milk, eggs, beans, and meat. He then teamed up with the economist Edgar Sydenstricker to survey the diets of southern wageworkers' families. They showed how the sharecropping system had impoverished tenant farmers, led to dietary deficiencies, and thus produced endemic pellagra.[49] That guilty wolf—the economic system of cotton production and the pattern of land ownership—had swallowed much of the South.

Alice Hamilton, Joseph Goldberger, and Edgar Sydenstricker were minority voices amid the growing majority focusing exclusively on bacteria. Only the minority continued to relate the problems of ill health and disease to the larger social environment. As most bacteriologists and epidemiologists concentrated on specific disease-causing organisms and the individuals who harbored them, the larger social environment became almost irrelevant.[50]

While the broader conceptions of public health required an understanding of economics and politics, the dominant model of public health knowledge was based almost exclusively on the biological sciences. This latter definition of the problems of health and disease in bioscientific terms moved public health closer to medicine and reinforced the medical profession's claim to a dominant influence in the field. Physicians felt that, since they were the experts in infectious diseases, they were uniquely qualified to become the ultimate authorities in the new, scientific public health.

By the second decade of the twentieth century, nonmedical public health officers were beginning to protest the increasing dominance of public health by medical men. By this time, the sanitary engineers were the only professional group strong enough to challenge the physicians' assumption that the future of public health should be theirs. Civil and sanitary engineers had created clean city water supplies and adequate sewerage systems. The provision of uncontaminated water was a major factor in declining death rates from infant diarrhea and other infectiou:

diseases. With the benefit of hindsight, we can say that the sanitary engineers, through the improvement of water supplies and sewage systems, had probably been the single group most responsible for the decline in infectious diseases affecting both adults and children.[51] If, as Chapin and others had complained, the nineteenth century emphasis on sanitary reform had led to much wasted or inefficient effort, few would have been willing to include sanitary engineering in this critique. In the early nineteenth century, most municipalities had given private water companies the authority to supply city water. Such companies provided water to the wealthier parts of cities, where the profitability of their initial investments could be assured, leaving poor areas to fend for themselves or make do with the often polluted water available from local pumps. Slowly and reluctantly, municipal authorities had come to admit the inadequacies of private water supplies and began to accept responsibility for providing all city inhabitants with fresh water.[52] Civil and sanitary engineers, who had learned to make surveys, take levels, construct water-tight masonry, and build dams, embankments, bridges, and tunnels, had the skills necessary to create adequate city water systems; the problems were less technical ones than those of persuading city taxpayers and property holders that such major capital outlays were justified municipal expenditures.

After providing public water supplies, the next problem was the disposal of wastes. Initially, the cities diverted waste water into cess-pools, storm water sewers, or street gutters, often causing serious problems of flooding, and the very pools of stagnant water thought responsible for generating disease. The cities then began to hire sanitary engineers to construct sewerage systems to carry away waste water. Ten cities had sewerage systems in 1860; by 1880, the number had grown to over two hundred.[53] At first, most cities simply dumped their raw sewage into the nearest available water supply: a river, lake, harbor, or tidal estuary. As the health conditions of upstream cities with sewerage systems improved, the conditions of downstream cities, now taking in untreated sewage with their water supplies, deteriorated.

Bacteriological and epidemiological research in the 1890s showed the relationship of typhoid fever to sewage-polluted water supplies. William Sedgwick at the Lawrence Experiment Station conducted research on methods of water analysis and purification and suggested intermittent filtration methods to treat sewage. Many cities also used sand and mechanical filters, thus reducing death rates from typhoid and other water-borne diseases. By 1900, the technology had been de-veloped to treat sewage wastes; the major problems were now political and financial.[54] Sanitary engineers continued to find new methods for analyzing pollutants and treating water systems to improve the quality of public water supplies.

As did the public health physicians, sanitary engineers debated alternate theories of disease etiology; they constructed sewerage systems in light of available knowledge and the financial constraints of municipal employers.[55] Thus, the sanitary engineers as well as the public health physicians claimed specialized expert knowledge that should be influencing the course of public health; both professional groups often fought among themselves and with the city authorities over the most appropriate actions. The professional competition between the sanitary engineers and the physicians became intense in the early years of the twentieth century as physicians reinforced their dominance in public health departments and as the sanitary engineers vociferously complained about the increasing "medical monopoly" of public health.

By 1912, fifteen states required that all members of their boards of health be physicians, twenty-three states required that at least one member be a physician, and ten states had no professional requirement for eligibility.[56] The medical profession was well organized and making a strong claim for dominance in public health. The sanitary engineers' counterclaim was an uphill battle; the physicians were willing to concede their responsibility for public sanitation and water supplies, but little else. A lively meeting of the American Public Health Association in 1912 was devoted to the professional struggle between physicians and sanitary engineers and their relative claims to competence as public health administrators.[57]

The central task in creating a new profession of public health would be to resolve these different approaches, and to weld unity of training, purpose, and function from diverse and often competing interests. Some resolution was needed of the tensions between public health and medicine, between the biological and social views of public health, between the physicians and the sanitary engineers, and between the bacteriologists and those who sought a broader definition of the field. Creating a more unified profession required decisions about the proper scope and content of public health, the kinds of knowledge and skillls, training, and credentials, needed by public health practitioners.

Most agreed that administrative ability was a central qualification for public health officials, but this seemed an innate personal quality rather than a skill to be acquired by training. Qualities such as wisdom, judgment, political savvy, and the ability to persuade reluctant legislatures to release funds marked the most successful public health administrators; no training programs were available to inculcate these qualities into the less successful. Special skills and competencies in bacteriology,

immunology, epidemiology, vital statistics, chemistry, and health education were given different priority, but, in any case, there were few
pathways for acquiring such knowledge. In short, the list of desirable
skills and qualifications seemed endless.

William Sedgwick suggested a possible resolution to the problem of
the future training of public health officers, his proposed "Y Plan" of
medical education:

The medical curriculum of today is for the most part a strong single track,
a narrow one-way road, leading straight to one great terminal,—the an-
cient, well-known, and famous metropolis of the medical degree. But since
1870 another great, though more modern, city has grown apart, but not far
from the original terminal and a strong branch road is now badly needed,
beginning half way up the line, which shall carry some of the many jour-
neymen to this new and thriving suburb of which the name is "Public
Health." . . . Instead of the present rigid medical curriculum which re-
sembles the capital letter I, we ought today to have a curriculum of equal
height and breadth, but shaped like the capital letter Y, of which the base
should still be substantially the first two years of the present curriculum—
anatomy, physiology, bacteriology, pathology, etc., but with the upper
parts diverging, the one arm or branch leading as now in the last two years
to the degree of Doctor of Medicine (M.D.) and the other in the last two
years to the Doctor of Public Health (D.P.H.).[58]

Sedgwick's scheme was one method for linking the professions of
public health and medicine, keeping them related although separate.
Medical schools, however, demonstrated little interest in the plan. The
unresolved problem of the relationship between the emerging profession
of public health and the well-established profession of medicine would
continue to dominate discussions of public health. Many of those
involved felt that public health should be a new career involving
elements of administration, medicine, and sanitary engineering. Public
health in England was known for its emphasis on administration,
Germany was admired for its scientific research productivity, and
Americans were proud of their accomplishments in engineering. But
how should these elements be combined to create a new profession of
public health?

One critical event in seeking at least provisional agreement on the
future structure of the public health profession was a conference held in
New York on October 1914 in the offices of the General Education
Board of the Rockefeller Foundation. The decisions taken on that
occasion would lay the basis for the future development of professional
public health education.

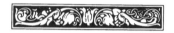

Competition for the First School
of Hygiene and Public Health

n the early decades of the twentieth century, the
Rockefeller Foundation intervened in the process of
the professionalization of public health. The officers of
the Foundation joined with several well-known public
health leaders in a deliberate effort to develop the new
science of hygiene and to create a professional basis for
public health practice. The central element in the plan was the establishment of a series of schools for public health research and the
professional training of public health officers. The first of these schools,
and in many ways the model for those that followed, was the School of
Hygiene and Public Health at the Johns Hopkins University in Baltimore. The decision to establish the first school of public health was the
result of a series of meetings between Rockefeller Foundation executives
and public health leaders during a three-year period from 1913 to 1916.
Decisions made then shaped the later development of the Hopkins
school and the professionalization of public health in the twentieth
century.

The contours of the "new" public health were largely shaped by a
small number of men who were in a position to marshal considerable
social, intellectual, and financial resources. The central figures in this
story include Wickliffe Rose, director-general of the International
Health Board of the Rockefeller Foundation; Abraham Flexner, secretary of the General Education Board; and William Henry Welch,
professor of pathology at the Johns Hopkins Medical School, the leading
"statesman" of scientific medicine. Also involved at critical points in
these deliberations were Hermann M. Biggs, health commissioner for
New York State; Milton J. Rosenau, professor of preventive medicine at
Harvard Medical School; George C. Whipple, professor of sanitary
engineering at Harvard University; Charles-Edward A. Winslow, of the
New York State Department of Health; William H. Howell, professor of

physiology at the Johns Hopkins Medical School; and Jerome D. Greene, secretary of the Rockefeller Foundation.

These men agreed that a new kind of public health service was needed, and that new educational institutions must be created to provide scientific training for a future generation of public health workers; yet they often differed in their conceptions of how best to accomplish this task. The process of planning for public health education was, therefore, a process of negotiation among men with different individual concerns, interests, and distinct perceptions of what public health should be. Their discussions resolved some of the fundamental questions about the future shape of public health education; others, left unanswered, would be the subjects of continuing debate: What should be the relationship between public health and medicine? What was the relative importance of fundamental scientific education versus practical and administrative training? Should public health education be primarily oriented toward physicians, or should a stronger emphasis be placed on training students from other professional backgrounds? Should public health be mainly concerned with the control of specific diseases, or should it embrace all determinants of the health and well-being of populations? These questions raised in the initial discussions about public health education not only are of historical interest, but remain unresolved today.[1]

Wickliffe Rose and the Rockefeller Sanitary Commission

Wickliffe Rose, originally a philosophy professor in Tennessee, had been the architect and organizer of the Rockefeller Sanitary Commission's campaign against hookworm in the southern states. A quiet man, Rose had a clear vision of the needs of public health and the iron determination needed to put his ideas into practice. Abraham Flexner described him as "a thoroughly intellectual type" and also as "a great general and strategist."[2] Rose had indeed the mind of a general, and he thought of the world as a field of strategy in the conquest of disease.[3] The general, however, needed an army: officers and soldiers who would be armed with the most effective and efficient methods of combating disease, possessed with zeal for the battle, and properly equipped for the seriousness of the task.

In 1913, Wickliffe Rose, fresh from the campaign against hookworm in the southern states, was ready to extend his sights to the rest of the world. For the international campaign, he needed three things: men, money, and organization. Money was hardly a problem; Rose had access to the Rockefeller millions, channeled through the International

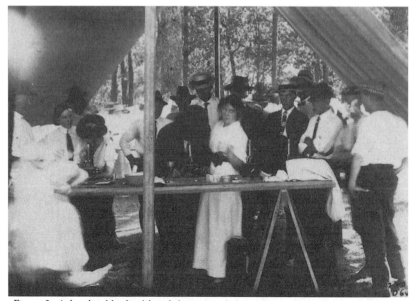

Figure 3. A local public health exhibit, intended to educate the population about hookworm disease, its nature, and prevention, Kentucky, circa 1910. Crowds gathered to see hookworms and hookworm eggs under the microscope. These exhibits were part of major hookworm campaigns carried out by the Rockefeller Sanitary Commission in the southern United States. (Courtesy of the Rockefeller Archive Center, Tarrytown, New York.)

Health Board. He had gained organizational experience in the South. Rose knew that the main problem was now to marshal public health personnel: for a well-orchestrated battle against disease, he could not rely upon part-time health officers, or physicians whose main income came from private practice.

In the hookworm campaign, Rose had first attempted to work through local health officials in each community. He had discovered, however, that public health was strictly a part-time avocation for these men, and that their primary interest was medical practice. He had also discovered that most public health officers were politically appointed and that they could not be counted on to support any activities that might challenge local political interests. He had thus come to the conclusion that a new profession was needed, composed of men who had been trained in the scientific foundations of public health, and who would devote their careers to the control of disease. Rose had decided that there must be two separate professions: medicine, for curing disease on an individual level, and public health, for preventing and controlling disease on a population level. Rose's assistant director-general, John A. Ferrell, expressed this distinction in the vigorous prose characteristic of that era:

The public health officer is an efficiency engineer in the most important department of human life—good health. He is a constructive searcher after truth. Instead of tampering and patching up the machinery here and there, he builds anew. He has to know the whole works, not merely one process; he deals with society as a whole, instead of with a few separate units. Translated into the terms of his calling, his task is to keep all the people well and strong, instead of concerning himself only with the unfortunates who come to him in dire necessity. Economically, he is a wholesaler, free and unrestricted in his operations, dealing in a commodity everybody wants, rather than a retailer whom, generally speaking, nobody really wishes to do business with.[4]

In the early twentieth century, as George Rosen has noted, the business ideal of "efficiency" was being widely applied to health and hospital services, and served to justify the reorganization and attempted rationalization of medical care.[5] The "efficiency criterion" was even more broadly interpreted: public health promised to be cost-effective on a grand scale, allowing the scientific management of health at the more fundamental level of the causes of disease. Good business sense suggested that it would be socially efficient to deal with the wholesalers of prevention rather than with the retailers of cure. Many of those concerned with public health couched their arguments in economic terms, calculating the economic benefits of public health expenditures as though they were interest rates on capital investments. In Germany, Max von Pettenkofer had developed the economic argument and analysis of the profit ratio of public health investments; in the United States, Wickliffe Rose and the Rockefeller philanthropies had the resources to test these ideas in practice.[6]

Abraham Flexner and the General Education Board

As the first step in the implementation of his plan, Rose turned to the General Education Board and to Abraham Flexner, whose "Flexner Report" of 1910 had been central to the reorganization of American medical education.[7] Long a friend and admirer of William H. Welch, Flexner had extolled the Johns Hopkins School of Medicine as the model for American medical education. Flexner was now embroiled in a struggle to institute full-time teaching of clinical medicine in the leading medical schools. He wanted professors to give full time to teaching and research, and not be permitted to earn income from private practice. Some medical school professors supported this idea, but others were violently opposed. To Rose, the need for full-time health officers had appeared in a similar light: real progress would depend on the separation of public health work from the competing loyalties of medical practice. On December 19, 1913, the Executive Committee of the International Health Board, of which Rose was director-general, passed a resolution "that the General Education Board be requested to consider the desirability of improving medical education in the United States, with a special view to the training of men for public health service."[8]

The Rockefeller philanthropies consisted of a number of independent trusts, each controlled by its own Board of Trustees. The General Education Board had been founded in 1902 to improve public education, especially in the southern states, and had later turned its attention to the universities and to medical education. The Rockefeller Sanitary Commission had been founded in 1909 to undertake the hookworm control program in the United States. When it began to conduct international programs, it was renamed the International Health Commission. In 1913, when it became part of the Rockefeller Foundation, it was again renamed as the International Health Board. (To compound confusion, in 1927 it would be renamed the International Health Division.) Of all the Rockefeller philanthropies, those devoted to public health and medicine were probably the most successful both in terms of public relations and practical social impact. The Rockefeller Foundation, refused a charter by the United States Congress in 1913 because of widespread political hostility and suspicion, gradually developed a reputation for its successful public health programs around the world, and the General Education Board played a major role in the scientific transformation of American medical education.[9] The Rockefeller Foundation and the General Education Board were financially and administratively separate, although their aims, activities, and personnel often overlapped, leading to some confusion among the applicants and recipients of Rockefeller grants, and even on occasion to territorial disputes between the officers of the different programs.[10]

As secretary of the General Education Board, Abraham Flexner began in January 1914 to explore the existing facilities for training health officers. He quickly discovered that Wickliffe Rose was not alone in his concern for professional training in public health. Hermann M. Biggs, the energetic commissioner of health in New York State, had for some time been bitterly complaining about the lack of properly trained men for health department work. By 1913, Biggs had maneuvered a bill through the state legislature that allowed the State Board of Health to set minimum qualifications for local health officers.[11] This bill was without immediate effect, for there were no applicants with special training in public health, and no training program available in New York State. The states of Massachusetts, Pennsylvania, and Maryland had similar legislation, but again it was ineffective because of the lack of trained people to fill the available positions. The legal framework had been created to remove public health from the control of local political forces by requiring professional qualification, but it remained meaningless until provision could be made for the education of the new professionals.

Existing training courses in public health were quite insufficient to meet the demand. In 1906, the University of Pennsylvania had started to offer special courses leading to degrees and certificates in public health, but no such degree was actually awarded until 1912.[12] By 1914, Alexander C. Abbott at Pennsylvania was graduating a handful of students from this public health program, which consisted of a one-year course combining sanitary engineering with bacteriology.[13] Abbott reported considerable difficulty in his attempts to gain the cooperation of the Philadelphia City Health Department for the practical training of his students. He commented to Flexner, with some feeling, that a necessary qualification for health officers was "the knowledge of people, how to handle them, and to use a slang expression, how to jolly them into doing what you want them to do even though it is against their own desires."[14]

Other universities had also run into problems in trying to begin programs in public health. E. P. Lyon of Minnesota had attempted to start a course for health officers but found that the jealousy of the different schools involved made cooperation impossible.[15] Still other universities were interested, but for various reasons had not been able to develop public health training. Edwin Jordan of Chicago described modest facilities for the study of public health, and William W. Ford reported from Baltimore: "Even with the most favorable interpretation of our facilities . . . it must be admitted that the subject of Hygiene or Public Health is in its infancy at Johns Hopkins, and that we would not be justified in maintaining for a moment that we have the opportunities for properly training men for a career in Public Health."[16]

By far the most developed and successful model for public health training at that time was the School for Health Officers run jointly by Harvard University and the Massachusetts Institute of Technology. By combining existing courses in Harvard and MIT with a number of new offerings, the School for Health Officers had produced an impressive catalog: seven courses in communicable diseases, eleven in sanitary engineering, ten in preventive medicine, twelve in personal hygiene, three in demography, nine in public health administration, and eighteen in sanitary biology and sanitary chemistry. Two or three years of academic work were required for a certificate in public health.[17] The Harvard-MIT School graduated a small number of highly trained health officers each year: five received certificates in 1914.[18] The director of the school was Milton J. Rosenau, author of the classic text *Preventive Medicine and Hygiene*.[19]

As soon as Rosenau heard of the General Education Board's interest in the training of health officers, he wrote to Flexner with a proposal for the establishment of a school, noting that "such a project might well be entrusted to Harvard University."[20] Rosenau's plan was essentially a description of the existing school, but with an added emphasis on research, building, and endowment. Perhaps the most curious part of this proposal was the budget which was a single sentence calling for $750,000 annually over a period of ten years—then an enormous sum, especially since the school was already running successfully with a budget of under $2,000 per year. (A copy of this memorandum in the Welch papers shows Rosenau's original figure corrected to $75,000 per year, which is probably what he had intended, but the error was not one calculated to endear Harvard to the General Education Board.)

While Rosenau wanted a school of public health to be established at Harvard, Charles-Edward A. Winslow thought one should be founded in New York. Winslow, however, visualized a school that would concentrate on training public health nurses, sanitary inspectors, and health officers for small towns: the rank and file of the profession. He argued forcibly that the laws recently passed in New York State called for many hundreds of trained men and women to work in areas such as industrial hygiene, infant mortality, and school inspection. This progressive legislation required many levels of professional workers, not just the highly trained elite.

Abraham Flexner was impressed both by the need for public health training and by the inadequacy of the existing facilities. He was, however, preoccupied with his medical school efforts, and made it clear that the whole question of public health training would have to wait. Jerome D. Greene of the Rockefeller Foundation suggested that Rosenau could be sent to Europe to study the problem: "It would seem to be not unlikely that Boston would be one of the places where a school would be set up. If that should prove to be the case, Rosenau would be head of the school and it would be quite important that he should have the knowledge that can only be got by studying the European experience."[21] Greene added in an emphatic note: "Mr. R. [Rockefeller] is in favor of considering this suggestion." Flexner stalled, however, and Rosenau was never approached; the plan to study the European experience was abandoned with the outbreak of World War I.

On May 28, 1914, Wickliffe Rose presented his own report on "Training for Public Health Service" to the General Education Board.[22] Rose felt that public health service was becoming a possible career for the first time in the United States. Recent legislation in New York had opened the possibilities of developing a new profession, one that would touch both medicine and engineering, and add new elements. The public health officer of the future would not be a practicing physician but would follow an "independent career." An opportunity for professional employment already existed; if a properly equipped school were in operation, there would be an immediate market for its graduates, "with the possibility of further demand keeping pace with a gradually increased supply." Existing American schools, however, were inadequate, and none of the men consulted seemed knowledgeable about European schools. Rose suggested further study of the question, and a conference to be held at the General Education Board offices, at which a concrete plan could be formulated to establish, on an experimental basis, one or two schools "at such places as Boston or New York."[23] Abraham Flexner planned such a conference for the following October. His initial invitation list included three from Boston (Rosenau, Whipple, Smith), three from New York (Biggs, Winslow, Park) and one each from Baltimore (Welch) and Chicago (Jordan).

Harvard University had already submitted a proposal for the establishment of a school for health officers. At this juncture, Columbia University submitted a proposal for a school in New York, formulated by a committee of twelve, headed by Edwin Seligman, professor of political science. This plan called for a combination of medical, engineering, and social sciences courses, leading to a doctor of science degree. Columbia proposed that the students admitted would hold either a medical degree or an engineering degree; the physicians would mainly take courses in sanitary engineering, while the engineers would mainly take medical subjects. Abraham Flexner now had to add a representative from Columbia to his invitation list for the October conference. Columbia's committee included a number of distinguished people such as Hans Zinsser, professor of bacteriology, and Mary Adelaide Nutting, professor of nursing, but Flexner rejected these names, and instead requested that Daniel Jackson, a junior faculty member from the engineering department, be sent as their representative. Columbia protested and asked that Seligman be invited to the conference,[24] but Flexner was adamant, and Jackson, who had neither an M.D. nor a Ph.D., received the invitation. It was a choice of Columbia's most junior man and also of a representative of engineering rather than the social sciences. Seligman protested in vain that "the broader social side was in danger of not being adequately represented."[25]

The Columbia plan was unusual in that it emphasized the importance of the social and political sciences for public health training. No other proposal was to give such central importance to the conception of public health as a social and political problem as well as a medical and engineering one. In the discussions that followed, three competing approaches to public health became evident: the engineering or environmental, the sociopolitical, and the biomedical. In the end, the biomedical conception dominated and sociopolitical and environmental concerns were relegated to a subsidiary role, just as Seligman had feared.

Yale University also wanted to start public health teaching in the medical school. Yale had been given an endowment to establish a chair of public health, and had written to Flexner for advice in selecting a candidate; Flexner suggested that the university postpone all plans until after the October conference. However, he invited no representative from Yale to the conference; the choice at this point seemed to be between Harvard and Columbia, with Boston as the favored location.

As Flexner drew up his plans for the conference, Wickliffe Rose was beginning to clarify his own idea of the necessary organization of public health training. By October 7, 1914, Rose already had the outlines of his plan to place schools of public health in strategic centers across the United States.[26] He sent Flexner a long list of men and organizations to be consulted, including, in addition to medical school representatives, the United States Public Health Service, the medical corps of the Army and Navy, state, city, and county health officers, food control officials, registrars of vital statistics, life insurance companies, industrial health managers, and sanitary engineers. Most of the men on Rose's list were never contacted; Flexner preferred to discuss the issue with a few trusted friends, and did not see the need to consult with so many different authorities. Flexner was not very interested in the opinions and concerns of practicing health officers, except those at the highest level. Daniel Fox has described Flexner, with some justice, as "a worshipper of heroes" and an educational elitist, a man with little concern for the problems of medical practice or the public's health.[27]

Hermann Biggs, however, had a conception of public health training that was closely tied to the practical needs of local communities. Biggs argued the need for short courses given in many different universities, supplemented by extension and correspondence courses, so that at least minimal training could be provided for the health officials of small towns and rural areas. In Biggs's view, the provision of graduate training for higher-level health officials was important but less urgent.[28] By the time of the conference in October 1914, Flexner had a variety of plans and proposals: Harvard and Columbia both wanted to establish schools; Biggs wanted a network of courses at different universities, Rose wanted a series of schools to be set up across the country, and both Abbott of Pennsylvania and Whipple of Harvard argued that no new schools would be needed if their existing facilities were expanded.

The General Education Board Conference: October 16, 1914

On October 16, the General Education Board held a one-day meeting in New York, bringing together eleven public health representatives and nine Rockefeller trustees and officers. The public health men were Alexander C. Abbott, professor of bacteriology at the University of Pennsylvania; Hermann M. Biggs, health commissioner of New York State; Frederick Cleveland, director of the New York City Bureau of Municipal Research; Daniel D. Jackson, assistant professor of engineering at Columbia; Edwin Jordan, professor of bacteriology at the University of Chicago; William H. Park, director of the New York City Public Health Laboratory; Milton J. Rosenau, professor of preventive medicine at Harvard; Theobald Smith of the Rockefeller Institute for Medical Research; William H. Welch, professor of pathology at Johns Hopkins; George C. Whipple, professor of sanitary engineering at Harvard; and Charles-Edward A. Winslow of the New York State Health Department.

Flexner began the meeting with a relatively safe question: What were the different types of public health officers for whom training was required? Biggs stated that there were three classes of health officers: executives, technical experts, and field workers. The "health officials of the first class," men with executive authority, included state and district health officers, and city commissioners of health. In the "second class" were the technical experts: the bacteriologists, statisticians, engineers, chemists, and epidemiologists necessary for research and the implementation of health department programs. Third were the "subordinates" or "actual field workers," the local health officers, the factory and food inspectors, and the public health nurses. This last and most numerous group were the "foot soldiers" in Rose's war against disease. George Whipple agreed: "I have also divided these health officers into three groups, like Gaul seems to be divided into three parts. We all agree on that."[29]

How, then, should these three classes be trained? Should the first class have broad, general training and the second class specialized training? William H. Welch solved this puzzle by emphasizing the importance of basic scientific principles: "Train them in the fundamental principles. The rest, of course, requires specialized training, but it almost takes care of itself, and is easily supplied."[30]

But who should be trained? The single most difficult question was whether public health officials ought to be medical men. If public health was to become a full-time career, was it reasonable to suppose that physicians would be willing to abandon their independence to become salaried employees? One consequence of the Flexner reforms in medical education had been a decline in the number of practicing physicians and a rapid increase in their incomes; it was hardly the most propitious moment to expect an influx of medical practitioners into public health, when, as Frederick T. Gates pointed out, "the attractions of practice are becoming so extraordinary."[31] Indeed, one effect of the General Education Board's previous intervention into medical education was to undercut the possibility of creating a new cadre of salaried physicians in public health.

Welch refused to see the situation that had thus been created; he insisted that public health work would be as attractive to medical men as the inducements of practice.[32] He further asserted that many physicians would be eager for graduate training in public health, and would see it as a "splendid opportunity." As Greer Williams has argued, Welch at that moment seemed to have lost his license to practice as a prophet, for physicians were to demonstrate little enthusiasm for public health training.[33]

Welch had stated that a qualified health officer should have a medical degree, hospital internship, and two additional years of special training in a public health school. Frederick Gates and Hermann Biggs argued against the requirement of a medical degree: Biggs realistically pointed out that he would rather have men "reasonably qualified to do the work" than wait forever for an unattainable ideal.[34] Gates, however, suggested that many medical men failed to establish successful practices; perhaps the failures in private practice might become students of public health? The idea of public health as a refuge for failed physicians hardly augured well for the new profession, but most of those at the conference felt that public health positions could only be filled by those with some medical qualifications. Even Theobald Smith, who argued that physicians were "absolutely color-blind to the preventive point of view," thought that the health officer needed an M.D. so that he could "stand on a level with the medical man."[35] As Abbott had explained, the health officer would be dependent upon the cooperation of the medical profession in his community; a nonphysician would find it doubly difficult to gain the respect and attention of local physicians.[36]

At this time, the increased activity of health departments in the identification and control of infectious diseases often brought health officers into conflict with private practitioners; many practicing physicians regarded public health with deep suspicion as a form of governmental encroachment on their freedom.[37] From the practitioners' point of view, it was better for public health officers to be medical men; they would be more likely to sympathize with other members of the profession. From the public health leaders' point of view, it was also preferable to have physicians as health officers, as otherwise the possibility of influencing local practitioners seemed almost nil. As soon as public health left the confines of sanitary engineering and took on the battle against specific diseases, it entered the territory of medicine; lacking strong state authority, public health officials had to cultivate the good will of the doctors. As John Duffy has argued, this attitude had the effect of making public health officers "cautious to the point of timidity" in the period between 1906 and the 1930s.[38]

The men at the 1914 conference found themselves unable to define clearly the relationship between medicine and public health, and they were swayed by Welch's benign assurance that no real conflict existed. Welch, however, was overly optimistic, and the issue, in different forms, would plague the future development of public health as a profession.

In the planning for public health training, this question was closely connected to another: What should be the relationship between public health and medical education? Welch initially spoke of public health as a department of a medical school, Rosenau proposed a completely separate school, and Biggs thought public health training should be independent of any existing institutions. Biggs and Winslow felt that association with a single university would severely limit the possibilities for field training, would seriously hamper the school's ability to influence legislatures and appropriations, and would make it impossible to standardize educational and professional qualifications.[39]

The meeting broke for lunch. When the conference reconvened, Flexner turned to Wickliffe Rose, who promptly laid out an elaborate and carefully articulated plan. Rose argued the need for a central scientific school of public health, well endowed for research. This school should be affiliated with a university, but must have its own independent identity, not be simply one department of a medical school. It must have its own building, grounds, endowment, and a faculty who would give their whole time to teaching and research. It should be located in a port city, "with its immigration element," but be within reach of opportunities for rural health work.[40] This school would select its students from across the country; its graduates would be carefully placed in strategic positions throughout the United States. The central school was, however, only the beginning of the plan. This central school would be linked to schools of public health to be established in every state; these simpler state schools would focus on teaching rather than on research. The state schools would in turn be linked to state health departments and medical schools, would give short courses for public health officers in the field, and provide extension services for rural health education. Both central and state schools would teach public health education methods and would seek to extend public health information to the entire population. Rose's plan brought together most of the elements of the morning's discussion; his description of the central school in a port city might have applied to Boston, New York, Philadelphia, or Baltimore. Biggs called the plan "admirable"; Theobald Smith found it "magnificent"; and Welch pronounced it "stirring and inspiring."

The discussion now turned to the organization of the central school. What would be needed that was not already in place? Rosenau found himself in a difficult position. As he was intent on demonstrating the Harvard-MIT School for Health Officers as the best model, he found it hard to answer questions directed at its inadequacies. According to Rosenau, his school lacked only money. For thirty or forty minutes, the other conference participants discussed the deficiencies of the Harvard-MIT School, while Rosenau grew increasingly uncomfortable. William Henry Welch made the most telling point: the new educational center must not be simply an administrative unit bringing together the departmental activities of existing schools; it must be an entirely new school, organized with an independent faculty. Flexner underlined the point: existing efforts "consisted simply in bringing together, in the form of a catalogue, things that are done elsewhere. . . . It is that sort of thing, apparently, we want to work away from, and not work toward." Rosenau could only protest, "We ourselves want to work away from it."[41]

Rosenau had come to the conference sure that the existing School for Health Officers was the best evidence of Harvard's commitment to public health education, but now his school was a negative example and a model to be avoided. By implication, Harvard's efforts in public health had been second rate. And the meeting was almost over. Wallace Buttrick, president of the General Education Board, suggested that Welch and Rose together work out a plan for the new school that could be mailed to all participants for criticism and suggestions. Magnanimous in victory, Welch agreed "if Rosenau and Biggs will join us." Flexner left the arrangements to Welch, and the meeting adjourned.

In retrospect, it appears that Welch had already taken charge of the project, that Rosenau had already lost his claim to the new school, and that neither Columbia nor Pennsylvania had made any strong showing. At the time, however, the idea that the new school might go to Welch at Hopkins must have seemed quite implausible to the other participants. In terms of its resources, Baltimore had the weakest claim on the proposed institute of public health, and, in terms of the overt competition between Boston and New York, Welch appeared as a disinterested party.

Immediately after the meeting the jockeying for position continued between Boston and New York. From Boston, Whipple wrote that he had been gratified to see how closely the ideal school outlined by Rose corresponded to their efforts: "It makes us feel all the more certain that we are on the right track."[42] Meanwhile, George Blumer of Yale announced plans to develop a School of Public Health following the Harvard-MIT model, while Flexner still advised waiting.[43] Edwin Seligman then produced a more detailed plan for a "School of Sanitary Science and Public Health" at Columbia University.[44] In addition to the two-year course of study for graduates of medicine and engineering, leading to a Doctor of Science degree, this plan called for a certificate in public health for nurses, sanitary inspectors, and local health officers. The budget asked for $60,000 a year, exclusive of research funds. With his proposal, Seligman enclosed a letter from E. H. Lewinski-Corwin arguing for the conception of public health as a social science. According to Lewinski-Corwin, most public health issues were not medical or technical problems, but questions of political economy:

Congestion of population in cities, the condition of tenement houses, the elimination of slums, recreation centers, alcoholism, prostitution, the standard of living, social insurance, the saving of human wear and tear in industry, the elimination of the insane and feeble minded, and many other similar problems affect the public health as much as the sewerage system, food inspection, and the quarantine of measles.[45]

Given this argument, social science and political economy should be at the center of the public health curriculum, along with "the principles of administration and efficiency," while medical and engineering skills were of secondary importance. But this social conception of public health was to receive little attention: the emphasis on medicine would displace both the social and the engineering approaches to public health.

While Harvard, Yale, and Columbia were making their appeals to Abraham Flexner, Wickliffe Rose was meeting with William H. Welch in Baltimore, and planning the proposed school. Welch had first promised to write up an outline in October, in time for a second conference.[46] By March, Welch was still saying that he would soon have the report ready.[47] By April, Rose was becoming increasingly anxious: the next General Education Board meeting was set for May 27, and Welch had still not written the report. By May 12, Rose had become still more anxious. Where was the report? By this time, Rose had produced his own memorandum entitled "School of Public Health": he only wanted Welch to add his ideas to the draft. At the very last moment, Welch produced a document titled "Institute of Hygiene," which was then presented at the General Education Board meeting as the "Welch-Rose report." By delaying until the last possible moment, Welch, probably quite unconsciously, had avoided another conference; even Rose did not have time to review the report before its official presentation.

There were actually two quite distinct versions of the famous Welch-Rose report: the first, written by Rose, and the second, rewritten by Welch. The longer Rose version was a plan for a national system of public health training, with a central school of public health as the focal point of a network of state schools. The central school would create "thoroughly trained and inspired leaders to mould public opinion and train the army of workers in the state's public health service."[48] The central school would also develop a new "science of hygiene" and establish public health service as "a distinct profession." Rose clearly differentiated medicine from public health: while one relieved the sick, the other protected the well; he asserted that "the science of protection is quite distinct from the science of cure."[49] Although the central school would be essential for creating this new science of hygiene, Rose's focus was on the state schools and extension courses. Here, his model was the agricultural extension courses and farm demonstration programs used by the Rockefeller Foundation to modernize agricultural production in the southern states.[50] The Smith-Lever Act of 1914 had placed these programs under the management of state agricultural colleges, and Rose wanted to reproduce this pattern in public health: "This lesson which has been learned by the teachers of agriculture through a long period of costly experimentation we shall adopt bodily in our system of public health education."[51]

These programs were based on the belief that real change in agricultural methods depended less on scientific research than on reaching the mass of the farming population: agricultural extension workers traveled from farm to farm personally persuading individual farmers to try new crop techniques, and organizing their children into clubs concerned with raising pigs, cattle, and poultry. In the same way, public health teachers would take instruction to "workers in the field" and would teach by practical demonstration. According to Rose, the central school would take the whole country as its "field of operations," sending out "an army of workers" to demonstrate the best methods of public health, and bring back their practical experience to be "assembled and capitalized" in research at the center of operations. In line with this conception, Rose had emphasized three of the more practical departments in the curriculum: epidemiology, public health nursing, and public health administration.

The orientation of Welch's version of the "Welch-Rose report" was quite different. The change in title was significant: the substitution of "institute" for "school" implied a main focus on research rather than teaching; the substitution of "hygiene" for "public health" meant an emphasis on science rather than on practice. Welch wanted an "institute of hygiene": a center for scientific research and the production of knowledge, not the command headquarters for an army of practical workers as envisioned by Rose.

In his introductory pages, Welch had summarized public health and hygiene in England and Germany by explaining that in Germany hygiene was taught as a scientific subject in the universities, while in England emphasis was given to practical public health administration.[52] Welch said that the ideal American plan would give due weight to both the scientific and practical aspects of public health, but he made obvious his own conviction that scientific research must take priority over practice. In fact, the Welch report dropped almost all mention of Rose's system of state schools, practical demonstrations, and extension courses. Enthusiastic paragraphs about the need for public health nurses and special inspectors disappeared; in Welch's version of the curriculum for the central school, he combined the three departments of epidemiology, public health nursing, and public health administration into a single "Division of General Hygiene and Preventive Medicine." He described the division as including "epidemiology, industrial hygiene, the principles of public health administration, and other subjects."[53] For Welch, the main divisions of the institute were to be the Chemical Division, the Biological Division, the Engineering or Physical Division, and the Statistical Division. Its main purpose would be to cultivate and advance "the science of hygiene in its various branches" and not to meet the immediate needs of the public health service: "It would be a misfortune if this broader conception of the fundamental agency required for the advancement of hygienic knowledge and hygienic education should be obscured through efforts directed solely toward meeting in the readiest way existing emergencies in public health services."[54]

In describing the institutional relationships of the new "school" or "institute" the differences between the Welch and Rose reports might appear minor, but they were to become highly significant in the eventual choice of its location. Rose stated that the school of public health was not to be a department of a medical school: "the two have divergent aims and must stand apart."[55] Nevertheless, the school of public health had to be close to a medical school "in the interest of economy and efficiency" so that basic medical courses would not have to be duplicated. Welch dropped Rose's phrase about the divergent aims of medicine and public health, and substituted the milder expression that the institute of hygiene should have "an independent existence." He then added a short paragraph stating that the institute must have access to the facilities of "a good general teaching hospital" for study and training in preventive medicine.[56] This was a critical point as the decision about the location of the new school would be largely based on evaluation of the medical schools and available teaching hospitals in Boston, New York, and Baltimore.

On May 27, 1915, the Welch version of the Welch-Rose report was presented to and accepted by the General Education Board, which then requested more specific proposals. Flexner now mailed the report to the original conference members for their comments and criticisms. Most of the responses were highly favorable; neither Rosenau, Theobald Smith, Whipple, nor the Harvard administration seemed to see its full implications. Meanwhile, the previous year, the General Education Board had turned down Harvard Medical School's application for funds on the basis that its "geographical full-time" plan for clinical teaching was unacceptable; at the same time, it had given 1.5 million dollars to Johns Hopkins.[57] The emphasis of the Welch-Rose report on the medical school and hospital teaching facilities rather than on public health experience or expertise could therefore have been read as an ill omen for Harvard, but this message was apparently not noticed. Instead, Whipple viewed the report as an endorsement of the Harvard plan: "The ideal of our School for Health Officers, which is much broader than its name implies, is very well set forth in the report of Dr. Welch and Dr. Rose."[58]

The New York men were more alarmed. Charles-Edward A. Winslow complained that the report was closer to the German than the English conception of public health, and should have placed more emphasis on practical fieldwork; he also wanted the title changed to the "institute of public health and hygiene."[59] William H. Park thought that part-time men from city health departments, school health departments, and industrial plants should be included in the teaching program.[60] Frederick A. Cleveland urged that emphasis be shifted "to make administration the big idea and statistics the ancillary one."[61] Edwin Seligman wanted the new center to be called a "school" rather than an "institute" and complained most pointedly about the emphasis given to the medical side of public health: "Nothing is said of the need of studying the substantial forces in our economic and social environment and the various plans for social and economic reform which frequently have a great influence on the health of the community. Again, such a matter as accident and sickness insurance, which usually occupies about half of any European book on social medicine, is not mentioned in the outline."[62]

Seligman agreed that connection with a medical school would be important, but argued for equal emphasis on the relation to a school of engineering and to other university departments: the majority of students would come, he thought, from departments of chemistry, biology, engineering, and from the social and political sciences, rather than from medical schools. In responding, Abraham Flexner said he considered the medical school relation to be essential: public health officers had to deal with the prevention and management of disease, and had therefore to gain their experience and understanding "in the laboratories and hospital of a medical school."[63] By this reply, Flexner demonstrated the distance between his conception of public health and that of the social and sanitary reformers; his was a "disease model" of public health practice. Flexner himself did not see Seligman's emphasis on social science as an alternative conception of public health, but as simply a self-interested position; he wrote to Rose that Seligman was "doubtless conscious of the fact that, on the medical school side, the position of Columbia is . . . vulnerable."[64] As Seligman was professor of political science, he had a "tendency to underrate the importance of the medical school." Rose answered mildly that Seligman was not underrating the importance of the medical school so much as objecting to the lack of emphasis on other departments, especially sociology. "We did recognize this relation and it could be expanded in much more detail."[65]

Rose did not share Flexner's adamant commitment to the medical model of public health, but it was Flexner who was to push forward the plans for public health education. In June 1915, Flexner wrote a memorandum to the Rockefeller Foundation proposing the next stages in the process: choice of location and a director for the "institute of hygiene." The director would be authorized to appoint professors for four divisions and a secretary, and then this group could detail plans of organization. The Rockefeller Foundation should provide support on an annual basis for five years; he anticipated the first year's costs to run around $20,000.[66] By this time, Flexner had probably already settled on his choice of Baltimore as the location, and on William Henry Welch as director of the institute. However, Jerome D. Greene of the Rockefeller Foundation thought the choice narrowed to Boston and New York, "with the chances very much in favor of New York, in view of the large opportunities here for both municipal and rural practice."[67] Hurriedly, Flexner replied that it would be "unfortunate" to restrict narrowly the number of possible locations before having examined "all fairly possible situations" and "unfortunate to gravitate towards any one place prematurely." He added what seems to have been a disingenuous note that "the factors are so many and so complicated that I have myself no idea as to what the ultimate decision should be."[68]

At this point, a rather embarrassing situation developed with Harvard University. On May 12, 1915, Harvard had submitted a proposal to the Rockefeller Foundation to support a School of Tropical Medicine at $50,000 a year for ten years.[69] By June 30, when the Harvard group met with the General Education Board to discuss their proposal, they had just read the Welch-Rose report, and rather abruptly changed their request to one for an "institute of hygiene" to include tropical medicine.[70] The General Education Board members then asked President Lowell to withdraw his original request and submit a new proposal; instead, he simply wrote a letter saying that "we should like to amend the petition by making it a part of a more general application for an Institute of Hygiene."[71] The Harvard proposal for tropical medicine was therefore dismissed.

Choice of a Location: The Site Visits

In September, Wickliffe Rose proposed to Flexner and Greene that they visit Boston, New York, Philadelphia, Baltimore, Washington, D.C., Chicago, and St. Louis, thus examining, as Flexner had suggested, "all fairly possible situations."[72] Boston was the first on the list; only four cities would be visited, as the tour stopped at Baltimore. The Rockefeller Foundation kept painstakingly detailed accounts of its activities; these site visits by Flexner, Rose, and Greene were recorded in hundreds of pages of stenographers' reports. For the first three days, the site subcommittee met at Harvard while Flexner directed interviews: instead of dealing with issues specific to public health, these discussions focused on the administrative relationships between the medical school and its affiliated hospitals. Flexner continually complained that Harvard did not control the hospitals it used for teaching. These hospitals were independent corporations, having cooperative relationships with the medical school. The medical school did not have the right to make hospital appointments or to reorganize hospital services since the independent hospital boards of trustees retained that authority.[73]

The need for medical schools to control hospital appointments was one of Flexner's most cherished themes, an important, though little discussed, part of the "Flexnerian reforms" in medical education. In the context of discussions about organizing a school of public health, however, Flexner's obsession with the administrative control of hospitals seemed rather out of place. He appeared to be looking for trouble; as President Lowell complained, Flexner was exaggerating Harvard's difficulties and underestimating its advantages.[74] In fact, Flexner paid little attention to the School for Health Officers and made one extraordinary omission: he failed to call on William T. Sedgwick, founder of the school, and the famed proponent of a separate educational track for public health. It seemed from his Harvard visit that Flexner was not especially interested in public health; he did not appear interested in nursing, social work, engineering, health promotion efforts, public education, or industrial health—only the administrative relationships among the medical institutions. Admittedly, Flexner in his opening speech to the Harvard faculty had already declared that he did not want to hear a recitation of resources and research accomplishments: "Harvard already has everything that exists. Our question is not what all this amounts to but how all this would fit with an Institute of Public Health if it were created."[75] Harvard appeared to have many advantages: a group of experienced public health teachers and researchers, a great deal of scientific talent, plentiful opportunities for fieldwork, and a progressive and cooperative city health department. All these resources, however, faded in comparison with the single issue on which Flexner turned the spotlight: Harvard did not control its teaching hospitals.

On his return from Boston, Flexner apologized to Sedgwick for his "unintentional and inadvertent" failure to invite him to the conferences on public health.[76] Sedgwick replied: "I am fortunately thick-skinned."[77] He continued, however, with a number of criticisms of the Welch-Rose report. As usual, the name was an issue: Sedgwick preferred an "American Institute of Public Health" and urged a less German, more American and democratic orientation.[78] The new institute should have "an almost absolute independence" to avoid being submerged by the medical school; it should articulate with federal, state and municipal organizations to "keep in vital contact with the traditions, customs and spirit of American Democracy."[79] Sedgwick especially emphasized the need for the new profession of public health to be independent of medicine: "coordinate, but not subordinate," and he wanted to maintain an even balance between the medical and engineering sides of public health, the new bacteriology and the older sanitary science. Flexner's interests, however, were entirely medical, and he continued to display a thinly veiled impatience with the older environmental approach to public health.

The visit of Flexner, Rose, and Greene to the University of Pennsylvania was brief. A. C. Abbott, who had been a friend and associate of Welch at Hopkins, gave the right answers to the question of hospital management, but he seemed to have little idea of how to establish the proposed school of public health. When asked how the school would be organized, for example, he simply replied, "I have not thought it out definitely."[80] The interview was in a low key: Pennsylvania seemed to have few resources in comparison to Harvard, and Abbott had modest ambitions. He declared that he already had ample facilities, and would just like an increase in staff: not the kind of inspiring vision that members of the General Education Board expected. When asked about the possibilities for tropical medicine, for example, Abbott replied that there would not be enough clinical material to justify a program. Rose, presumably trying to be helpful, suggested that the United Fruit Company might arrange to bring cases of beriberi or sleeping sickness to Philadelphia, but Abbott sensibly protested that these would not get through the quarantine.

Abbott gave the impression throughout the meeting that he was unprepared to host a new institute of hygiene; he was ready to discuss an extension of his current work, but little more. Reading the transcripts, one cannot help feeling that this visit was really a formality, that Flexner had included Pennsylvania in the site visits so as to extend the committee's sights beyond Boston and New York—in the direction of Baltimore.

The third visit, to Columbia University, was a more extensive one. Beginning with the School of Engineering, however, Flexner found Daniel Jackson unprepared for his searching organizational questions. The dean of engineering, admitted to be "autocratically influential," had not been consulted in the program planning, nor had arrangements been made for him to see the visiting committee.[81] The question whether a school of public health would be located with the engineering school at 116th Street or at the medical school (then at 59th Street) had never been discussed; neither had the institutional status of the school as an independent organization. With Edwin Seligman, Flexner explored the complicated administrative structure of Columbia University, pushing the idea of an independent institution with its own board of trustees and financial autonomy—a conception that the president, Nicholas Murray Butler, was bound to oppose, as he was engaged in a lengthy battle to centralize the administrative organization of the various schools and colleges associated with Columbia.[82]

Columbia had two strong cards to play in the competition for the new school of public health: the first was an excellent program in public health nursing run by Mary Adelaide Nutting, and the second was a progressive and cooperative City Health Department. Haven Emerson from the New York Department of Health explained that they were already doing research with a variety of different agencies, from the Metropolitan Life Insurance Company to the Association for the Improvement of the Condition of the Poor, and would welcome research workers from an institute of hygiene.[83]

While Nutting and Emerson offered strong support, the medical school provided little basis for optimism. Governed by an oligarchy, the school demonstrated no unified organization; in some cases, the medical school simply appointed as professors men who had previously been nominated to the surgical staffs of the hospitals; in other cases, nominations were made by agreement between university and hospital managers. Neither plan remotely resembled Flexner's idea of the proper relationship of a university, medical school, and its teaching hospitals. The medical professors, meeting at the Century Club, appeared to have little comprehension of public health work or of its possible implications. Most were convinced that public health officers should be medical men, but beyond this, had few suggestions. It became clear that Columbia's strength lay in engineering, nursing, the social and political sciences, and in the opportunities for practical fieldwork: all issues much less important in Flexner's mind than the quality of the medical school and hospitals.

The last site visit was Baltimore and the Johns Hopkins University, and here Flexner's dreams had been realized. Both the medical school and the hospital were heavily committed to the research ideal. As at Columbia, the medical school faculty at Hopkins had almost total power over the running of the medical institutions, but Flexner explained the difference: "They have a tremendous organization, a thoroughly homogenous one, sympathetic to their authorities to start with. They have not got a lot of old fogies here."[84] At Hopkins, in theory the medical school and the hospital were independent corporations, but in fact they had interlocking boards of trustees and tended to act as a single unit.

The hospital Board of Trustees had always in practice simply followed the advice of its medical board, composed of professors from the medical school. As Judge Henry D. Harlan, chairman of the Board of Trustees of the hospital, explained, they gave an annual dinner for the medical faculty "and we ask them to tell us frankly what their slightest desires are with reference to their different departments."[85] Flexner was reassured that there would be no difficulty in using the hospital for research and training, or in opening up special hospital departments if desired.

William H. Welch then met with the committee and reinforced the favorable impression already created. He noted additional advantages of Baltimore: that property was cheap, that its proximity to the southern states offered advantages for public health work, and that closeness to Washington would facilitate cooperation with the United States Public Health Service. Welch promised that the school could be flexible in taking students with or without a medical degree.

Welch minimized the difficulties at Hopkins: there were few facilities for the study of infectious diseases, but a small amount of material, "thoroughly studied," would be better than "an ordinary infectious disease hospital." The Hopkins hospital had never focused on occupational diseases, but a special hospital service could be organized. The medical school was across town from the Homewood campus, but a bus could easily be arranged to transport students.[86] All difficulties seemed to fade in the light of Welch's optimism and enthusiasm.

Theodore Janeway of the medical school was equally optimistic. Baltimore, he claimed, had many diseases not available in New York: amebic dysentery, pellagra, and hookworm from the South, and tropical diseases from Cuba and the West Indies. Baltimore, too, had more occupational disease than New York, including chromium and arsenic poisoning.[87] John Howland argued: "There is enormous opportunity for the study of infectious diseases here in Baltimore on account of the Negro, because they have infectious diseases of all kinds all the time."[88]

After their medical school visit, the committee received "the heartiest, most hearty welcome" from an ebullient Mayor Howard Jackson, who enthusiastically announced, "We have a high death rate here and there is an admirable field for efficient research work."[89] The mayor and Dr. John Blake, health commissioner for the city, were especially proud of Baltimore's new water filtration plant and sewerage system. The City Health Department employed full-time sanitary officers and part-time physicians. As Mayor Jackson explained, "We do regard party lines in appointments, but the man must be on the job all the time, and he must give the highest percentage of efficiency that we can find."[90]

Clearly, the City Health Department was run on the older political lines, and not according to the ideals of the new professional and scientific public health. William Howard, the assistant health commissioner, was, however, one of the new men, and he was in charge of the bacteriological laboratories. He represented the promise of the future professionalization of public health practice in the city.[91] The Maryland State Health Department, with Welch as president of the board, already employed full-time health officers, not subject to political removal.

The School of Engineering on the Homewood campus seemed to be adequate, if unexciting. Several faculty members had interests touching on public health, the main ones being ventilation, air purification, heating, and lighting. Flexner dismissed an interest in scientific management with the words "they promise everything and do nothing."[92]

A final visit to the medical school brought the group to William Howell, professor of physiology, whose only criticism of Hopkins was the often quoted "it is too poor to start with."[93] J. Whitridge Williams summed up the advantages of Baltimore: "If this school comes here the best thing we have to offer you is Dr. Welch. I feel sure that Dr. Welch with very little urging will take it on his shoulders to develop it. . . . Another thing, we have 100,000 darkies here with all their diseases, and their mortality twice as high as the whites, and three times as much tuberculosis, and four or five times as much syphilis."[94]

The visitors were evidently persuaded; within a week, they had submitted their report to the General Education Board with Baltimore as the heavy favorite. Harvard, Columbia, and Pennsylvania were criticized because of the organization of their medical schools and hospitals, and especially because medical professors tended to be locally prominent practitioners rather than academic researchers. The resources of the Johns Hopkins University in engineering, the sciences, and sociology were declared to be "modestly developed" though "modern in spirit." The City Department of Health was "far inferior to that of Boston, New York, or Philadelphia" though "the attitude of the authorities assures the University a free hand in utilizing its resources and possibilities, whatever they are."

The real advantage of Hopkins was its medical school, with a small faculty "animated by high ideals and very efficiently led." In summary, the report concluded: "The general resources of the University and of the community are inferior—in some respects much inferior—to those found in New York, Boston and Philadelphia; the Medical School fulfills the requisite conditions in the highest degree anywhere obtainable."[95]

The decision in favor of Baltimore produced considerable bitterness between Hopkins and Harvard. Abraham Flexner has been accused of rank favoritism for Hopkins, of hating Harvard, of being "Welch's matchmaker," and of dogmatic conviction that Hopkins was the only medical school worthy of respect.[96] Certainly, Charles W. Eliot, the former president of Harvard, was infuriated by the decision. He wrote to Flexner:

The more I consider the project of placing the proposed Institute of Hygiene at Baltimore, the less suitable and expedient I find it. Johns Hopkins is a small and weak university compared with either Harvard or Columbia; and Baltimore is a provincial community compared with either Boston or New York. In comparison with either Boston or New York, it conspicuously lacks public spirit and beneficent community action. The personality and career of Dr. Welch are the sole argument for putting the Institute in Baltimore—and he is almost sixty-six years old, and will have no similar successor. This is the first time that a proposed act of a Rockefeller Board has seemed to me to be without justification or reasonable explanation. My lifelong interest in the great problems of public health and sanitation will account in your mind for this frank statement.[97]

Flexner replied that the Welch-Rose report, earlier endorsed by the Harvard men, had pointed to the School of Medicine as the single most important factor in locating the institute of hygiene. "Viewed from this angle the personality and present activities of Dr. Welch, helpful as they might be at the outset, are not so essential as the character of the medical school organization, a thing which will surely endure."[98] Eliot was not to be pacified; he responded: "I cannot imagine that the present organization of the Medical Department of Johns Hopkins should 'surely endure.' It is one man's work in a new and small university made comparatively independent of community action by large bequests from one benefactor. It seems to me that the whole situation at Johns Hopkins University is sure to change materially with time and growth."[99] Eliot went on to suggest a totally new scenario: that the General Education Board add research in hygiene to the functions of the Rockefeller Institute for Medical Research, and then "endow departments of preventive medicine in half a dozen of the better medical schools." It was hardly the right time to start producing entirely new proposals, but Eliot's anger was clouding his judgment. To Jerome Greene, he then complained that Welch and Flexner between them had decided the location of the institute.[100] Greene responded that this impression was gratuitous: "In our Committee Dr. Rose occupies a very impartial and judicial position, and there is no doubt of his emphatic leaning toward Johns Hopkins. The conclusive factors in his mind seem to be, first, the unanimity of spirit and administration at Hopkins, and the perfect contentment of the staff with the conditions under which they work as contrasted with the decentralization, disunity and discontent (I regret the unintentional alliteration) at Harvard." Greene added that Baltimore's strategic position on the border between the North and the South was an extra advantage, and he warned Eliot: "The attitude of the President [of Harvard] and the Corporation has made it difficult, if not impossible, for me to have any further relations of an official nature with the University."[101]

There can be little doubt that Flexner was biased toward Hopkins, and that his admiration for Welch verged on adoration. Both Abraham Flexner and his brother Simon had long been friends of Welch, and must have known that Welch had been dreaming of an institute of hygiene ever since, as a young man visiting Germany in 1884, he had seen Pettenkofer's institute in Munich. In his autobiography, Abraham Flexner recalled the site visits and decision in the following terms: "Someone in each of these centers had more or less vague ideas, but one man alone possessed the requisite knowledge and vision. I reported to Rose that it was immaterial where the school was located; it mattered only who directed it. The only possible director, in my opinion, was Dr. Welch; the school might be placed wherever he wished."[102]

It seems entirely plausible to suppose that Flexner had reached this conclusion early in the deliberations, well in advance of the actual site visits. It is also possible to read the transcripts and questions as an orchestrated effort to present Hopkins in the most favorable light, and to emphasize the disadvantages of the other universities. Even if one admits, however, that Flexner was less than impartial, the questions remain: Why did Wickliffe Rose and Jerome Greene endorse the decision to place the new institute at Hopkins? Why did the other two committee members agree that the organization of the medical school should be the single determining factor in choosing a location? Why the overwhelming importance given to the management of hospitals, when most public health activities took place outside the walls of those institutions?

From Jerome Greene's letters, it is clear that Wickliffe Rose had the deciding voice. Flexner clearly had his mind set on Baltimore; Greene had been impressed by Harvard; Rose was regarded not only as the most impartial of the three, but also as the man who best knew from intimate experience the practical side of public health work. And Rose had decided on Baltimore. The reason for his choice, though never fully articulated in public, seems to have been that Rose perceived a contra-diction between the aims of public health and the interests of the medical profession. Rose was entirely serious in his ambition to elimi-nate disease from the earth; he believed that in controlling infectious diseases, he would eventually put much of the medical profession out of business. As Rose saw the situation in the South: "A physician has to make a living but that depends on the prevalence of disease. Insofar as this function [prevention] is successful it diminishes the prevalence of disease and therefore diminishes his work and his income."[103]

In his work in the southern states, Rose had found that the local medical profession often opposed public health initiatives. Even in New York, the City Health Department had been under attack by physicians for infringing upon professional activities; the Rockefeller Foundation had attempted to fund health department personnel but had been forced to withdraw by strong medical opposition.[104] Many physicians saw the Rockefeller activities in public health as an assault on the small (medi-cal) businessman, and Rose understood their point of view; it was, indeed, his ultimate ambition to undercut the practice of medicine through the prevention of disease.

To Rose, therefore, the medical practitioners represented, in theory and often in practice, the potential opposition to the new profession of public health. For this reason, the influence of powerful local prac-titioners on the faculty of the medical schools at Harvard, Columbia, and Pennsylvania might constitute a threat to the survival of a new school of public health. Johns Hopkins was different: there, the medical professors were full-time men, committed to research and teaching rather than to private practice.[105] These men would not be economically threatened by public health activities. They might be sympathetic to the new school or they might be indifferent, but in any case, they were unlikely to destroy the fledgling institution by overt or covert opposition.

Rose therefore backed Flexner strongly in his advocacy of Hopkins. Of the two men, Rose was less immediately obsessed with the details of management and administration of medical education and more con-cerned with the ultimate objectives of public health, but the interests of Flexner and Rose coincided in the desire to prevent physicians in private practice from setting the policy of medical schools. For each of them, therefore, Hopkins provided the ideal model of medical education.

In April 1916, the Executive Committee of the General Education Board accepted the site visit report of Flexner, Rose, and Greene. At this point, Abraham Flexner was replaced on the subcommittee by Simon Flexner—probably in response to Charles Eliot's accusation of

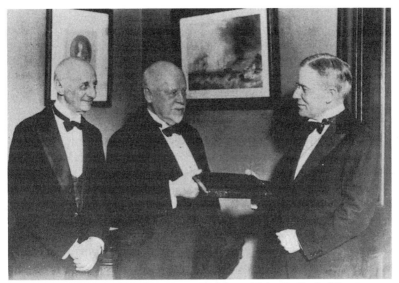

Figure 4. Simon Flexner, William Henry Welch, and John D. Rockefeller, Jr., at a dinner to celebrate Welch's eightieth birthday, Baltimore, April 1930. Rockefeller is presenting a book, *William Henry Welch at 80*, a collection of the tributes, speeches, and addresses given around the world on Welch's birthday. (Courtesy of the Rockefeller Archive Center, Tarrytown, New York.)

bias, as it would have been exceedingly difficult for anyone to question Simon Flexner's integrity and judgment. The new committee was sent off to consult with the authorities at Johns Hopkins, and to formulate more detailed plans for the proposed institute of hygiene. On April 22, Simon Flexner, Rose, and Greene met with Frank Goodnow, president of Hopkins, William H. Welch, and William H. Howell, then professor of physiology at the medical school. This group agreed that Welch should be director of the institute, that he would have to retire from "all other labors and responsibilities," and that his principal associate would be "an investigator of high rank in the physiological field." Because of Welch's advanced age, it was important to select someone who could take over the administrative burden of running the future school. Indeed, Welch had more of a reputation as a planner and a spokesman than as a practical manager. William Howell was therefore chosen to undertake the "executive management" of the institute.[106] The Rockefeller Foundation was to pay for the expenses and physical equipment of the institute for a period of five to ten years, at which time an endowment would be required. Welch and Howell agreed to prepare a plan of organization that could be formally presented to the Board of Trustees of the Rockefeller Foundation. No official decision had yet been made, but

Competition for the First School / 53

on April 30 the *Baltimore Evening News* broke a story that the General Education Board intended giving $3 million to the Johns Hopkins University for a "bureau" of public health research.[107] President Goodnow hastily denied the rumor.

Planning the Institute (or School) of Hygiene

In planning the institute of hygiene, Welch worked with William Howell, and also consulted with William Ford in the medical school. Ford argued that the new enterprise should be called a "school" and not an "institute" of hygiene, for although research would be important, a main aim, as with the medical school, would be the training of students.[108] The argument about the name was now a familiar one; Welch and Howell titled their report "Suggestions Regarding Organization of an Institute or School of Hygiene," although their text consistently referred to an "institute."[109] Ford suggested a basic two-year course for public health officers resulting in a degree or diploma of public health, and including three months of practical fieldwork. The subjects to be covered in the first year were biology, chemistry, demography, political economy, social economics, sanitary law, and mechanical and electrical engineering; and in the second year, physiology, sanitary engineering, municipal economics, epidemiology, diagnosis of the exanthenata, entomology, medical zoology, and industrial diseases.[110]

Although Ford emphasized the idea of hygiene as a part of medicine, he thought that sanitary engineers could take this training if supplemented by additional courses in the medical school. The principal departments of the school would be biology, chemistry, physiology, and demography. Demography, he felt, would be a special problem because there were no experts in vital statistics in America qualified to organize a department; he thought a young medical man would probably have to be trained for the post.[111]

The organization proposed by Welch and Howell was considerably simpler than Ford's scheme. Welch and Howell proposed two main divisions: a Physiological Division, and a Medical-Biological or Pathological Division.[112] They emphasized the importance of physiology as "the science and art of healthy living" in contrast to the study of disease and of pathogenic organisms. In this emphasis, they said, they wanted to reflect the broad conception of Pettenkofer, founder of the first hygienic institute in Munich, rather than the narrower vision of the bacteriological laboratory. The Physiological Division would be divided into two parts: the chemical section and the physical or environmental section. The first would deal with the chemical analysis of food, water, soil, and sewage, and with the nutritional analysis of foods. The second would deal with environmental influences on health, including the effects of ventilation, temperature, moisture, pressure, and radiation; also the influence of exercise and fatigue, bathing, clothing, and lighting. Both "personal hygiene" and "public hygiene" would be the subjects of research and instruction. The physical section was to have a budget of $9,050, and the chemical section was allotted $11,300.

The Pathological Division embraced the study of "communicable and other preventable diseases, so far as relates to their prevention." It too would be divided into sections: a bacteriology section and one for protozoology and medical zoology. Epidemiology was to be placed in the first section; occupational and industrial diseases were either to be given to one of the staff assistants or included with epidemiology in the bacteriological section. The rationale for including epidemiology and occupational health within bacteriology was none too clear, but the report suggested that this arrangement might be a temporary one.

Protozoology would include the study of protozoa and other animal parasites; within this section, noted the report, would fall many of the problems with which the International Health Board was most concerned, especially tropical diseases. Demography and vital statistics would be placed in a small independent unit. The budget for bacteriology was estimated at $13,450, for protozoology at $9,000, and for demography and vital statistics, $4,250. The School of Engineering would teach sanitary engineering, requiring one assistant at a salary of $1,500 or $2,000.

The proposal also asked for appropriations for a small library, for a hygienic museum, and for special lecturers, fellowships, and scholarships. Welch's relative disinterest in fieldwork was shown by the absence of any budget for practical training. Administrative expenses of the institute were set at $7,580, and the total operating budget, exclusive of the director's salary, estimated at $59,630. Welch had been asked to provide an annual budget between $50,000 and $60,000 and he wrote to Simon Flexner, "I came as near the limit as I dared."[113] In addition, the costs of the building and equipment were estimated at $200,000.

On June 12, 1916, the Executive Committee of the Rockefeller Foundation approved the plan, appropriating $267,000 for the operation of the new school at the Johns Hopkins University. They gave the school a name representing a compromise between those who wanted a "school of public health" on the English model and those who wanted an "institute of hygiene" on the German model. The new school thus gained its unwieldy title: the School of Hygiene and Public Health, implying that it would be both an institute for basic scientific research and, at the same time, a school for practical training in public health. The day after hearing the news Welch read the announcement at the university's commencement exercises, and concluded in his stirring style:

The dreams which many of us in the medical faculty have long cherished are now about to be realized. The opportunity which this great benefaction places in the hands of the Johns Hopkins University is most inspiring. . . . May we not confidently anticipate that in this new field the results will not fall short of the achievements of the University in the other fields which it has cultivated so successfully?[114]

The new mayor of Baltimore, James H. Preston, expressed great pleasure that the school had come to Baltimore, promised his "hearty cooperation," and declared his expectation that health conditions in the city would soon be improved.[115] Unintentionally, the mayor had raised yet again the question of the name of the proposed school by referring to it as "the Rockefeller School of Hygiene and Public Health." That same day, Welch wrote to Jerome Greene asking if the addition of Mr. Rockefeller's name to the school would be acceptable to him and to the foundation?[116] Greene replied: "I can hardly exaggerate my own personal feeling that this would be unwise, and I know it has never been expected or thought of. . . . Any name that might imply a unique or anomalous relationship to the other parts of the university would be a positive handicap."[117] The name of the new school remained, therefore, simply the "School of Hygiene and Public Health" of the Johns Hopkins University.

In the competition for the first school of hygiene, William Henry Welch had always seemed to be above the fray. Although Welch had treasured the dream of an institute for research in hygiene even before the opening of the Hopkins School of Medicine in 1893, he had not publicly declared his interest in the proposed school; instead, he left Columbia and Harvard to compete openly for funds and recognition from the General Education Board and the Rockefeller Foundation. Only during the actual site visits did Welch overtly argue the case for Hopkins; his earlier concern over organizational issues had appeared to be purely disinterested. A talented organizational strategist, Welch had remained the "statesman" while others argued their particular interests; now the prize had fallen directly into his lap. As principal author of the Welch-Rose report, Welch now had the agreeable task of putting his own recommendations into practice, with assured funding for five to ten years, and the virtual promise of an endowment.

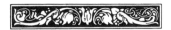

Working It Out: William Henry Welch and the
Art of Negotiation

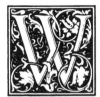 illiam Henry Welch had dreamed of developing an institute of hygiene for over thirty years, ever since his visit to Max von Pettenkofer's institute in Munich in the 1880s. In 1884, Welch wrote from Germany to Daniel C. Gilman, president of the Johns Hopkins University: "I have been particularly impressed with the hygienic institute which is the pride of the medical school in Munich. I hope that we may have a similar institute in Baltimore . . . hardly another department would attract in greater degree the favor of the general public than such a hygienic institute."[1] Welch's original plan for the Johns Hopkins Medical School included just such an institute, one that would be closely associated with the medical school, but devoted to research on the special problems of sanitation and hygiene. At the time of building the medical school, there had been no money, and perhaps little enthusiasm, for Welch's concept of a research-oriented institute of hygiene. Twenty-two years later, Welch had both the money and the enthusiastic backing of leaders in the public health movement and the Rockefeller Foundation.

In partial contrast to Welch's dream of a research institute, the International Health Board of the Rockefeller Foundation was interested in founding and funding a training center for public health leaders from around the world. Their vision included short training courses for health officers in the field, education for public health nurses and engineers as well as physicians, a training center for tropical health specialists, and a recruiting center for international field officers. The International Health Board agreed that research was needed on specific problems in hygiene and public health, but their major orientation was toward practical health programs: the first necessity was to teach men and women how to implement the knowledge already available. In this view, research was subsidiary to the primary task of organizing and

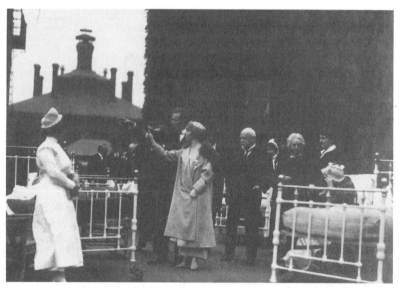

Figure 5. Queen Elizabeth of Belgium visiting the Johns Hopkins Hospital, October 31, 1919. From the left, Winford H. Smith, director of the hospital (pointing); Queen Elizabeth of Belgium, Frank J. Goodnow, president of the university (in top hat), and William Henry Welch, director of the School of Hygiene (1917–26) (hands in pockets). The Johns Hopkins nurses, patients, and visitors are standing on a bridge between hospital wards, where patients were taken on balmy days to enjoy fresh air and sunshine. (Courtesy of the Alan Mason Chesney Medical Archives of the Johns Hopkins Medical Institutions.)

staffing international disease control programs.

The School of Hygiene ultimately represented a compromise between the visions of Welch and the International Health Board: a compromise worked out in extensive negotiations over the period between 1916 and 1922. These negotiations concerned each of the major aspects of the new school: the selection of faculty, the admission of students, and the structure of the curriculum. The symbol of and reward for the completion of a satisfactory compromise was the award in 1922 by the Rockefeller Foundation of $6 million for the school's endowment and building construction. This chapter details the process of negotiation over the school's first five years during which Welch and the Rockefeller Foundation worked out a mutually acceptable organizational plan intended to satisfy both Welch's vision of a specialized research institute of hygiene and the International Health Board's interest in a practical training program for national and international health officials.

The first and most important decision facing the fledgling institution was the selection of a faculty. This choice was not simply one of picking individuals, but of picking the disciplines that would comprise and define the basis of scientific education in public health.

Welch and the Rockefeller Foundation had already agreed on the first faculty member: William Howell moved from the Hopkins School of Medicine to become head of the department of physiological hygiene. The choice of Howell seemed ideal from a number of different perspectives. As a physiologist, Howell represented an inclusive vision of public health as concerned with the promotion of good health and not

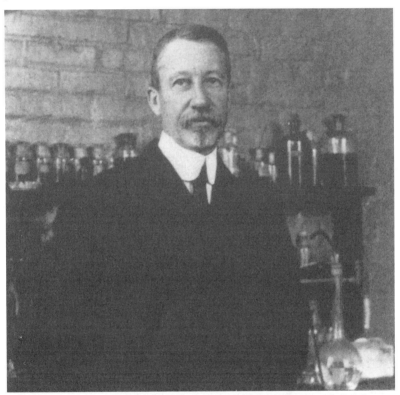

Figure 6 William Henry Howell, professor of physiological hygiene (1917–31), assistant director (1917–26), and director of the School of Hygiene, (1926–31). Here Howell is standing in his physiological laboratory in the School of Medicine. Photograph by Frederick L. Gates, advisor to John D. Rockefeller, Jr., circa 1911. (Courtesy of the Alan Mason Chesney Medical Archives of the Johns Hopkins Medical Institutions.)

William Henry Welch and the Art of Negotiation / 59

simply the control of specific diseases: his would be the task of broadening health research beyond the often narrow perspective of the bacteriologists. Second, Howell already had national and international stature as a leading physiologist, so his appointment enhanced the prestige and legitimacy of the new school. An excellent administrator, Howell was willing to take on day-to-day responsibility for running the school. A trusted personal friend and colleague of Welch, Howell was to take Welch's vision of the school and make it a reality. The only struggle over Howell's appointment was that of persuading the medical school to let him go; Abraham Flexner and the Rockefeller Foundation insisted, over medical school protests, that Howell devote himself full time to the new institution.[2]

Welch and the Rockefeller Foundation agreed that they next needed to appoint a bacteriologist. By consensus, bacteriology was a central discipline in any conception of public health: bacterial diseases were major causes of death both nationally and internationally. They disagreed, however, over the individual to be appointed. Welch wanted William W. Ford, his colleague from the medical school, while Simon Flexner urged him to consider J. W. Jobling or Hans Zinsser.[3] In this case, Welch prevailed, and Ford was appointed associate professor of bacteriology in April 1917.

Bacteriology and sanitary engineering were the twin pillars of public health. Bacteriology represented the achievements of laboratory research; sanitary engineering the practice of providing clean water supplies and treating sewage wastes. Although associated with the older environmental view of public health, sanitary engineering practice had been responsible for much of the improvement in health and the dramatic decline in infectious diseases since the mid-nineteenth century. Welch and the representatives of the Rockefeller Foundation agreed that sanitary engineering must be represented in the School of Hygiene and Public Health. Within the university, they agreed, the School of Engineering should take responsibility for its teaching. Granville Reynard Jones was already offering courses entitled "Elements of Sanitary Engineering," "Advanced Sanitary Engineering," and "Sanitary Engineering and Water Analysis" and these could readily be offered to new students at the School of Hygiene. Charles Tilden, professor of civil engineering, represented the School of Engineering in planning discussions with Welch, Ford, and Howell. Frank J. Goodnow, president of the university, also agreed to contribute a course of lectures on sanitary law and public health. By January 1918, the new school thus had an informally organized faculty of six: Goodnow, Welch, Howell, Ford, Jones, and Tilden.

The School of Hygiene had initially been expected to open in October 1917. The process of planning, however, took longer than expected, and the school did not open until October 1918.[4] William Henry Welch was, as usual, involved in a plethora of activities and devoted only a small part of his attention to the organization of the school. In fact, by July 1917, Welch had volunteered his services for the war effort to William C. Gorgas, the surgeon general, and had been appointed a major in the Officers' Reserve Corps. For the next year, Welch was largely preoccupied with the urgent tasks of visiting army training camps, inspecting their often wretchedly poor sanitary facilities, and recommending immediate improvements to help in the war effort.[5]

Although Welch had temporarily forgotten the School of Hygiene, Flexner had not. On February 15, 1917, after eight months of silence, Abraham Flexner wrote impatiently to President Goodnow:

In view of the close approach of spring without any official announcement regarding the development of specific plans for the new Institute of Public Health, may I say that, while we have no desire to urge action without proper deliberation, we have the feeling that the time has come when successive steps ought to be taken looking to the establishment and opening of the proposed Institute. . . . It would be a satisfaction to us if we could be assured that we shall from now on receive formal reports of progress at regular intervals—say weekly.[6]

Flexner's irritated letter provoked a burst of activity. The Advisory Board of the School of Hygiene was formed with President Goodnow, Welch, Howell, and Tilden.[7] The efficient Louise Durham was appointed secretary, and a cataloger was employed to take charge of books both for the School of Medicine and the School of Hygiene. Members of the Advisory Board discussed the curriculum, selection of faculty, and the admission of students.

George E. Vincent, who had just assumed the presidency of the Rockefeller Foundation, traveled to Baltimore on March 13 to assess the progress.[8] Vincent returned to New York full of enthusiasm: "Drs. Welch and Howell have the broadest and most complete conception of what the proposed school should be. This institution will connect itself in most fruitful ways with the International Health Board and the various public health agencies throughout the country."[9] He even told Simon Flexner that the initial budget had been too low, and that the foundation should consider another budget "based upon a somewhat larger conception of the scope and purpose of the school."[10] He wrote to Welch: "I can see great opportunities for the new school. I hope I shall not bore you with my enthusiasm."[11]

Welch was delighted to submit a larger budget. He was also delighted to have his broad conception of the scope of public health supported and backed by George Vincent as he could now proceed to make several unconventional choices of new faculty. Welch wanted, for example, to appoint Elmer Verner McCollum professor of chemical hygiene. McCollum was engaged in experimental studies of animal nutrition at the College of Agriculture at the University of Wisconsin. There, he was one of a small group working under Stephen Babcock, founder of the nutritional research that was reordering dairy practice in the United States and Europe. Welch and Howell were thus reaching outside the boundaries of public health as usually understood to bring in the relatively new field of experimental nutrition. They were among the first to grasp its possible implications for human health.

At the University of Wisconsin, McCollum had started doing nutritional studies on young cows to determine the food rations that would best promote the growth of cattle and other economically important farm animals. It was critically important for scientific agriculture to understand the nutritive value of different foodstuffs; McCollum had taken the important, but at the time, eccentric step of selecting the rat as his experimental animal. Because rats had a short life span, and because they could easily be fed and housed, McCollum was able to conduct many more nutritional experiments and obtain much faster results than other investigators.[12] In a series of elegant experiments between 1912 and 1915, McCollum and his co-workers had discovered a fat-soluble vitamin, later called vitamin A, and a water-soluble vitamin, which he called vitamin B. These results were of immense importance in establishing the experimental study of nutrition, with implications reaching well beyond the feeding of farm animals.

Although the connection between animal experiments and human nutrition may seem obvious today, few saw it at the time. In McCollum's own words: "In the agricultural field, experimenters in animal feeding for profit were looked to with respect as sources of information by exceptionally intelligent farmers, but such knowledge was considered by only a few to be of importance in solving problems of human nutrition."[13] William Howell, recognizing the contribution that nutrition could make to the promotion of health, had originally intended to include it in his own department of physiological hygiene; he was, however, so impressed by McCollum's work that he and Welch decided to make him head of a separate department of "chemical hygiene."

McCollum was amazed and delighted by the invitation:

Out of the clear sky I had been appointed to a professorship in the most notable research university in the country. . . . I could scarcely realize that I, a worker in an agricultural experiment station, with no medical training and no contacts with public health, was the first professor selected to take charge of a department in the new and exciting adventure of training medical and nonmedical students to reduce or control, and perhaps to eradicate, the great scourges in the form of diseases which afflicted mankind. I was filled with enthusiasm about my future."[14]

In order to bring McCollum to Baltimore, Howell and Welch had to arrange for the transportation and housing of an extensive rat colony. McCollum's letters to Howell were filled with details about the care and feeding of rats, the building of animal cages, and the training of assistants to prepare rations and keep records. Over the summer, the rats were moved into the basement of the School of Medicine, and the nutrition experiments continued with little interruption.[15]

The choice of McCollum as professor of chemical hygiene had thus broadened the concerns of the new school well beyond the traditional bases of public health: sanitary engineering and bacteriology. Welch now started hunting in a new direction, for someone to represent the theory and practice of "vital statistics." Statistics in public health departments was usually a dull bureaucratic task, a mere compiling and filing of death and disease reports. Instead, Welch wanted someone who could provide a general theoretical and philosophical approach to quantitative methods as applied to human health and disease. In Welch's view, a good teacher should be able to demonstrate the underlying principles of a subject; the applications were a matter of detail and would flow almost automatically from a solid grounding in the underlying theory.

Again, Welch found the person he wanted in experimental agricultural science. Raymond Pearl held a Ph.D. in biology from the University of Michigan and had studied statistics with Karl Pearson at University College, London. From 1901 to 1917, he had been a biologist, eventually chairman of the department of biology at the Maine Agricultural Experiment Station, where he studied the heredity and reproduction of poultry and cattle. Pearl was one of the few people in the country who was applying statistical methods to biological problems, being especially concerned with heredity, eugenics, and population studies. In 1917, he had been chosen as chief of the Statistical Division of the United States Food Administration, responsible for wartime planning of food production and distribution.

Welch had known Pearl for several years and felt that he would contribute quantitative skills and a new set of theoretical concerns to the School of Hygiene. Welch persuaded George Vincent of the Rockefeller Foundation that Pearl could bring distinction to the school and would be worth the high salary he was demanding.[16] When Vincent agreed, Pearl was appointed professor of biometry and vital statistics. Pearl insisted on this title because he saw "biometry" as the fundamental science and "vital statistics" as its application.[17] A student of Karl Pearson, editor of the journal *Biometrics*, Pearl emphasized the science of quantitative biology and wanted to distinguish himself from those who merely gathered the statistics of health and disease.

Pearl now suggested that Lowell Reed be appointed associate in biometry and vital statistics. A mathematician who had taught math and astronomy at the University of Maine, Reed had then gone to Washington to become director of the Bureau of Tabulation and Statistics of the War Trade Board. Reed's mathematical and statistical training was stronger than Pearl's, but Reed had less knowledge of biology. When Pearl later set up his Institute of Biological Research, Reed took over as head of the department of biometry and vital statistics where he spent twenty years convincing doctors and public health workers of the importance of quantitative methods.

For his next appointment, Welch accepted the recommendation of the Flexners that Carroll Gideon Bull be chosen as associate professor of immunology. Bull was an associate in pathology and immunology at the Rockefeller Institute for Medical Research in New York and had impressed Simon Flexner with his talent for experimental research. Welch retained the title of head of the departments of bacteriology and immunology, but was pleased to have promising younger researchers develop the research programs and take charge of teaching.

The International Health Board was especially interested in the appointments to be made in tropical medicine, since it expected that many of its staff members would be trained at Hopkins for international health work. Simon Flexner urged Welch to hire one of the more prominent graduates of the Liverpool or London schools of tropical medicine to build a major program in this field; instead, Welch delayed, and hired three relatively young and unknown men—Robert Hegner, William Cort, and Francis Root.

Welch had deliberately chosen biological researchers rather than clinical men. He could have turned to the schools of tropical medicine, either the English schools, or those at Harvard and Tulane University. Instead, he had gone across town to the department of biology at Hopkins. There he found Robert Hegner, author of two popular zoology textbooks, working on interesting problems in the variation and heredity of free-living protozoa.[18] This work had no immediate application to tropical medicine, but Hegner's passion for research and prolific writing abilities impressed Welch, who promptly hired him to head the new program in medical zoology. Hegner suggested an old friend, William Cort, whom he had known from the summer teaching program at the University of Michigan's Biological Station, to develop research work in helminthology. Although not a physician, Cort had done research on parasites, amebic dysentery, and hookworm, and thus seemed an appropriate person for the job. Hegner then suggested Francis Root, a colleague in the biology department, to begin a program in medical entomology, the study of insect vectors in disease. Root actually had no training in entomology: with Hegner, he had been working on protozoa. He did have a personal interest in field collecting, was fond of birds and dragon flies, and professed himself willing to take on the new field. The choice of these younger, relatively inexperienced men worried the staff of the Rockefeller Foundation who feared that insufficient attention would be given to tropical medicine, but Welch felt that these young investigators would be able to develop an innovative research program. In fact, the choices worked out extremely well. Hegner, Cort, and Root worked closely with the International Health Board in the areas of malaria and hookworm control; later, they were joined by Donald Augustine and Gilbert Otto in helminthology, William H. Taliaferro and Justin Andrews in protozoology, and Lloyd Rozeboom in entomology.

Almost half of the first faculty appointments at the School of Hygiene were women. All of the senior appointments went to men, but women filled many of the junior appointments. Included were Helen Parsons, Martha Koehne, Mathilde Koch, Nina Simmonds, and Florence Powdermaker in chemical hygiene (later renamed biochemistry), Sylvia Parker and Amy Phillips in biometry and vital statistics, Linda Lange in bacteriology, Ida Pritchett in immunology, and Ruth Stocking Lynch in protozoology. The pay scales for junior faculty appointments were so low that these young women were often paid less than students on fellowships, and they rarely stayed at the school for more than a few years. One of those who did stay was Janet Howell Clark who had been instructor in physics at Bryn Mawr College and Smith College, and who came to the School of Hygiene to continue her research on the health effects of ultraviolet radiation. Clark was William Howell's daughter and one of the first women in the United States to make a career in radiation science. Another young woman on the faculty was J. Ernestine Becker, trained at Cornell University, and one of the first women in the United States to study the biochemistry of nutrition. She would become the assistant and later the wife of Elmer McCollum.

The earliest faculty appointments had all been made in fields considered by Welch and Howell to constitute the scientific basis for public health research and education. None of the faculty had ever been a public health officer or had any direct experience of public health practice. George Vincent and the International Health Board had, however, been hoping for a much stronger emphasis on public health practice and popular health education. To this end, Vincent, on more than one occasion, suggested the faculty appointment of Selskar Gunn, the editor of the *American Journal of Public Health*.[19] Vincent called Gunn's work on popular health education "a model of imagination, ingenuity and efficiency."[20] Welch resisted the pressure toward popular health education:

The school . . . must not feel directly and immediately responsible for public health administration or for a knowledge of public health matters throughout the nation. . . . The work of formulating schemes of training, teaching and research will more than tax the time and strength of the highly specialized staff which the school must possess. These men must not be disturbed at the outset by having to do popular work or by being part of a large organization part of which is meant to do popular work.[21]

Welch's relative lack of interest in popular health education may be contrasted with the enthusiasm of Charles-Edward A. Winslow, a public health leader who became professor of public health at Yale University in 1915 and president of the American Public Health Association in 1926. In 1923, Winslow described popular health education as the keynote of "the new public health":

The dominant motive in the present-day public health campaign is the education of the individual in the practices of personal hygiene. The discovery of popular education as an instrument in preventive medicine, made by the pioneers in the tuberculosis movement, has proved almost as far-reaching in its results as the discovery of the germ theory of disease thirty years before.[22]

Welch responded during a formal lecture at Harvard two years later:

The great discoveries which have revolutionized preventive medicine and which continue to enrich it with life-saving knowledge have come from the laboratory worker and are achievements of the experimental method of research. . . . I should be inclined to characterize "the new public health" with somewhat less emphasis than is customary upon the mere technique of popular education, important as this is.[23]

Welch was also relatively uninterested in practical public health administration. When he was insistently urged to appoint a faculty member to teach public health administration for health officers, he invited his old friend, Sir Arthur Newsholme, to come from England as resident lecturer. English public health was known for its focus on administrative skills, just as the German system was famous for its concentration on research; and Newsholme was an eminent representative of the British approach. Since 1908, he had been principal medical officer of the Local Government Board of Great Britain, the main official responsible for planning medical and public health services. He had been closely involved in providing services for the prevention and treatment of tuberculosis, the diagnosis and treatment of venereal diseases, and the welfare of infants and young children. He had retired from his government post in 1919, a few months before the Ministry of Health Act brought sickness insurance, school health, and public health work under a single centralized administration. Newsholme brought to the School of Hygiene an English administrator's view of public health, and he took for granted the idea that students should be responsible for medical services as well as strictly preventive work. A strong advocate of "socialized medicine," Newsholme argued that preventive and curative medical services should be organized, financed, and administered by the state: "We aim to fit the many to survive, not only to secure the survival of the fittest."[24]

Sir Arthur Newsholme's appointment was conceived as only a temporary expedient; as a distinguished elderly gentleman, recently retired, he was mainly interested in visiting the United States and seeing his old friend William Henry Welch. It was to be a pleasant reward for many years of hard work rather than a new career. Sir Arthur divided his time between writing his autobiography, teaching, and driving up and down the East Coast in his new Ford automobile. When Newsholme retired from his position and returned to England, Welch asked Wade Hampton Frost, the professor of epidemiology, to serve as head of public health administration in addition to his other responsibilities, perhaps an indication that Welch did not consider this job an onerous one.

Frost, a somewhat reluctant interim head of the department of public health administration, was eager to devote his whole time to epidemiology. Wickliffe Rose of the International Health Board then urged Welch to offer the appointment in public health administration to Hermann Biggs, the dynamic commissioner of health of New York State. Welch asked Biggs if he would be interested in the appointment, but Biggs declined the offer. Although he supported the research ideal, Biggs was more interested in practical politics and in administrative and social reform. Disease, he said, continued to afflict humanity "because it is extensively fostered by harsh economic and industrial conditions and by wretched housing in congested communities. These conditions and consequently the diseases which spring from them can be removed by better social organization."[25] Committed as he was to the principle of short training programs and extension courses for practicing health officers, Biggs may well have viewed the research-oriented Welch school as largely irrelevant to the pressing needs of public health practice.

In 1922, Allen Weir Freeman was invited to become resident lecturer in public health administration. This appointment satisfied both Welch's interests and those of the International Health Board. Freeman had done epidemiological research; he was also a good practical organizer and administrator. A graduate of the Johns Hopkins Medical School in 1905, Freeman had found that he disliked private practice, and had become medical inspector for the City Health Department of Richmond, Virginia. From there, he became assistant commissioner of health of Virginia and state director of the hookworm program of the Rockefeller Sanitary Commission. Much of his work in Virginia concerned typhoid fever, hookworm, and trachoma, and is vividly described in his autobiography *Five Million Patients*.[26] In 1915, Freeman accepted a newly created position of epidemiologist in the Public Health Service; he worked in Kansas, Iowa, Ohio, and New York before becoming commissioner of health of Ohio in 1917.

In Ohio, Freeman became known for reorganizing the state's local health service. He pushed a bill through the legislature to divide the state into rural health districts, each with a full-time health officer. The bill eventually cost the state almost a million dollars and was considered the most advanced piece of health legislation of the time. Howell invited Freeman to Hopkins to lecture on his reorganization of the state public health services and afterward offered him an appointment as visiting lecturer in public health administration. Since the new governor of Ohio, Harry L. Davis, was determined to abolish Freeman's job and appoint his own men to run the state government, Freeman was glad to accept an academic position. The School of Hygiene now had one member of the faculty who was more enthusiastic about teaching practical public health administration than about research. After three years as a lecturer, Freeman became professor and head of the department of public health administration.

In September 1919, Welch succeeded in making a faculty appointment that helped establish epidemiology as one of the fundamental disciplines of public health in the twentieth century. He appointed Wade Hampton Frost, an officer in the United States Public Health Service, resident lecturer in epidemiology. It is appropriate to say that

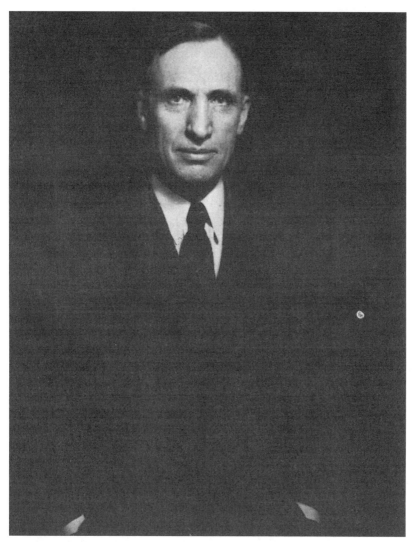

Figure 7. Wade Hampton Frost, resident lecturer (1919–21), professor of epidemiology (1921–38), and dean of the School of Hygiene (1931–33). Frost, who came to the School of Hygiene from the United States Public Health Service, made major contributions to the theory and practice of epidemiology. (Courtesy of the Alan Mason Chesney Medical Archives of the Johns Hopkins Medical Institutions.)

Welch "succeeded" in this appointment because he exerted the full weight of his influence to persuade Rupert Blue, then surgeon general, to release Frost from his duties in the Public Health Service. Welch and Blue reached a compromise agreement: Frost would remain an officer on active duty in the service, but be "loaned" to the School of Hygiene.

Wade Hampton Frost had come from a prominent southern family, trained as a physician, and then became an officer in the Public Health and Marine Hospital Service. He worked on the yellow fever epidemic in New Orleans and, at the Hygienic Laboratory, participated in research on typhoid fever, septic sore throat, cerebro-spinal meningitis, and poliomyelitis. In 1913, he was put in charge of a major study of stream pollution and water purification based in Cincinnati. He also studied a polio epidemic in New York, and, when the war began, organized the Bureau of Sanitary Service of the Red Cross.

In November 1917, Frost contracted tuberculosis and was sent to a sanatorium; on his return to active duty in 1918, he began a statistical and epidemiological study of the influenza epidemic with Edgar Sydenstricker. By 1919, Frost had thus gained considerable experience with both laboratory and field investigations, had studied many major infectious diseases, and had displayed marked talents for both administration and research. With Sydenstricker, he had developed new methods of handling morbidity surveys and had begun to develop statistical techniques for epidemiological research. Welch decided that Frost was the ideal person to teach epidemiological methods in the School of Hygiene; he could offer a sophisticated approach to methodology, introduce students to the techniques of practical field studies, and provide an important link with the Public Health Service.

Promoted to full professor in 1921, Frost became the first professor of epidemiology in the United States. For his epidemiological teaching and research, he had access to the large volume of statistical data gathered by the Public Health Service. Although an officer in the service for another eight years, Frost declined the suggestions of Surgeon General Hugh S. Cumming that he accept a high administrative post.[27] Preferring research to administrative duties, he finally resigned from the Public Health Service in 1929, retaining institutional affiliation solely with the School of Hygiene.

Welch and the Advisory Board made a number of part-time and unpaid appointments to the school's faculty. Though these appointments were usually largely honorary, some had a major impact on the school's development. One, for example, was Abel Wolman, appointed assistant in sanitary engineering in 1921 when he was assistant engineer at the Maryland State Department of Health. Although Wolman initially only taught on a part-time basis, his intellectual energy and enthusiasm immediately fired the interest and imagination of the students in the problems of environmental health.

Another remarkable, but unpaid, member of the early faculty was Charles E. Simon, who organized the first formal course on filterable viruses in the country and did much to establish this field as an independent area of research.[28] The son of a prominent Baltimore merchant, Simon had studied medicine in Germany, the University of Maryland, and Johns Hopkins. He opened his own diagnostic laboratory and, in addition to assisting local physicians, undertook research on problems of immunity, financed by small grants from the Rockefeller Institute. In 1912, he published *An Introduction to the Study of Infection and Immunity*, and in 1919, *Human Infection Carriers: Their Significance, Recognition, and Management.*[29] In 1919, Robert Hegner suggested that Simon be nominated "fellow by courtesy" in protozoology. The next year, Simon, appointed "lecturer at no salary," assisted in teaching the course on medical zoology. While working with the department, he developed a special interest in the study of the filterable viruses, organized the first course on this subject in 1922, and became resident lecturer in filterable viruses.

In his autobiography, Allen Freeman provided vivid images of early faculty members attending a meeting of the Advisory Board:

President Goodnow with his stooped massive frame, his great head and his heavy moustache was a formidable figure to look at, but he was in reality a most kindly and understanding executive. To his left sat Dr. Welch, the director of the school. He looked much the same as in medical school days, except that the years had thinned and whitened his hair and rounded his figure until he had come to look like a most intelligent and benevolent oracle. On the chairman's right as secretary of the board was Dr. Howell, the assistant director: small, precise, grey, gentle and kind as ever. In the chair to the left of Dr. Welch, the chair that had come for some reason to be regarded as a place of special privilege, sat Raymond Pearl. He was a great hulking figure of a man with thick black hair growing in a straight line across his forehead. His knowledge was colossal and covered surprising fields. With his powerful voice and impressive manner he was a hard man to stand up to in an argument.

Next to Pearl sat McCollum, in those early days so thin as to be a poor advertisement for his own theories of nutrition. He had the figure and voice of his native Kansas, but his hands were long and delicate as was fitting to the great experimenter that he was. He had little to say and sat often with his eyes closed as if asleep. But it was never safe to assume that he was not fully aware of all that went on. Next came Gregory, the picture of the successful businessman and with the precise and practical mind of

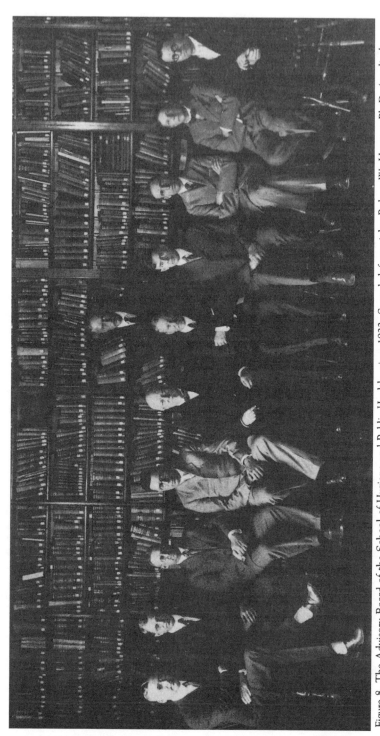

Figure 8. The Advisory Board of the School of Hygiene and Public Health, circa 1922. Seated, left to right: Robert W. Hegner, Ph.D. (medical zoology); Allen W. Freeman, M.D. (public health administration); John H. Gregory, S.B. (sanitary engineering); Raymond Pearl, Ph.D., LL.D. (biometry and vital statistics); William Henry Welch, M.D., LL.D. (director of the school); William Henry Howell, Ph.D., LL.D. (assistant director (physiology); Elmer V. McCollum, Ph.D. (chemical hygiene); Wade Hampton Frost, M.D. (epidemiology); William W. Ford, M.D. (bacteriology); Carroll Gideon Bull, M.D. (immunology). Standing: Frank J. Goodnow, LL.D. (president of the university). (Courtesy of the Alan Mason Chesney Medical Archives of the Johns Hopkins Medical Institutions.)

the good engineer. Beside him sat Bull, intense and eager with the soft brown eyes of the dreamer. Across the table and next to Dr. Howell was Ford who had been one of Dr. Welch's assistants in the medical school and had come with him to teach bacteriology in the new institution. Next came Frost with his slight frame and face of an Indian chief. His mind was crystal clear and his kindness and courtesy almost old fashioned in their perfection, but he had a wit as penetrating and corrosive as strong acid. Then Hegner with a solid and conservative exterior that hid a restlessness and imagination that were to take him all over the world.[30]

Students: Domestic and Foreign

Consistent with their different conceptions of the purpose of the school, William Henry Welch and the men of the International Health Board had different conceptions of the ideal students to be trained. As in the case of the selection of faculty, the selection of students was a process of negotiation and compromise between the ideas of Welch and those of the International Health Board. Welch had the authority to decide the criteria for student admissions, but the International Health Board had the money to offer student fellowships. For Welch, the process of coming to terms with the International Health Board was a relatively easy matter; the larger problem was in fitting his ideals to reality. The applicants flocking to the School of Hygiene in the 1920s were not necessarily those he had had in mind.

For his planned institute of hygiene, Welch wanted highly trained young medical scientists. Ideally, they would be graduates of "class A" medical schools, trained in modern, post-Flexnerian schools with high scientific standards. Welch was prepared to admit students who were not medical school graduates as long as they had had adequate scientific training in the basic biomedical sciences: physics, chemistry, biology, gross and microscopic anatomy, physiology, physiological chemistry, pathology, and bacteriology. Welch was looking for young doctors and scientists, fresh from medical and graduate programs, ready for further training in research methods.

The International Health Board had a somewhat different set of priorities. It expected the school to provide advanced scientific training in public health, but it also wanted the school to train its present and future staff members, to give advanced degrees to experienced men in the field, and to bring field staff in for specialized short training courses. The officers of the International Health Board expected to select international students for training, and then send out the best to head their health programs and become faculty for schools of public health around the world.[31]

The officers of the International Health Board assumed they could go to the School of Hygiene for additional scientific training as required; ideally, such training could be taken during their regular vacations in the United States. Welch and Howell did not want the school to be a drop-in center for international health officers, but a place where a small, carefully selected elite would spend several years in residency training for research careers. The compromise allowed for both kinds of students. Those admitted for short courses were designated "special students" while doctoral candidates were required to spend two years in residence.[32]

The category of "special student" was later expanded to cover several classes of students: those who did not fulfill all the admission requirements for degree programs and those who only wanted to spend brief periods of time at the school, taking one or two courses. The "special student" category represented a compromise resolution of a fundamental contradiction: the school was offering full-time research training extending over several years, but attracting mainly people who wanted short, practical courses.

The Advisory Board decided to offer three degrees: Doctor of Public Health (Dr.P.H.), Doctor of Science in Hygiene (Sc.D.), and Bachelor of Science in Hygiene (B.S.). These degrees corresponded to the three levels of public health workers discussed at the General Education Board Conference of October 1914: the executives, the specialists, and the fieldworkers. The Dr.P.H. degree was open to graduates of an approved or "class A" medical school who also had a degree in arts or sciences, as evidence of a liberal education. Johns Hopkins Medical School students were allowed to enter the Dr.P.H. program after three years of medical training; all students spent a summer of practical fieldwork "in an organized public health service" to fulfill their degree requirements.[33] They were to be the executives of public health.

The public health specialists were to be trained in the Sc.D. program. Initially, the requirements for the Sc.D. degree included a degree in the arts and sciences and two years in an approved medical school, or adequate courses in all the preclinical medical sciences. The long list of required courses was soon found to be unrealistic and was gradually reduced to include only biology, physics, and chemistry. Once admitted, Sc.D. students were to spend three years in the school before presenting "a dissertation embodying the results of an independent investigation."[34] At first, all Sc.D. students were required to publish their dissertations, but as the numbers of students increased, and the *American Journal of Hygiene* was swamped with student papers, this rule was withdrawn as impractical.

Applicants for the B.S. degree were required to have had two years' work in an approved college, with adequate courses in biology, physics, chemistry, and organic chemistry. Two years of additional course work at the School of Hygiene prepared graduates for employment in health departments as laboratory workers, bacteriologists, and public health inspectors. (No special arrangements were made for public health nurses, nor was nursing training recognized in any of the entrance requirements for degree programs.)

In 1919, the faculty met to decide on a suitable designation for students taking courses for less than two years and agreed that a certificate of public health (C.P.H.) could be awarded on completion of one year of courses. Students receiving the C.P.H. were either required to have the M.D. degree *or* "previous training in the physical and medical sciences."[35] The Dr.P.H. could thus be awarded after two years of study, the Sc.D. after three years, and a C.P.H. after one year. Tuition fees for all programs were set at $250 per annum; some scholarships covered tuition fees, six research fellowships offered stipends of $1,000 plus tuition, and generous Rockefeller Foundation scholarships carried a stipend of $2,000 plus tuition.[36]

What kinds of students actually applied to the school? Most of the first twenty-five applications came from people well advanced in their careers. These included a retired U.S. Navy surgeon, a pharmacist, several professors of biology and physiology, several state health officers, and field directors of the International Health Board. Most applicants were rejected—some because they had not graduated from an approved medical school, some because they lacked a liberal arts degree, and some, perhaps, on grounds of age. James A. Nydegger, a surgeon with the United States Public Health Service, was rejected for lack of a "preliminary chemical and physical knowledge," but nonetheless was invited to the school to lecture on his experiences in public health.

These applicants were eminent men, with established careers, yet they often lacked one or more of the stated admission requirements. These requirements had been written for recent medical graduates— men and women who had been through medical school since the Flexner reforms, and had therefore acquired a "modern" medical scientific training. Applications from recent medical graduates were, however, few and far between. Instead of appealing to young graduates fresh from medical school, the School of Hygiene was attracting older men who had worked, often for many years, in public health, without having acquired formal qualifications. Thus, the first candidate for the Dr.P.H. degree was John A. Ferrell, then director of the International Health Board for the United States, a man who may very well have known more about public health practice than any of the assembled faculty.

For the first class admitted on October 1, 1918, four doctoral students had been selected, two candidates for the B.S. degree, and two special students. Of the four doctoral candidates, three had been sent by the International Health Board. In addition to John Ferrell, Dr. Francisco Borges Vieira and Dr. Geraldo de Paula Souza were brought from São Paulo, Brazil, where the International Health Board was intending to open a school of public health for Latin America; they were to be two of the first faculty of this Brazilian school. Welch had selected the fourth Dr.P.H. student, George Huntington Williams. Welch, a close friend of the Williams family, had personally encouraged the young man, then a fourth year medical student at Johns Hopkins, to embark on a career in public health.[37] Williams would later become commissioner of health of Baltimore City.

Classes for this first group of students started quietly. The nation was at war, and an influenza epidemic was sweeping across the country. In Baltimore, the commissioner of health had prohibited all unnecessary public meetings. The School of Hygiene, therefore, had no formal opening; classes began quietly in an old physics laboratory on West Monument Street.

For the first year, all students took the same schedule of courses: administrative law, history of hygiene, bacteriology, public health organization and sanitation, statistics, physiological hygiene, metabolism and diet, and clinical lectures on tuberculosis and venereal disease. Since the students had very different levels of previous training, they did not like having to attend all the same classes together. Huntington Williams, for example, was annoyed at having to take a class in bacteriology that repeated the material he had just covered in the third year of his Hopkins Medical School course. At the same time, another of the first students who had come to take the B.S. degree spent most of the first year in the medical school taking courses in anatomy, physiology, and histology, trying desperately to catch up with more advanced classmates.[38] These early students were the guinea pigs for professors trying to find the right combination of subjects and levels for teaching public health.

It was a small and intimate group in the early days, but the student body soon began to increase. By 1921, there were 23 students; by 1922, 96; and by 1923, 123. Much of this rapid growth was due to the special students, who came for one or two courses but did not register for a degree. The number of candidates for the specialized Sc.D. was growing rapidly, the Dr.P.H. program was growing slowly, and registration for the B.S. degree was slowly declining (see table). The B.S. program was

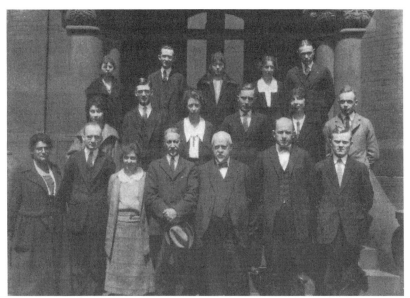

Figure 9. William Henry Howell and William Henry Welch with the Sc.D. graduating class of 1923. From the left, front row: Rachel E. Hoffstadt, D. L. Augustine, Claire McDowell, W. H. Howell, W. H. Welch, B. D. Reynolds, H. M. Powell. Second row: Shulamite Ben-Harel, E. R. Becker, Anna M. Baetjer, N. R. Stoll, Bertha Langwell, J. C. Swenarton. Back row: Henrietta Lisk, L. R. Cleveland, Mary Gover, Florence K. Payne, J. M. Scott. (Courtesy of the Alan Mason Chesney Medical Archives of the Johns Hopkins Medical Institutions.)

Students, 1918–1922

	1918–19	1919–20	1920–21	1921–22
Candidates for Dr.P.H.	5	14	22	20
Candidates for Sc.D.	1	9	19	31
Candidates for C.P.H.	—	5	4	11
Candidates for B.S.	2	9	8	4
Special Students	10	47	47	75
Total	**18**	**84**	**100**	**141**

Source: The table was compiled from figures in the reports on the School of Hygiene and Public Health, 1918–19, 1919–20, 1920–21, 1921–22, RG 1.1, Ser. 200, Rockefeller Foundation Archives of the Rockefeller Archive Center, Pocantico Hills, North Tarrytown, New York.

Note: The numbers of students registered varies slightly with different official reports, presumably because the student body fluctuated somewhat over the course of the academic year.

soon discontinued. The Dr.P.H. offered a broad, general program, the Sc.D. a specialized course of study. Dr.P.H. students took required courses in all the departments, while Sc.D. students concentrated on courses in the area of their special interest. The many early Sc.D. candidates who were to go on to distinguished careers in their disciplines included Edgar Sydenstricker, Anna Baetjer, Hugo Muench, Ella Hutzler Oppenheimer, Homer Smith, Norman Stoll, Martin Frobisher, Jr., Robert Riley, and Andrew Warren.

Although the overall growth in student numbers appeared strong, the faculty was concerned about the slow growth of the Dr.P.H. This program was expected to produce the new leaders, the executives, of public health, but recent medical graduates were hard to attract, and the demand for Dr.P.H. graduates far exceeded the supply.

Across the country, public health leaders agreed with Welch and Howell about the need to draw more medical students into public health. State health officers were unable to start budgeted programs because they could not find competent directors for the work. Endless surveys and papers reiterated complaints about the lack of physicians with public health training.[39] According to John A. Ferrell, the first Dr.P.H. graduate of the Hopkins school, more than seven thousand full-time health officers were needed to staff state and local health services. If twenty years were allowed for the development of public health services, this meant that three hundred such men would be needed each year.[40] To fill these positions, Ferrell calculated that about 10 percent of all medical graduates should be specializing in public health: only a tiny fraction of this number were actually doing so. In 1921, when Ferrell was making his plea for more trained health officers, the Hopkins school was training twenty-six of the needed three hundred.

Most writers on public health in the early 1920s agreed that there were tremendous opportunities in public health, but few well-trained people available to meet the need. "The health movement has risen like a flood and is overflowing the banks of the medical profession," declared George Whipple, professor of sanitary engineering at Harvard University.[41] "The lack in the whole scheme of things at the present moment is the lack of personnel," said Charles-E. A. Winslow.

We stand, I believe, at the beginning of a new phase of human history, a phase in which the physical and mental health and efficiency of the human being will be transformed by science as the physical background of civilization has been transformed in the past half century. In the name of the need that confronts us for the personnel to carry on this work, I believe we have the right to say boldly to the college men and women of America that we need them in this great business.[42]

The Rockefeller Foundation tried to encourage student applications by offering generous fellowships of $2,000 a year; in 1920 this figure was larger, as mentioned, than most junior faculty salaries (approximately $1,500) and about twice the normal secretarial salary (approximately $1,000). It was also larger than the average salary of practicing local health officials in the United States and Canada. A questionnaire sent to the more important local and state health officers in 1919 had reported their average salary as $1,383 a year.[43] Student fellowships at the School of Hygiene were thus a real inducement to study. Two of the young women hired as junior faculty, Ida Pritchett in immunology and Florence Powdermaker in biochemistry, actually applied for, and were awarded, student fellowships. The students awarded Rockefeller Foundation fellowships included Kenneth Maxcy, who later became a professor of epidemiology at the school; Reginald Atwater, later the executive director of the American Public Health Association; and Garland H. Bailey, an eminent figure in immunology. John B. Grant, another Rockefeller Fellow, had to cut short his student research when the International Health Board sent him to the Peking Union Medical College to become the first professor of public health and community medicine in China. Lewis Hackett, Bob Watson, Fred Soper, later the world authority on yellow fever, and Frederick Russell, director of the International Health Division, were among the Rockefeller fellows who became international leaders in public health. The International Health Board sent a steady stream of students to the school from Asia, Latin America, and Central America. Each year it sent about one-third of the students so that the school always had a strongly international student body.

Welch and Howell were under constant pressure from the Rockefeller Foundation and other agencies to conduct special short courses for public health workers, to admit part-time students, and to admit students who did not fulfill all the formal entrance requirements.[44] Welch submitted to most requests from the International Health Board and the Rockefeller Foundation, but resisted many of those from other sources. At the Rockefeller Foundation's request, Sir Arthur Newsholme directed a six-week course in 1920, attended by health officers from Maryland, Pennsylvania, Virginia, North Carolina, South Carolina, Kentucky, Costa Rica, and Puerto Rico.[45] The course provided an introduction to bacteriology, medical zoology, vital statistics, and administration, and was enthusiastically received. Drs. Hegner, Cort,

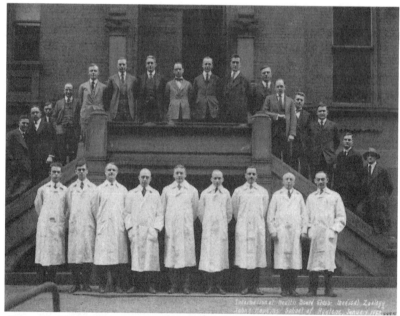

Figure 10. The 1922 International Health Board class with the faculty of medical zoology. Students, top row, from left: Docherty, Rector, Weston, Johnson, Wilson, Mieldazis, Craig, Mazoon, Tiedemann, Boyd, Lenert, Bedell, Knight, Taylor, Cox, Conrad (assistant). Faculty and instructors, front row, from left: Francis O. Holmes, Elery R. Becker, William W. Cort, William H. Taliaferro, Robert W. Hegner, Donald L. Augustine, Francis M. Root, Charles E. Simon, William A. Hoffmann. (Courtesy of the Rockefeller Archive Center, Tarrytown, New York.)

and Root also created a special intensive course for field directors of the International Health Board. This course consisted of classwork and laboratory exercises in medical zoology, especially relating to malaria, hookworm, and other parasitic diseases, and the schedule was arranged to fit the vacation period of field directors working in tropical countries.

Requests for other special short courses flooded the school's administrative offices. During the war, the school was asked to provide courses for the Students' Army Training Corps and the Sanitary Corps of the Army; after the war, the United States Public Health Service wanted short courses for its trainees; technicians in state diagnostic laboratories wanted courses in bacteriology; and health officers from the South wanted courses in medical zoology. While refusing to create a whole range of specialized short courses, Welch and Howell agreed to allow these students to enroll in one or more of the regular classes as "special students."[46] Welch also permitted members of the health departments of Baltimore City and the State of Maryland to attend courses without paying tuition, if recommended by the Baltimore commissioner of health or the secretary of the State Health Department. This policy proved an excellent method of creating friendly and cooperative relationships with local health departments.

Other groups of potential students were, however, excluded. A black physician from Baltimore, Dr. B. M. Rhetta, had asked that he and other black physicians be allowed to take the public health course: "We have said that these men are working in the public schools. We do not need to say to you that if any physicians need special training, we do. We do not need to say that such training would help us markedly in meeting actualities found in a people, who are in special need. . . . The Health Commissioner endorses this request."[47] After consultation with the faculty, William Howell responded that the school was unable to grant the request because a state-supported institution was required to maintain separation of the races, possibly the only occasion on which the school claimed to be a state-supported institution. It seems unlikely that the State of Maryland could actually have stopped the university from admitting black physicians to its courses, although the hospital, and city and state clinics were, of course, all segregated at this time. The easier option would have been to create a special course for black physicians, but the faculty apparently rejected this possibility. Howell wrote: "If it were not for the additional burden placed upon the teachers, the [Advisory] Board, I believe, would feel disposed to arrange a separate course for Negro physicians."[48]

Public health nurses also were unsuccessful in asking the school to provide special courses. Gertrude Howling, director of the Instructive Nurse Visiting Society, asked William Howell to provide extension courses for public health nurses attached to the army. Howell replied that such courses were of doubtful legality under the university charter, and would take too much of the instructors' time.

Welch rejected a similar request from F. F. Russell of the International Health Board, that the school offer special courses for laboratory technicians in state health departments, in the following terms: "It would hardly be in conformity with our general policies to undertake to provide special courses for technicians who lack fundamental training in general bacteriology and command only routine technical procedures."[49] In general, Welch maintained his original view that the School of Hygiene was a research institute, providing high-level education for an elite corps of public health professionals, and that it should not, or could not, undertake to provide training for lower-level public health workers. The school's most enthusiastic advocate of special training courses was Elmer McCollum, a laboratory scientist. It was McCollum, for example, who arranged for a special course to be offered for public school teachers on nutrition and diet, with the idea that teachers trained in nutrition would be able to improve the health of school-children.[50]

The school's original announcement had promised that special lectures would offer "useful knowledge" to the general public.[51] Thus community groups or charitable agencies frequently asked the school to give popular health education lectures and courses. When the National Congress of Mothers requested public lectures on maternity, J. Whit-ridge Williams, professor of obstetrics in the School of Medicine, agreed to offer a lecture course for mothers.[52] The farm community of Better-ton, Maryland, then asked for speakers to explain child health, and especially the weight gains of small children, but was told that the School of Hygiene did not do public education, and that it was properly the responsibility of the county health organization.[53] Similarly, the school declined requests to take up industrial hygiene, social hygiene and eugenics, oral hygiene and personal hygiene. Welch and Howell reiterated their basic priorities: the School of Hygiene was a research institute and should not be expected to take on the task of popular health education.

George Vincent of the Rockefeller Foundation had been hoping for a stronger emphasis on public health practice and popular health edu-cation, and pushed Welch and Howell as far as he could in this direction. Under pressure, Welch and Howell showed some willingness to compromise: they agreed to public education projects that conformed with their main priorities, that were relatively easy to undertake, and that did not threaten to distract faculty or students from their main task of research.

Vincent set out his suggestions in a long memorandum to Welch in November 1917. Vincent wanted the school to attract a leading health educator to the faculty and begin publication of popular health mate-rials.[54] He thought the school should publish a journal of public health, written for both laymen and specialists, giving "authorized popu-larizations" of research work, and accounts of public health plans and progress. He suggested that the school take over the *American Journal of Public Health* by adding Selskar Gunn, its editor, to the school's faculty. He wanted the school to publish an international public health yearbook—an encyclopedia of public health information—for dis-tribution to newspapers and libraries. He suggested a series of textbooks on public health for schools and colleges, and publicity materials for public health campaigns, including popular manuals, posters, slides and photographs, exhibits, charts, models and diagrams.

These recommendations were much more than either Welch or Howell wanted to contemplate. When Welch disagreed with a suggestion, he usually just ignored or postponed it. He postponed the idea of hiring a health education specialist and quietly ignored the request for popular health publications. Welch wanted to start a new journal, but a journal for scientific research, not for popularizations.

Instead of responding to the insistent suggestions for popular health publications, Welch offered a series of talks on public health, the De Lamar lectures. This lecture series brought in out-of-town celebrities and leading lights in public health.[55] The first series of speakers included William T. Sedgwick of the Massachusetts Institute of Technology, the man who had started the Harvard-MIT School for Health Officers, Victor C. Heiser of the International Health Board, George Whipple of Harvard, Simon Flexner of the Rockefeller Institute, W. F. Willcox of Cornell, William H. Park of the New York City Health Department, Milton J. Rosenau of Harvard, Charles-E. A. Winslow of Yale, Hermann M. Biggs of the New York State Health Department, and Wickliffe Rose, director general of the International Health Board. The speakers for the 1920 series included Charles Chapin, Haven Emerson, Charles W. Stiles, Livingston Farrand, Hugh Cumming, Hideyo Noguchi, and Carlos Chagas. The De Lamar lectures were a great intellectual, social, and gastronomic success: after the lectures, speakers and selected faculty were treated to splendid dinners, organized by Welch, at the Maryland Club.

Another of Welch's efforts was less successful: the hygienic museum. Originally, the museum was intended to provide a focus for public health education in the school, but no one seemed to put much time or attention into its organization or promotion. The museum housed a rather random and eccentric assortment of objects: an exhibit on hookworm presented by Wickliffe Rose; a large collection of insects presented by G.A.K. Marshall, director of the Imperial Bureau of Entomology of the British Museum of Natural History; two specimens of the Haygood Pit Privy presented by the State Board of Health of Georgia; and 30,000 trematodes presented by Charles Barlow. What the public thought of this collection is, unfortunately, not recorded.

As the Rockefeller Foundation continued to push the school toward a more practical orientation, it held one large negotiating chip: Welch and Howell wanted money for a new building. As a matter of principle, of course, the Rockefeller Foundation did not attach "strings" to its grant awards nor did it try explicitly to influence the policies of private universities. Its officers did, however, clearly indicate to Welch and Howell the directions in which they thought the school should be moving. They agreed to consider the question of buildings after "a comprehensive plan for the development of the School both for the present and for the future . . . had been worked out."[56] They also clearly suggested that future planning for the school should include its extension into new fields—specifically, industrial hygiene, tropical diseases, and short courses for training public health officers. Since the school had neither a permanent building nor an endowment, it was doubtless the better part of wisdom to pay careful attention to these suggestions.

The foundation representatives argued that the school should do more applied and practical work and see its mission as tripartite: research, teaching, and service. The plan of the agricultural colleges was again produced as a model, involving research, extension work, and popular education. The need to establish short courses for health officers was emphasized "to meet the immediate pressing need of this country for better qualified men."[57] Similar intensive, short courses were suggested for public health nurses and social service workers; the foundation again endorsed Vincent's suggestion of the publication of a journal to present special topics in hygiene to a lay audience. It now raised the issue of teaching industrial hygiene and tropical medicine. Despite the fact that it had declined to give specific support to industrial hygiene as "too controversial," the foundation wanted this subject to be developed. At Harvard, local corporations and large industrial plants supported an extensive program. George Vincent wrote Welch: "I have wondered whether some good men are not emerging, one of whom might soon be secured for your staff in Baltimore."[58] The foundation also wanted the school to teach general tropical medicine in addition to the specialized research courses in helminthology and parasitology.

Foundation representatives were willing to help Welch with the problem of recruiting students for the degree of Doctor of Public Health. They suggested that the school revise its admission requirements by expecting two years of college work in the sciences, rather than a four-year liberal arts degree. They also offered a new carrot: thirty-five new scholarships including stipends and tuition.

The Advisory Board of the School of Hygiene discussed these suggestions at a special meeting in October 1919, and agreed they seemed reasonable. The faculty established a committee "to draw up a plan of organization for the School of Hygiene and Public Health, which would include, in addition to the departments already provided for, the new activities suggested by Rockefeller representatives in Industrial Diseases, or Industrial Hygiene, Tropical Medicine, Intensive Courses for Health Officers, Instruction in Social Service, Instruction for Public

Health Nurses."[59] The committee members were Pearl, Welch, News-holme, and Ford; Pearl, as chairman, asked each department head for a plan, to include "the immediate needs of the department, the expansion which is necessary to care for the present rapid development of the school, and an outline of the future plan of organization . . . allowing for the expansion of each department on a broad, comprehensive basis."[60]

Sketching the Future: Facts and Fantasies

The plan for the school submitted in 1919 was written in draft form by Raymond Pearl and then edited and amended by Welch. In Pearl's draft, the existing departments represented "the fundamental scientific basis of all applied hygiene."[61] Next came the applied fields, especially industrial and tropical hygiene. Pearl suggested a hospital for clinical instruction and research, containing wards devoted to occupational, nutritional, tropical, bacteriological, and venereal diseases. Finally, he proposed a department of applied health and public education to conduct extension courses for nurses and social workers and to publish popular health educational materials.

Welch's final draft of the report suggested a much more modest development of applied hygiene and public health education. He proposed a slow and gradual expansion into a few new areas, picking up each of the issues previously discussed with representatives from the foundation. In answer to their plea for shorter periods of training for public health officers, he promoted the one-year course leading to a Certificate of Public Health, and promised an even shorter three-month intensive course for "incumbent health officers . . . not in a position to leave their work for any extended periods."[62] Welch held the line on providing special training for public health nurses and social service workers by pointing to the controversies over the whole future direction of nursing education. As usual, his tactic was postponement: "In view, however, of the survey of this whole field now under way by Miss Goldmark and the expectation that this will lead to important recom-mendations in a field concerning which much diversity of opinion exists, it has been deemed best to await the publication of Miss Gold-mark's studies before making proposals."[63] Here, Welch was referring to the study on nursing education, to be known as the Goldmark Report (1923), which would criticize hospital training schools and advocate the development of university-affiliated schools of nursing.[64]

Welch offered only vague and general promises about the school's involvement in popular health education. The school would continue to sponsor public lectures; instruct students in methods of educating the public; and issue publications of general and popular interest. When the school moved into its new building, its museum, open to the public, would contain models, charts, diagrams, lantern slides, photographs, and public health exhibits. Welch included a plan for the *American Journal of Hygiene*, a series of specialized monographs, and a series of reprint collections, but no popular journal. As usual, Welch resisted the pressure to promise any extensive program of popular education.

For future expansion, Welch addressed four areas of "applied hygiene": child hygiene, mental hygiene, industrial hygiene, and tropical hygiene. The last two received the most attention. Welch proposed four areas of development in industrial hygiene: studies of fatigue and personal hygiene, studies of malnutrition in various industries, studies of clinical cases of occupational diseases in cooperation with the Johns Hopkins Hospital and local industries, and toxicological studies of occupational diseases. In tropical hygiene, Welch proposed studies of climatology, clothing, housing, and sun exposure, and clinical studies of tropical diseases. He promised that the shipping companies of Baltimore and the Public Health Service hospital for immigrants and sailors would provide clinical material for students in tropical medicine.

The reports from the department heads in 1919 gave a detailed account of the operation and organization of the school at the end of its first year, and they also provide insight into the personalities and aspirations of their authors. William Howell's report for the department of physiological hygiene was modest, even self-effacing. Howell planned three main lines of investigation in the department, each the responsibility of a junior faculty member. Reynold Spaeth was to develop a course on industrial hygiene and industrial efficiency; Arthur Meyer would teach a course on air quality and ventilation; and Janet Clark would teach a course on the physiological effects of radiation. As head of the department, Howell would direct the research work, give a lecture course on personal hygiene, and run a weekly journal club for discussion of new research.

Elmer McCollum offered a similarly modest description of the work of the department of chemical hygiene. The main research involved nutritional studies on the rat colony; four younger associates—Helen Parsons, Nina Simmonds, Martha Koehne, and Mathilde Koch—assisted in the laboratory. McCollum would teach an intensive course on nutrition, and David Klein, an associate professor, would teach a course on the chemical analysis of food and water, and on the detection of food and drug adulterants. The extension work of the department included McCollum's study of the nutritional status of children in

Baltimore's schools and orphan homes, and public lectures on nutrition.

Wade Hampton Frost's plan for the department of epidemiology emphasized the need for cooperation with other departments and agencies. Frost planned a course on general methods of epidemiological analysis, a set of laboratory exercises using original records and official statistics, and fieldwork surveys with the State Health Department and the Baltimore City Department of Health. Most of the epidemiological research would be done with, and for, the Public Health Service, with some special projects undertaken for the City and State Health Departments.

By contrast with these modest plans and proposals, Raymond Pearl's report for the department of biometry and vital statistics was both grand and grandiose. His research was to deal with "large and fundamental problems"; the department would be "unique" and would "lead the world." It would conduct intensive genetic and environmental studies of the important causes of death, including acute respiratory infections, cancer and heart disease, to provide "great advances in knowledge of the fundamentals of public health in the next half century."[65]

Pearl asked for a huge staff of fieldworkers: sixteen in the first year, ten more in the second year, and eight more in the third. He wanted two Ford automobiles and a large budget for travel expenses. The teaching plans of the department were also ambitious; Pearl proposed basic and advanced courses in five areas: statistical methods, the construction of mortality tables, the history of disease, anthropometry and the principles of eugenics.

Pearl's report made an eloquent appeal for the use of quantitative methods in public health work, and complained that vast sums of money were being wasted by men not trained in statistical methods. His report included a critique of the malaria control work done by the International Health Board as "entirely inconclusive and essentially worthless." (Welch tactfully removed this section from the draft submitted to the Rockefeller Foundation.)[66]

William Ford gave the department of bacteriology a thoroughly practical orientation. Students were to be trained in the techniques used in diagnostic and public health laboratories for the isolation, identification, and cultivation of pathogenic bacteria. Ford proposed establishment of a model diagnostic laboratory for examinations of water, milk, throat cultures, and blood cultures, thus providing a bridge between laboratory studies and epidemiological fieldwork. Carroll Gideon Bull's department of immunology was directed at more fundamental research on the mechanisms of natural immunity. The department's future plans for applied research included the evaluation of existing immunological materials, an effort to discourage the commercial exploitation of vaccines, and the independent production of vaccines and sera as necessary.

Two departments offered teaching programs with no research component. Sir Arthur Newsholme's course in public health administration covered a broad field, including some statistical and epidemiological methods. Newsholme's own work in this period was largely historical and autobiographical, concerning his own reflections on a long career in public health administration.[67] In the department of sanitary engineering, John Gregory, a working engineer, taught courses on water supplies, water purification, and sewage disposal.

Perhaps the most ambitious plan came from the department of medical zoology, led by Robert Hegner and William Cort. Their report included a wish list for almost indefinite expansion. In Baltimore, twenty-eight instructors would each have a private office and a laboratory; in all, eighty-two rooms would be needed for the department, including student laboratories and lecture halls. Branch laboratories, each with its own staff, were proposed in Panama, Caracas, Guayaquil, and other Latin American cities. A "laboratory ship" would sail to sites of tropical disease outbreaks, sending results to permanent laboratories in Baltimore and Norfolk, Virginia. An educational director for public education would have "a laboratory railroad coach" at his disposal. Research expeditions would be sent to Brazil, Equador, and the Amazon Basin. Cort and Hegner evidently intended to travel in style, and to pattern their activities after those of the International Health Board. As their report correctly concluded, the department would be unique, "since there is no other institution in the world that would approach it in size and comprehensiveness."[68] In accord with the importance of this operation, the salaries of all staff were to be greatly increased.

The budget submitted with the school's report of 1919 was large enough to cause consternation at the Rockefeller Foundation.[69] Until this point, William Welch had prepared budgets every six months on the basis of the expected needs of the school, and the foundation had simply appropriated the funds requested. The sudden expansion of the budget from operating costs of about $100,000 to $300,000 reflected the department heads' submitting their own budgets, untempered by the caution of Welch and Howell. In addition to the departmental funds, Welch had asked for money to finance a small diagnostic laboratory, a museum, a photographer, an artist, and general travel funds for fieldwork.[70]

The Rockefeller Foundation issued an ultimatum: the school would have to restrain its expenditures. The school's future was up for negotiation. Simon Flexner complained that several of the departments were already outspending their equivalents in the School of Medicine. He criticized the business administration of the school:

The school as at present organized takes no account of a kind of central business control which might, I believe, be introduced in the interests of economy. . . . This control should include standardization of salaries and wages of all persons not on the scientific staff, some voice in the number and quality of technical assistants employed by the scientific workers; the making of all purchases in the open market, a system of store room checks and balances . . . a competent business head to assist in preparing the budgets.[71]

In December 1919, the president and secretary of the Rockefeller Foundation spent two days in Baltimore conferring with Welch, the department heads, and the president and the trustees of the Johns Hopkins University. Wickliffe Rose and Simon Flexner followed up with more meetings in Baltimore. A weekend conference in January 1920 was attended by President Vincent, Edwin Embree (secretary of the foundation), Victor Heiser, Simon Flexner, William Welch, and Starr J. Murphy (treasurer of the foundation). The outcome of these negotiations was that the school agreed to accept a fixed, though large, annual budget of $250,000 per year. The foundation officers claimed that the budget restriction was in the institution's best interest: "Rapid growth was resulting in great increase of the budget and was probably not conducive to sound development of departments and their interrelation to the whole institution. . . . If a definite limit were fixed there would be a more gradual and a more carefully studied growth."[72]

Welch acknowledged that the school could thrive on the $250,000 proposed, and he agreed to implement immediately some of the extension work desired by the foundation. As part of the negotiated agreement, Newsholme and Frost would offer a six-week course for public health officers; Hegner and Cort would offer a course in medical zoology for officers of the International Health Board; and the Rockefeller Foundation would provide an additional $10,000 in fellowships for recent medical graduates studying for the Dr.P.H.

The full round of negotiations between Welch and the Rockefeller Foundation would not, however, be complete until the foundation agreed to give the school a new building and an endowment—the one a visible symbol of permanence, the other providing long-term financial security. This accord would be the final reward in a successful series of agreements between the negotiating parties, who had some, but not all, interests in common.

The first classes at the School of Hygiene had been held in temporary quarters in an old physics laboratory at 310–312 West Monument Street, left vacant when the Arts and Sciences faculty moved to a new campus at Homewood in 1915. William Howell renovated the laboratories for bacteriology and chemical hygiene; the other classes were given in existing School of Medicine laboratories. The plans for a new building were to be postponed, and postponed again; for seven years the school operated from a series of temporary offices and laboratories. As the number of faculty and students increased, departments expanded into other vacant buildings, the faculty constantly complaining of cramped quarters and inadequate facilities, and frequently moving in the restless search for additional space.

Originally, the Advisory Board had hoped that a new building could

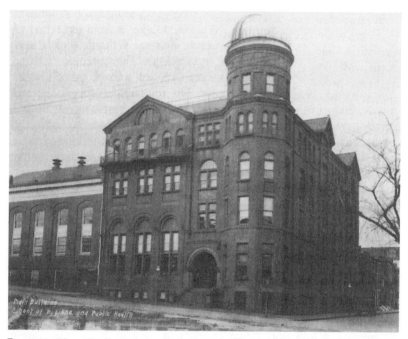

Figure 11. The old Johns Hopkins University physics laboratory at 310–312 West Monument Street served as the temporary headquarters of the School of Hygiene and Public Health from 1918 to 1925. As the school expanded, some of the faculty moved across the street into McCoy Hall. When that building was destroyed by fire, they moved into 625 St. Paul Street and an old biological laboratory at the corner of Eutaw and Little Ross streets. (Courtesy of the Rockefeller Archive Center, Tarrytown, New York.)

be erected before the first class of students arrived. On June 12, 1916, the Executive Board of the Rockefeller Foundation had voted $50,000 for purchase of land and $200,000 to construct the new building. The site of the school had been tentatively chosen as the southeast corner of Wolfe and Monument streets, immediately across the street from the School of Medicine and hospital.[73] In 1916, the cost of this property was estimated at $30,000. Jerome Greene of the Rockefeller Foundation also suggested that the university should gradually acquire the entire block of property enclosed by Monument, Wolfe, McElderry, and Chapel streets.[74]

In July 1916, the university began to acquire options on the land between Wolfe and Monument streets, and the local neighborhood was in an uproar. R. Brent Keyser, a member of the Board of Trustees of the university, explained to Greene, "We have not attempted to get prices on any other location, as we were advised that to do so would probably not make the price on that block any lower, but probably still further rouse the whole neighborhood."[75] Local homeowners were rapidly raising their prices and some were insisting on cash purchases for their houses; under the circumstances it was in the university's interest to buy the property as quickly as possible.[76]

Having acquired the land, the university hired the architectural firm of Archer and Allen to draw up plans and estimates for a new building. The entry of the United States into World War I had, however, delayed all civilian construction as every available architect and draftsman was put to work on war projects. In October 1917, President Goodnow broke the news that it would be impossible to construct a new building before July 1919.[77] The war had not only delayed construction but also greatly inflated the price of building materials. Revised estimates suggested that the building costs would be increased by 50 percent, from $200,000 to $300,000.

In March 1918, Archer and Allen sent the university an architectural sketch of the building, and in July, an estimate of $530,000 prepared by the Bennett Building Company. President Goodnow was "rather appalled." So was George Vincent, who wrote: "I am afraid this is another case of optimistic architects leading their patrons into temptation."[78] Vincent was almost as unhappy about the architectural style of the proposed building as about the price, and he quoted an English publication's review of the design: "It seems to us that an old Greek architect would have used the same material at the same expense and produced a building which would be a delight to the eye; modern science seems to require a formal, military barrack kind of building."[79]

Vincent continued to grumble about the expense of the proposed building, but as the costs of labor and construction materials continued to escalate, he finally approved the plan. President Goodnow asked the War Industries Board for permission to build, but was refused in view of the national shortages of steel and labor.[80] The building plans were thus shelved until after the war.

As the faculty continued to complain about overcrowded conditions, more old biological laboratories belonging to the university were partially renovated for use. McCoy Hall housed the department of biometry and vital statistics, with Pearl's mouse colony in its basement. In 1919, a fire completely destroyed the building, wiping out Pearl's "private scientific library of fifteen thousand pamphlets and books" and killing his experimental mice.[81] These mice had been part of a series of experiments on longevity; since Pearl had claimed that they would live three times longer than normal mice, he was particularly upset about their untimely demise.

In January 1922, President Goodnow and Welch decided that the time was again right to appeal for a new building and they brought their architectural plans to New York to show George Vincent. By now, the cost of the proposed building had again doubled, to more than a million dollars. Each year, the foundation was spending a sum equal to the original projected cost of land, building, and operating costs on the upkeep of the school, and each year the cost of the proposed building was rising. On January 26, 1922, three foundation officers—Richard Pearce, Frederick F. Russell, and Edwin Embree—traveled to Baltimore to argue that, if the Johns Hopkins School was to be a model for other schools in the United States and abroad, it was important "that it be a model which can be copied not only from [the] standpoint of curriculum and work accomplished, but from the standpoint of economical housing and administration."[82] Could the costs of the proposed building be reduced? Could the lecture rooms be reduced in number? Could large student laboratories be combined? Could the School of Hygiene share laboratory space with the School of Medicine? Welch and Howell defended the details of their building plan, giving way only on a couple of large lecture rooms, a combined media preparation room, and a few private laboratories.

On February 1, Embree, Goodnow, Welch, and Howell met with members of the Johns Hopkins Board of Trustees. Embree announced that the foundation officers were prepared to recommend an appropriation of $6 million of which not more than $1 million could be spent for land, buildings, and equipment, with the remainder for endowment.[83] The $5 million endowment represented the annual maintenance of $250,000 capitalized at 5 percent; $1 million was a somewhat conservative estimate of the building costs, reflecting the suspicion that Welch and Howell's building plans were grander than really necessary. This appropriation would complete the foundation's financial obligations to the school; the trustees would be responsible for raising any further funds needed for its development.

On February 24, 1922, the Executive Committee of the Rockefeller Foundation accepted these recommendations and appropriated $6 million for the School of Hygiene, voting "its appreciation of the splendid record already made by this unique institution and its confidence in the ability of the school to continue to make notable contributions to education and leadership in public health."[84]

This gift exceeded all previous Rockefeller grants; as the *Baltimore Sun* announced in banner headlines: "Rockefeller Foundation in Biggest Donation of Kind on Record Provides Permanent Endowment."[85] Goodnow, Welch, and Howell were delighted. Goodnow announced that the school would eventually establish a "model" community, to be administered from the standpoint of public health and hygiene, on principles developed as a result of research.[86] Welch declared that "the good fortune of Baltimore and of Maryland in possessing this School of Hygiene and Public Health should be a stimulus and incentive to make the health administration of the State, the counties and the cities an example worthy of imitation in safeguarding the health of the people."[87]

Three more years were needed to complete the new building across from the Johns Hopkins Medical School on Wolfe Street. The result was a formal and imposing eight-story construction, faced with light-colored brick and limestone. At last the faculty had space for offices, research labs, and experimental animals, together with ample room for student teaching and research.

The first floor boasted a large auditorium, a museum, a library, a lounge, a reading room for students, and the administrative offices of the director and associate director. Each department was allocated one floor, its rooms arranged according to the wishes of the department head, into private offices, seminar rooms, and laboratories. Going up in the elevator, one passed epidemiology and public health administration, biometry and vital statistics, medical zoology, bacteriology, immunology, physiological hygiene, chemical hygiene, and, under the roof, filterable viruses. The construction of the new building was extensively reported in the *American Journal of Hygiene*, the *Revue d'Hygiène*, the *Medical Journal of Rio de Janiero*, *España Medica*, and the *British Medical Journal*. The last publication declared it "carefully designed, well built, attractive in its layout, pleasant as a working place and admirably adapted to the purposes which it has to serve."[88]

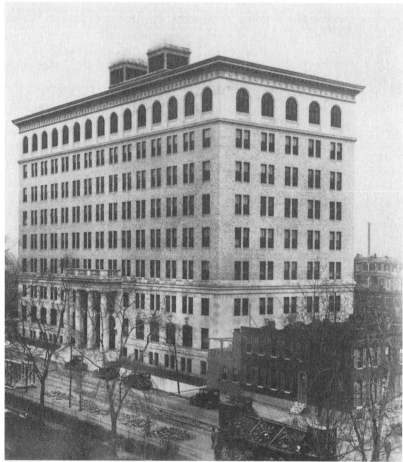

Figure 12. The new building at 615 North Wolfe Street in 1926. (Courtesy of the Alan Mason Chesney Medical Archives of the Johns Hopkins Medical Institutions.)

The *Baltimore Sun* was more interested in the popular health exhibits and demonstrations organized to celebrate the opening of the building: "One of the most extensive exhibits of the enemies of health and cleanliness ever gathered together" was about to be opened to the curious public. The *Sun* reporter continued with enthusiasm:

In the department of entomology there will be a special demonstration of disease-carrying insects. These will include tsetse flies which carry the deadly African sleeping sickness; rat fleas, of the type that still spread the bubonic plague through Asia, and an assortment of midges, flies, lice, and even the lowly bedbug. Living exhibits of mosquitoes, of the types which carry yellow fever and malaria, will be shown in all stages of their live development.

There will also be a demonstration of the smallest disease-producing organisms known to man, the filterable viruses. These, it is said, cannot be seen under even the most powerful microscopes, but their presence is demonstrated by their effects. The effects of the bacteriophage, a submicroscopic germ, which eats certain larger germs, also will be shown.

One of the exhibits which already has attracted attention throughout the world is the rat colony in which Dr. E. V. McCollum, professor of bio-chemistry, tests the favorable and adverse effects of diet. It was through the feeding of rats in this colony, it is said, that cod liver oil was discovered as a preventive and cure for the disease of rickets in children.[89]

The new building was formally opened on October 22, 1926, during the celebration of the university's fiftieth anniversary. Dr. Andrew Balfour, director of the London School of Hygiene and Tropical Medicine, gave a stirring opening address on "Hygiene as a World Force." "I believe that today you are opening and consecrating not a school but a temple, a shrine with infinite possibilities," declared Balfour; "how wide and far-reaching is the sovereignty of hygiene, a dominion to which the limits have not yet been set and which will undoubtedly make its presence felt in many countries where today man grovels in filth and is a prey to pestilence. . . . The pursuit of wealth and the pursuit of pleasure are but evanescent compared with the pursuit of hygiene as a world force."[90]

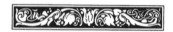

Creating New Disciplines, I:
The Pathology of Disease

hrough their selection of the first faculty, William Welch and William Howell had already established the general framework for professional public health education in the new school; they had decided the disciplines and departments to be represented, and had picked the men whose general approach, philosophy, and research accomplishments they most admired. These first professors of the School of Hygiene were responsible for developing their fields as fundamental disciplines of public health. Welch had always believed that the proper way of running a scientific institution was to pick the "best men" and then give them the freedom and resources to work in their own way, with minimal central direction or planning. The structure of the school reflected this philosophy: each professor had his own budget, and was responsible for organizing the research and teaching in his discipline.

The departments were largely autonomous. Each had only one full professor; the professors were free to cooperate with each other or not, as they saw fit, to select their own staffs, and to determine the intellectual direction of their departments. Some department heads favored a tightly structured unit with a single intellectual focus determined by their own research interests; others favored a more loosely organized structure, with junior faculty and students free to pursue independent research.

The organization of the school in its early years thus produced a loose federation of departments, each dominated by the personality and interests of its leading professor. Although Welch and Howell set the overall direction of the school, the particular character of public health education at Hopkins can also be described as the work of a small number of individual faculty who were, by necessity, responsible for developing and articulating the contributions of their own disciplines to the "new" public health.

96

The "new" public health incorporated a range of scientific disciplines with different objects of study and methods of analysis. Both Welch and Howell had been eager to include disciplines concerned with the promotion of health as well as those investigating the causes of disease. They conceptualized the former group as "physiological hygiene" and the latter as "pathological hygiene" and established strong bases for both within the school from the beginning. This chapter examines the early research in the disciplines centered on the causative agents of disease—pathological hygiene. The next chapter explores the disciplines taking individuals and their health as their object of analysis—physiological hygiene.

The disciplines represented in the various departments were at different levels of development. Some were well-recognized components of public health; others seemed eccentric choices. In general, the closer the original discipline to the biomedical sciences, the more uniform the opinion that it "belonged" in public health. The disciplines investigating the causes of disease were among those universally accepted as a basis for the new public health, as, for example, bacteriology. A few medical schools had included immunology in bacteriology departments, but it was here, for the first time, awarded status as a separate department. Next came the fields already established within zoology: such as protozoology, helminthology, and medical entomology, now linked in the department of medical zoology. The task of medical zoology would be to show the usefulness of these established bodies of knowledge and methods of inquiry to the problems of public health. One branch of this subject, the study of the filterable viruses, was completely new; here, the faculty were contributing to the earliest stages of a scientific field.

The articulation of the disciplines in the 1920s laid the foundations of public health training until World War II and, to a large extent, even to the present. The specific health problems addressed would change over time, and the methodological tools of research would become more sophisticated, but the structure of the disciplines elaborated in this period would continue to provide the basis of public health research and education. Here, the focus on the particular research being undertaken at the School of Hygiene of necessity neglects the important contributions of scientists working at other institutions. Science is a cooperative endeavor, building on the research of many individuals, but a full description of the development of any one discipline is beyond the scope of this book. What follows, then, is a glimpse inside the laboratories, offices, and classrooms of the School of Hygiene in the 1920s.

The disciplines of "pathological hygiene" involved the hunt for the pathological agents of disease, whether bacteria, viruses, insects, protozoa, or parasitic worms. These disciplines primarily involved biological research. The successful laboratory researches of the bacteriologists were now extended to a variety of types of organisms involved in the transmission of disease. Laboratory-based scientists searched for the specific organisms involved in each of the infectious diseases, tried to identify and classify them, to describe them, to follow their life cycles, to investigate their habits and modes of living, to explore ways in which they could be isolated and, if possible, eliminated. As the field of bacteriology had produced prolific discoveries in the 1880s and 1890s, the fields of protozoology, helminthology, entomology, and filterable viruses now yielded rich findings applicable to human disease. As in other disciplines, there was some tension between pure research and its applications, but this tension was minimal; most of the laboratory research seemed quickly to find application in practice.

The hub of pathological research in the School of Hygiene was the department of medical zoology; by 1926, Wickliffe Rose could call it "probably the most active and scientifically productive department in the School."[1] The faculty and students were pouring out volumes of research papers on hookworm, malaria, and other infectious diseases. Students, many of them members of the International Health Board staff or associated with IHB programs around the world, came to learn the methods of investigating the disease-producing and disease-carrying organisms. Some stayed for a few weeks, some for a few months, and some for a few years; many later staffed teaching and research programs on infectious diseases in their home countries. Medical zoology in this period could have been named "tropical diseases" as it was oriented to the infectious disease problems typical of less developed countries.

The leading faculty were Robert Hegner, William Cort, and Francis Root. Hegner and Cort were lively, energetic, sociable, and outgoing, and they helped create a department known for its friendliness and practical jokes. Root, by contrast, was shy, quiet, and reserved, and less boisterous than the others.[2] Hegner came from a small town in Iowa, Cort was a country boy from Colorado, and Root hailed from Ohio; a midwestern faculty who encouraged other young scientists, many from small towns and from the Midwest, to develop careers that would take them around the world.

Hegner defined medical zoology in the following terms:

Medical Zoology is the study of animals that cause human disease, are of direct injury to man, or that disseminate disease producing organisms. . . . From a public health standpoint, the most important species of protozoa and helminths are those parasitic and pathogenic to man. The phenomena presented by the parasitic species, however, can only be inter- preted on the basis of a knowledge of free living species or those living in lower animals which are accessible for both observational and experimental studies.[3]

Hegner thus defined medical zoology as the province of the biologist and declared the relevance of his own early research on free-living protozoa. He believed that there was no essential difference between free-living and parasitic species, and that the parasitic forms had undoubtedly evolved from free-living relatives. He also suggested that a close relationship between parasites (as between the parasites of man and apes) could be used to establish the common ancestry of their hosts.

Parasitology, for Hegner, involved fundamental biological questions. It was a vast and largely unexplored field. Most of the many thousands of species of protozoa and helminths had never been adequately described or studied. Hegner claimed that the discovery of new species of protozoa was an easy business, since so little was known: "Students who have only an elementary training in biology may undertake a problem in pro- tozoology and within a few months may acquire a more extensive and intensive knowledge of the particular subject he is studying than anyone else on earth."[4] It was, he said, easy to be a pioneer in the field; anyone with an inquisitive mind and the instincts of a naturalist could go exploring for new parasitic protozoa. He might also have added that the pioneer needed physical energy and a sense of adventure, judging from his own accounts of excursions to catch crocodiles in the Philippines and hunt monkeys in Panama and Costa Rica—all in order to study the species of protozoa they carried.[5] These adventures brought results, for Hegner himself became the sole or senior author of descriptions of twenty-six new species and two new genera.

As Hegner pointed out, zoologists in parasitology directed their attention to the parasitic organisms, while researchers paid attention to their human hosts. Ideally, the two sides of the subject should be brought together in a new biology of host-parasite relationships. While the zoologist followed the different stages in the life cycle of the parasite, the physician could follow the corresponding clinical signs of infection:

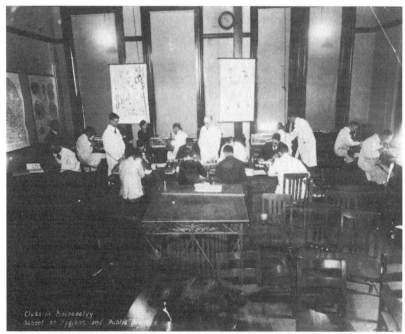

Figure 13. Robert W. Hegner (standing, center), teaching a class in protozoology, circa 1921. (Courtesy of the Rockefeller Archive Center, Tarrytown, New York.)

incubation, symptomatology, convalescence, latency, and relapse. Together, they could raise questions about the factors that allowed infection to take place and determined whether the parasite managed to establish itself or be rejected by the host.[6]

Hegner and his colleagues found that the diet of the host was an important determinant of whether intestinal parasites could become established. They found that some of McCollum's rats—the ones fed on high protein diets—were free of trichomonads. As a result of further experiments, they were able to recommend that people suffering from flagellate diarrhea or *giardia* should eat as much cottage cheese as possible. The casein in cottage cheese apparently created an intestinal environment hostile to the survival of the parasite.

Most of Hegner's experiments were conducted with animal hosts. He found young chicks especially useful, calling them "veritable living test tubes for the cultivation of protozoa." The students collected some of their own experimental animals and parasitic organisms. George Chu, a Chinese teaching assistant, kept a colony of snakes which wandered on occasion into other offices and laboratories. Gerald Winfield, another teaching assistant, was responsible for finding a good supply of experimental animals infected with living parasites to dissect in the laboratory.

Well . . . the best way to get rats was to go out to the city dump. The dump was essentially a huge ashpile and the rats had built huge nests where 15 or 20 of them would live. They had a system of entry or escape tunnels. . . . If you got out there with an old piece of iron pipe 6 or 8 feet long, you could wreck most of the tunnels and force the rats to come running out of one tunnel. . . . You could get a cage of 25 or 30 rats without any trouble. . . . We had a wonderful time. . . . We got on the streetcar. . . . It was about quitting time and the streets were filling up with people. When we changed streetcars in the middle of the city, I had to turn the cage sideways to get on, but we had forgotten to wire the tray at the bottom of the cage. Bang! The tray went out and a half dozen rats with it. . . . The screams came as the rats hit the sidewalks and one of them ran up across the car. It was just a trail of screams. In two minutes the rats were all down in the sewers and gone.[7]

Hegner built a major teaching and research program on the relation of parasitic protozoa to public health problems, especially tropical diseases: African sleeping sickness, Chagas disease, amebic dysentery, intestinal flagellates, and malaria, among many others. Students who had completed the basic courses were encouraged to undertake original research on parasitology and tropical diseases. Their published papers covered a wide range of organisms and disease problems: bird coccidiosis and malaria, trypanosome infections, amoebiasis, intestinal flagellates, herpetomonas of insects, hookworm disease, schistosomes, ascaris, rat nematodes, intestinal flukes, sand flies, dengue fever, and many species of mosquitoes.[8]

Hegner's own work focused especially on intestinal protozoa and malaria, but his publications also ranged widely over the whole field of medical zoology. He was enormously prolific: by the time of his death in 1942, his bibliography totaled some 236 titles, including 13 books. The books included several written with William Cort and Francis Root on parasitology and methods of field diagnosis, and a delightful set of popular lectures called *Big Fleas Have Little Fleas, or, Who's Who among the Protozoa*.[9] This popular work communicated Hegner's delight in protozoology, his ease in explaining technical material, and his robust sense of humor. The text, illustrated with cartoons by Betsy Bang, was sprinkled with instructive poems "such as a gray-haired and feeble protozoologist might dedicate to the fascinating microorganisms that have been his constant companions during long years of toil and trouble."[10] Here is a sample of Hegner's excursions into poetry:

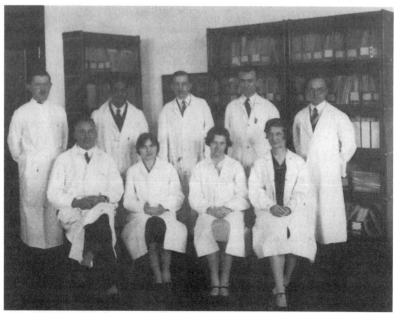

Figure 14. Robert W. Hegner and members of the staff in protozoology, 1926. Front row, from left, Robert W. Hegner, Catherine Lucas, Elizabeth Sanders, Septima C. Smith. Back row: Justin M. Andrews, unidentified, Reginal D. Manwell, Herbert L. Ratcliff, Charles W. Rees. (Courtesy of the Alan Mason Chesney Medical Archives of the Johns Hopkins Medical Institutions.)

Where did you come from protos dear?
Out of the everywhere into the here.
When protos grow up, what do they do?
Each one divides, and then there are two.
Don't little protos long for sex?
You'd be surprised; they vex and vex.
How did the parasite habit evolve?
From free-living ancestors, that's easy to solve.
How did the protos become so prominent?
Mass reproduction rendered them dominant.
Why do the protozoologists weep?
The're too many protos and too little sleep.[11]

Hegner obviously loved to travel and he happily seized opportunities to work in several countries during his professional career. He was exchange professor of parasitology at the London School of Hygiene and Tropical Medicine and spent a year setting up a program in medical zoology at the University of the Philippines. There, he developed a research program for the study of monkey parasites and he later developed another at the Yerkes Experimental Station in Florida. He spent time in Panama and also helped establish a department of protozoology at the Institute of Hygiene and Tropical Medicine in Mexico City. He transmitted his enthusiasm for protozoology to his students in other countries, and they helped expand the research effort on the problems of parasitic diseases and insect vectors in tropical climates, thus applying the basic biological knowledge developed in the laboratory to the practical control of infectious diseases.

Perhaps Hegner's best-known work was on the biology of the malaria parasite *Plasmodium*. In 1920, Hegner noted that although brilliant work had been done on malaria, much was still unknown: there was no adequate method for the detection of malaria carriers, no certainty about the form of the parasite in carriers, no clear knowledge about how the parasite entered the human bloodstream or the blood corpuscles, no understanding of where and how the parasite existed during the dormant phase between relapses, and no agreement about the best methods of therapy for malaria.[12] Hegner proposed studies in each of these areas. In 1921, Wickliffe Rose asked him to discover better methods for the

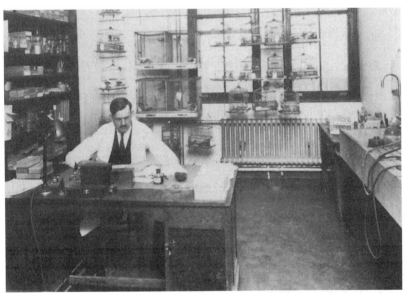

Figure 15. Ernest Hartman (Sc.D., 1926), in the research laboratory for bird malaria studies, 1925. Canaries were used to study host-parasite relationships and the mechanism of infection and to evaluate possible therapeutic agents for treating human malaria. (Courtesy of the Alan Mason Chesney Medical Archives of the Johns Hopkins Medical Institutions.)

The Pathology of Disease / 103

diagnosis of malaria: "The present blood examination as a basis for diagnosis has decided limitations. . . . The percentage of failure to find the parasite is so great as to make the microscope valueless as a means of diagnosing malaria in dealing with large masses of people in malaria control."[13] While Hegner was working on this problem, the International Health Board came up with an even more urgent project: to study the relative effectiveness of different quinine derivatives in malaria prevention and treatment. The Rockefeller Institute supplied the chemicals to be tested and Hegner studied the effects of these drugs on infected canaries.[14] The aim was to find an agent that could destroy all the parasites in the bodies of the experimental animals and hence prevent relapse.[15]

Any drugs found successful in treating bird malaria were supposed to be tested on human beings in the United Fruit Company hospitals in Honduras and Guatemala.[16] (The series of drug tests on bird malaria failed to identify any sufficiently promising new therapeutic agent. Some of the derivatives had beneficial effects but were less effective than quinine; others, powerful in killing the parasite, were also toxic to birds, and by extension, would probably be toxic for humans.) While working on bird malaria, Hegner and his students studied the effects of the parasites on the blood, their tendency to invade immature red blood cells, and the effects of gases, sugar, and other substances on the activity of the parasite. They also investigated the natural course of malarial infection in birds, the periodicity of the infection, and the relationship of relapse to host resistance.[17]

In his later years, Hegner continued to study the host-parasite relationship as it was influenced by changes in the host environment, by feeding experimental animals varied diets, for example, or by exposing them to changes in temperature.[18] He also extended his investigations into the complex biological cycle of the malaria parasite, and continued to argue that, although the problems of malaria control seemed infinite, there was no justification for pessimism. The mechanism of malaria transmission was so complicated and delicate that it could not long resist continued sabotage; with persistence, energy, and money, he believed, malaria would eventually be eradicated.[19]

From Bugs to Worms

William Cort was one of the International Health Board's main hookworm experts and a central figure in hookworm research. When he began work in 1919, hookworm experts thought they already knew enough about the organism to control the disease. Practical experience, however, had shown them wrong: the parasite successfully resisted all efforts to eradicate it from any but the most isolated island populations; in most cases, those freed from hookworm quickly became reinfected. Cort began to study the parasite in the field, taking the first steps toward what is now called an ecological approach to the disease. Beginning in 1921, Cort and his associates conducted field research in Trinidad, Puerto Rico, Panama, Egypt, and China, and published a huge volume of work on the hookworm parasite and existing methods of control.

Cort pushed field research to observe the activity of larvae in the soil, to count the numbers of eggs in the stool of infected hosts, and, in general, to study the biology of the hookworm from every possible point of view. During the winter months he continued research in the laboratory in Baltimore using dog hookworm. Cort and his colleagues also had human hookworm to work with because they had injected themselves in the field. "All this work was relevant," said Cort, "because, in spite of a good deal of literature on the subject of hookworm, this was the first really intensive study of its biology."[20]

Cort began his research when the Rockefeller Sanitary Commission for the Eradication of Hookworm Disease had just finished its work in the southern states with what were then considered remarkable results. The International Health Board had begun extending the program worldwide, entering upon joint contracts with agencies in the tropics guaranteeing to eradicate hookworm. Experience showed such promises to be uncautious and unrealistic. As field administrators encountered frustrations, they began to doubt whether they had enough basic knowledge about hookworm.

In this atmosphere, Cort began formulating his questions. Precisely where did people contract hookworm? How many hookworms lived in the soil? Did domestic or wild animals help disseminate infection? At a time when precise hookworm studies in field laboratories were almost nonexistent, Cort set himself the task of organizing such studies and developing in the laboratory the basic knowledge needed for more successful field operations.[21]

Cort's work followed a progression over a twelve-year period as he traveled around the globe peeling back the layers of complexity to understanding hookworm infection, transmission, and control. In his first field research on a sugar plantation in Trinidad in 1921, Cort wrote that he had found

the place which comes nearest to the lower regions . . . the edge of a sugar cane field on the side of a hill about 10–12 a.m. Can you imagine Dr. Payne, an assistant and myself walking up and down the rows counting the fresh human stools deposited that morning. . . . The field shows numerous hookworm larvae in almost every soil sample taken near the edge. . . . We are planning to get the manager to put in adequate latrines and then carry on an educational campaign and follow the reduction in soil pollution and soil infectivity.[22]

In the first stage of his research, Cort concluded that the educational campaign conducted by the International Health Board, combined with mass treatment programs, had practically eliminated hookworm infestation in Puerto Rico within a period of six weeks. This finding was exactly what Wickliffe Rose, director of the International Health Board, wanted to hear: "I need not say how gratifying it is to have the assurance which this study gives that the measures which have been employed and are being employed in many countries are not altogether in vain. No more important study in the field of hookworm control has been made."[23]

In the wake of this initial success, Cort planned a series of field investigations in tropical countries; unfortunately, he soon discovered that his first conclusions had been premature. Continued research showed that with existing methods it was impossible to eliminate hookworm in any large area; hookworm could only be eradicated in small and isolated populations. As many fieldworkers were to discover, the initally positive effects of control efforts were soon diminished or even negated by the constant problem of reinfection.

From 1921 to 1931 Cort did detailed studies, many of them quantitative, on the life cycle of the hookworm, including methods for measuring the intensity of larval infestation of the soil and for measuring the intensity of hookworm infection in people.[24] He traveled to China in 1923 with his assistant, Norman Stoll, to study local problems in hookworm control. Stoll had developed a simple method for measuring hookworm infestation by means of egg counts, thus saving time and expense in hookworm control programs. Cort and Stoll found that hookworm was not so universal in China as had been suspected; it was endemic only in the silk-growing areas. They also discovered that the use of night soil in cultivating rice did not spread hookworm because the eggs were unable to hatch under water in the rice paddies; its use in silk growing was, however, dangerous because of the method of cultivation: "In the late summer they poured night soil around each mulberry tree to push the growth of the leaves. Then about two weeks later they went into the mulberry groves to pick the leaves to feed the silk worms. In other words, they made a good hookworm culture around every mulberry tree and about two weeks later after the hookworm larvae had had time to develop in the soil they walked in it barefoot."[25] These findings meant that hookworm control programs could now be more effectively targeted in silk-growing areas.[26]

In China, Cort also began to confront the economic and political problems in trying to create an effective disease-control program:

The goal of our research project was to find a practicable control method for hookworm disease. . . . We tried many schemes to render the nightsoil harmless before it was spread, but most of them were too expensive to appeal to the Chinese landlord. Finally we hit upon the simple solution of having nightsoil stored for some days before use on the land and found that this considerably lessened the danger of hookworm transmission. If there had been a strong and stable government to enforce the storage of nightsoil, great strides could have been made in hookworm control. But just at that time, civil war broke out and all progress in the field of public health came to a halt.[27]

Despite the accumulating mass of information concerning the biology and ecology of hookworm, practical control of hookworm disease was still not very successful. After a final field trip to Panama in 1926, Cort began to focus on the human hosts. With a constant exposure to hookworm infection, why did some individuals suffer much more than others? Why did only some of those infected display symptoms of disease? After conversations with Hegner and others, Cort began to study the problem from a new perspective, that of host resistance. He and his students began to investigate the resistance of dogs to infection with dog hookworm, a different but closely related parasite. Gilbert Otto and William Cort found that healthy dogs developed immunity to repeated hookworm exposures, but when placed on a deficient diet, the dogs lost their resistance and acquired heavy hookworm infestations. When well fed, the dogs again became hookworm resistant. By a mechanism not then understood, proper functioning of the dog's immune system depended on proper nutrition.

Cort became tremendously enthusiastic about the idea that "it may be actually possible to cure hookworm infestation and disease by putting the patients on an adequate diet."[28] In 1931, he met William Porter of the University of Virginia Medical School, who found that he could cure the symptoms of both anemia and hookworm by giving children liver extract. This meeting confirmed Cort's conviction that he was "on the trail of one of the most important developments in hookworm disease," that it was really a dietary deficiency disease. To test this hypothesis, he suggested large-scale nutritional experiments with human hookworm. In a rather backhanded compliment, Charles Stiles, the man who had first directed national attention to hookworm disease, wrote to Cort: "I want to congratulate you on what I consider by all odds the most important piece of work you have yet done on hookworms, worth more than all your other painstaking work on hookworm put together." Stiles went on to object to the economic cost of improving the diet of the poor: "Acknowledging the full importance of diet in hookworm disease, the important question arises from the standpoint of the field worker, how much does the improved diet cost, and since we are dealing with very poor families this has been the stumbling block in emphasizing the diet in the field."[29]

Cort wanted to pursue the relationship between diet and hookworm disease but, in 1933, just as he was ready to begin a major new research project, he lost his funding. The depression was in full swing and the International Health Board budget had been cut; it was now moving out of the field of hookworm control.

Beginning in 1935, Cort was able to get small grants for laboratory research on dog hookworm, but he was unable to carry out his planned work on human nutrition and its relationship to hookworm disease. Cort confirmed his findings for dog hookworm and continued to suggest, though he could not prove, that "a general improvement of a population group especially through an adequate diet" was necessary to control human hookworm. Although Cort felt enormously optimistic that this insight provided the answer to the hookworm problem, many field-workers thought it provided no solutions. If hookworm was a disease of malnutrition and poverty, then none of the available biological and sanitary methods could eradicate the disease.

Unfortunately, Cort was right: to solve the hookworm problem, it would be necessary to deal with poverty and hunger. People needed good food to increase their resistance to hookworm; they also needed shoes and sanitary latrines to prevent constant reinfection from the soil. In this case as in many others, research could clarify the depth of the problem but could not provide easy solutions. Hookworm remains a problem in tropical countries today.

Though hookworm was the parasite investigated over the longest period of time, it was not the only subject of research. Ascaris and other parasitic diseases were studied in the southern states in the summer months. Students also followed their own independent research inter-ests. Claude Barlow's investigations of the human liver fluke were glowingly reported in 1925 by the Baltimore Sun as "a human and pulsing story" and "a story of patient and unremitting toil, of perseverance in the face of repeated discouragement, of seemingly insuperable obstacles overcome, of personal heroism unsurpassed on any battlefield since the first Egyptian pharaoh led an army against the Hittite chiefs."[30] Barlow, a medical missionary in China, had found the people heavily infected with the liver fluke, *Fasciolopsis buski*, whose mode of transmission was then unknown. Barlow decided to study the parasite. He investigated it in China as far as his minimal equipment allowed, then sailed for Hopkins to extend his research. Before leaving China, he swallowed thirty-two live parasites. By thus carrying the experimental material in his body, he could avoid being challenged by customs and immigration officials.

After intensive study, both in Baltimore and China, Barlow was able to close the life cycle of the parasite, including the transmission of the microscopic larvae of the liver fluke by the raw water chestnuts eaten by Chinese agricultural workers. Barlow again experimented on himself in outlining the course of human infection. In 1922, he swallowed 132 live cysts and, in the four months of illness that followed, recorded every symptom and stage of the disease. He tested various remedies, noted the effects of each, and, as the newspapers reported, he "came out of the ordeal with a weakened body, but a strengthened conviction that he had found how the disease was caused and how it was spread."[31]

During World War II, Barlow continued parasitic research using his own body as his experimental laboratory. This time he brought home schistosomiasis to study the course of the disease. For this work, he was awarded the Medal of Honor. Despite his rather gruesome research methods, Barlow displayed the curiosity and playful creativity of a child let loose in a world of strange and wonderful discoveries. This same kind of feeling seemed to pervade much of the research done on the fourth floor and spilled over into practical jokes, Dr. Cort's W. C. Fields' imitations, excursions to Baltimore's Skating Palace, and even the animated discussions of research at the Friday luncheons.

A World of Mosquitoes

Francis Root, given responsibility for teaching and research in medical entomology, immersed himself in this new field and emerged as a specialist in the taxonomy and identification of mosquitoes. Mosquitoes were especially important in public health as the transmitters of malaria and yellow fever. Some species of mosquitoes spread these diseases while others were harmless, and each species had its own particular range, habits, and behavior. In order for disease control programs to be effective, it was important to be able to sort out the vectors from the nonvectors and to direct attention to the few dangerous disease-carrying species rather than to the control of all mosquitoes. The principle of "species sanitation" meant the identification and destruction of the disease-carrying species, leaving harmless species alone.

Root worked mainly with malaria control programs. Since malaria control workers in the field were often unable to differentiate one mosquito from another, they had to rely on the services of a few knowledgeable and experienced taxonomists. In the 1920s, taxonomic work was a matter of patient microscopic observation; only those with extensive experience could weigh the small differences among closely similar species and correctly identify individual specimens. International Health Board officers from the malaria control programs captured mosquitoes and sent difficult specimens to Baltimore for Root to identify. Although Root complained about the mangled specimens arriving from Latin America, he was usually able to identify them; his letters to field directors were full of patient instructions as to the best methods for distinguishing species.[32] Root dissected out thousands and thousands of mosquitoes in order to determine which species actually transmitted malaria; the work required only simple equipment but infinite patience. Root's work on the *anopheles* mosquitoes included the description of the most dangerous malaria vector in Latin America, *Anopheles darlingi.*

In 1925, the International Health Board asked Welch if he would allow Root to spend six months in Brazil demonstrating methods for identifying mosquitoes and discussing the problems confronting malariologists. Welch responded:

Our men in the medical zoological group are crazy to get into the field and I sympathize with them. There is nothing quite so worthwhile as giving coming young investigators the best chance for their development and for winning their spurs. The more I see of Root the more I am impressed with his ability and zeal. He is rather retiring and reserved and I shall be glad to see him given the opportunity.[33]

Root conducted extensive studies of the Brazilian mosquitoes, the blood-sucking arthropods of Honduras and Costa Rica, the sand flies of the West Indies, and the mosquitoes of Venezuela and Grenada. Despite his professional concern with mosquitoes, Root much preferred dragonflies, the subject of his first published article.[34] Whenever he went to a new area of the United States or Latin America, Root always first investigated the character of its dragonflies, before settling down to a serious study of its mosquitoes or ticks.[35]

Root continued to assist the International Health Board with malaria control programs until his early death in 1934. He was remembered for his "disciplined energy and efficient skill," "kindly smile," and "complete lack of ostentation."[36] He was an outstanding lecturer, being well organized and warm and sympathetic to students. Root was succeeded by his former student, Ottis Causey, who had been professor of biology in Bangkok, and would later join the International Health Division of the Rockefeller Foundation in Brazil. When Lloyd Rozeboom in turn succeeded Causey, he shifted the program in entomology from purely microscopic taxonomy to experimental taxonomy, by which species were differentiated by cross-breeding experiments. The aim remained the same: to understand mosquito populations better so that malaria control work could be carried out more effectively.[37]

The Smallest of All Disease-Producing Organisms

In planning the scope of pathological hygiene, no one at first thought of including filterable viruses. These smallest of disease-producing organisms were just beginning to be recognized, and their enormous importance for human disease was not widely realized. The department of filterable viruses at the school was created through a series of accidents and the personal dedication of Charles E. Simon. Simon had completed extensive medical training in Philadelphia, Baltimore, Paris, and Basel, but found that psychological problems prevented him from establishing a successful medical practice; he then turned to a career in medical research, setting up his own diagnostic laboratory and devoting himself to teaching, writing, and experimental work in the field of immunology.[38]

Simon came to the School of Hygiene in a most unorthodox manner. He had been professor of clinical pathology and experimental medicine at the University of Maryland at the outbreak of World War I, but his outspoken pro-German sympathies had made it impossible for him to continue working there. In 1919, he found refuge in the Hopkins department of medical zoology.

Despite a lack of financial support, Simon devoted himself to the School of Hygiene and began to teach in the new field of filterable viruses. Filtration was the method by which microorganisms were separated from the fluids in which they were contained; the viruses, being much smaller than bacteria, could pass through all known filtering agents—hence, the name "filterable viruses."[39] Simon's first formal course on this subject, offered in 1922, was said to be the first of its kind in the world.

Simon poured his soul into his teaching. He traveled to laboratories in Germany, Austria, Switzerland, and Denmark, seeking their latest experimental materials and results, and he hounded investigators throughout the United States with requests for slides and tissue cultures.[40] Everything he obtained was turned into raw material for his

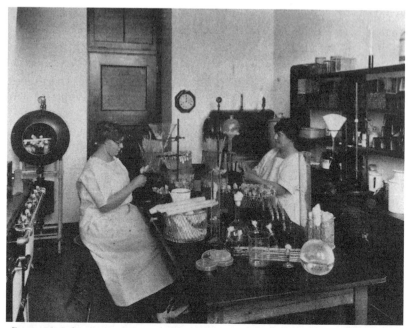

Figure 16. Laboratory assistants in the media room, preparing materials for the students, circa 1926. Miss Imwold is seated at right. (Courtesy of the Alan Mason Chesney Medical Archives of the Johns Hopkins Medical Institutions.)

course and for student research projects. Simon collected so much material that by 1923, he told Welch: "We are now in the possession of what is probably the largest collection of material bearing on diseases caused by filterable viruses that exist[s] in the world."[41]

The students were delighted with these efforts and presented Simon with a formal "appreciation," which read:

As members of the First Class of *Filterable Viruses* of Johns Hopkins University (and, we understand, of any institution in the world) we wish in this formal way to express our profound esteem and gratitude for the insight given us by the breadth of its subject material. And, we feel that this course was admirably organized and presented.

Just as impressive is the scope of the experimental investigational field disclosed by even so brief a survey of a new world.

These were the more forceful in that we were privileged to enjoy this laboratory course for only six short weeks. We dare to suggest that the lecture material and laboratory experiments, pertinent to the subject, seem easily sufficient for a major course in the School of Hygiene.

We wish therefore to take advantage of the historic opportunity afforded us as students in this initial teaching enterprise in Filterable Viruses, to present these sentiments over our signatures, to the teacher of the course, Dr. C. E. Simon and to the Director of the School, in which such a forward-looking course was first given, Dr. W. H. Welch.[42]

Simon's course explored a "new world" of scientific research including investigations of smallpox, poliomyelitis, influenza, typhus, rabies, and herpes. It was so successful that it first expanded into a division of filterable viruses and soon after, the department of filterable viruses. Simon was made full professor. Despite this formal recognition, few fully realized the importance of filterable viruses, or, in modern terminology, of virology. Simon was given two small rooms at the top of the School of Hygiene, next to the elevator apparatus, for his research and that of his students.

Research on viruses could be an adventurous business in the early days. One of Simon's students, Howard Andervont, spoke of his research on fowl plague, better known as Hühner, a highly contagious and fatal infection of chickens: "Unfortunately, this work had to be discontinued because it was discovered that Simon had imported the fowl plague virus illegally, to say the least, into this country, without the knowledge of the Department of Agriculture."[43] Andervont had taken this highly contagious and fatal virus out to his home in Ohio where he had transferred it at regular intervals into chickens. Luckily, he had then buried the carcasses of the chickens, upon Dr. Simon's suggestion, at least two feet deep. When the Department of Agriculture discovered this venture, its officials were understandably upset. Fortunately, there were no chickens in the immediate neighborhood of Andervont's home and no real damage was done.

Andervont also remembered working on the *Rous sarcoma* virus at the School of Hygiene.

We were on the roof of the new School of Hygiene building taking the feathers out of the [experimental] chickens with no other purpose in mind but that we would put them in an autoclave and have some chicken for food. Who should come out suddenly but Dr. Welch and Dr. Goodnow (President of the Johns Hopkins University at that time). Dr. Welch showed him the view and on the way out asked us what we were doing. We said we were working on the Rous sarcoma virus and explained the purpose and the results we were getting. When they left to get the elevator, Dr. Welch let Dr. Goodnow go first, turned and said: "I hope it tastes good, boys."[44]

After a short career at the School of Hygiene, Simon died in 1927, leaving a rich legacy. He had started the first teaching program in filterable viruses, compiled an enormous store of research materials, and left a group of enthusiastic students to extend the work he had begun.

Of all the disciplines institutionalized in the School of Hygiene, bacteriology was probably the most widely recognized as a foundation of the "new" public health. The germ theory of disease was celebrated: a rapid succession of bacteriological discoveries over fifty years seemed to promise the solution to all the problems of infectious disease. Rarely had any research program been so fruitful in terms of the application of scientific knowledge to human health.

But by the 1920s, the very success of bacteriology in the preceding half century meant that fundamentals of the field had already been well established; the most dramatic period of rapid discoveries was over, and the subsequent period of "normal science," of consolidation and extension of bacteriological techniques and methods, was less glamorous, less studded with startling breakthroughs and discoveries. The department of bacteriology in the School of Hygiene trained students in the essentials of the field but did not, in this early period, develop a national or international reputation for research. The necessity and utility of bacteriological studies were never in question; professors of bacteriology did not have to campaign for the recognition of their field, nor did they have to struggle to attract students; everyone agreed that public health officers needed to be trained in bacteriological methods of analysis.

From 1918 until 1923 William Henry Welch held the title of head of the departments of bacteriology and immunology. Welch was not active in either department; the major responsibility for bacteriology lay with William W. Ford who had transferred to the School of Hygiene from the Johns Hopkins Medical School. Ford had earlier graduated from the medical school, studied at McGill University and the Institute for Infectious Diseases in Berlin, and returned to teach on the Hopkins faculty in 1903. As was Welch, Ford was interested in the history of medicine; he wrote a lively and popular text on the history of bacteriology, published in 1939.[45] Ford had helped Welch and Howell in planning the School of Hygiene and continued to be actively involved in the major committees and administrative work; he became full professor and head of the department of bacteriology in 1923. A rather reserved person, he mixed relatively little in the social life of the school. He gave his students and staff a great deal of freedom and independence to determine their own research interests.

Ford's research involved two main areas: the poisonous mushrooms and the bacteria found in heated and pasteurized milk.[46] The mushroom research combined clinical reports, experimental research on animals, and chemical tests for active principles; Ford produced a comprehensive survey of about forty "suspicious" or "doubtfully edible" mushrooms with an account of their chemical constituents and physiological effects. Ford's work on the bacteriology of milk was directed at the widespread problem of summer diarrhea in children. He believed that the problem was related to pasteurization and argued that, under normal circumstances, the lactic acid bacteria in milk inhibited the growth of organisms responsible for decomposition and putrefaction. When the lactic acid bacteria were killed by heating, the spore-bearing organisms remaining could still produce decomposition and bacterial toxins. When pasteurized milk was kept too long, it could therefore produce diarrhea in children.

Students in the department of bacteriology were taught to organize and administer public health laboratories and to identify the pathogenic organisms responsible for human diseases. They were shown how to differentiate pathogenic bacteria from closely similar, but harmless, organisms. They identified bacteria by morphological, cultural, and biochemical reactions and were trained in the bacteriological methods of examination of air, soil, water, sewage, milk, and foods.[47] The department sponsored a joint research seminar with the department of

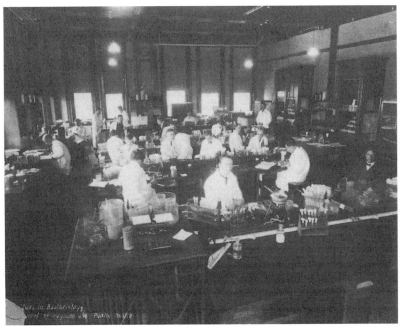

Figure 17. Class in bacteriology, taught by William W. Ford (in bow tie, far right), circa 1921. (Courtesy of the Rockefeller Archive Center, Tarrytown, New York.)

The Pathology of Disease / 115

immunology and also offered a teacher's course in elementary bacteriology for public school teachers in Baltimore.

Ford's associates in the department of bacteriology in the 1920s were Percy D. Meader, George H. Robinson, Linda B. Lange, Samuel Reed Damon, Martin Frobisher, Jr., and Calista P. Eliot. Each member of the department pursued his or her own interests. Meader concentrated on pathogenic anaerobes and Robinson on the spirochaetes. Linda Lange worked on the susceptibility of rats and guinea pigs to tuberculosis, and studied the influence of diet. (Lange, an early feminist, complained about discrimination against women in science, and later willed her money to encourage other women scientists.) Extending Ford's work on food toxins, Samuel Damon published a comprehensive text on *Food Infections and Food Intoxifications*. [48] Martin Frobisher studied the effects of low surface tension on bacteria and carried out extensive studies of diphtheria. During the war, he became acting head of the department and managing editor of the *American Journal of Hygiene*. He later left Baltimore to work on yellow fever in Brazil. Calista Eliot worked on phagocytosis and on the bacteria found in oysters, the latter subject being of special interest to the seafood industry of Maryland. Later, she worked to improve typhoid vaccines through a method of selecting the bacteria most effective in producing antibodies.

One of the most significant, and certainly the most lucrative, pieces of research in the department was begun by a voluntary research worker. Veader Leonard worked with the new chemical disinfectant, hexylresorcinol, and found that when given orally, it had a bactericidal action on infectious material in the genito-urinary tract. The pharmaceutical company of Sharp and Dohme then gave the school $5,000 a year to continue this work under Leonard's direction, in effect more than doubling the department's research budget. Leonard, Frobisher, and several students published a series of papers confirming the clinical usefulness of hexylresorcinol and studying its properties. [49] The immediate clinical applications of this work were quickly recognized by the pharmaceutical companies and the medical community. Several of the younger faculty members left the School of Hygiene to work directly for Sharp and Dohme because the company paid more attractive salaries than did the university.

When Ford died in 1937, Kenneth F. Maxcy, who was mainly interested in epidemiology, took over the department for a brief period until he became professor of epidemiology; Maxcy was in turn succeeded by Thomas B. Turner who worked on the bacteriology and epidemiology of syphilis, and turned the department into an international center for research and training in venereal disease control.

One department concentrated on the resistance of human and animal hosts to invading pathogens: immunology was the effort to discover and elucidate the mechanisms of this resistance. Though Welch was the formal head of the department of immunology, Carroll Gideon Bull really directed the teaching and research work of the department. Bull had come to Baltimore from the Rockefeller Institute for Medical Research in New York, where he had been studying the Welch bacillus. (In 1891, Welch had discovered the causative organism in gas gangrene, then called the Bacillus welchii, and now named *Clostridium perfringens*.) Infections from this organism were especially problematic in hospitals where they could prove fatal to surgical patients. Bull had produced an antitoxin for fighting gas gangrene, used on the western front in World War I.[50] This antitoxin could render men or animals resistant to the effects of the toxin and arrest progression of the disease.

In addition to his work on the Welch antitoxin, Bull studied the natural immunity to pneumonia found in domestic chickens and pigeons. Domestic fowl were immune to infection by pneumococci, whereas rabbits and mice showed almost no resistance. Roscoe Hyde, who became associate professor in the department in 1923, also investigated this phenomenon. Working with a doctoral student, Clennie Bailey, he discovered specific antibodies in the blood of chickens that conferred resistance when given to mice and produced immunity to the disease.[51]

Bull was interested in studying the significance of hereditary factors and diet in the acquisition of immunity to infectious diseases, and he wanted to investigate the epidemiological factors involved in the natural diseases of different species. He studied the numerous brain lesions found in "normal" laboratory rabbits and reported that up to 50 percent of stock rabbits had brain lesions.[52] Though this finding helped clear up many conflicting reports of the experimental reproduction in rabbits of the characteristic lesions of syphilis, poliomyelitis, and encephalitis, a source of healthy "normal" rabbits was still needed. In 1925, the department established a rabbit colony on the Magothy River.

Members of the department of immunology worked closely with faculty in the departments of bacteriology and epidemiology. In the 1920s, the three departments cooperated in a study of diphtheria in Baltimore and examined the entire school population to determine the frequency of diphtheria carriers. The faculty and students studied cultures from 8,000 schoolchildren and opened a summer diphtheria

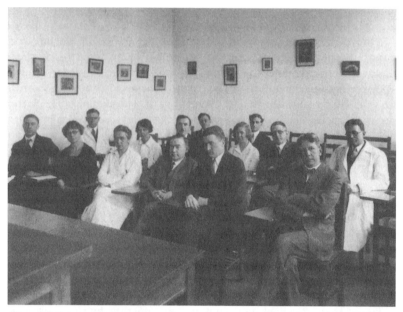

Figure 18. Joint seminar in bacteriology and immunology, taught by William W. Ford and Carroll Gideon Bull, circa 1925. Front row, from left: G. Howard Bailey, Elizabeth I. Parsons, Linda B. Lange, Percy Meader, William Feirer, William W. Ford. Second row: S. Reed Damon, unidentified, Roscoe R. Hyde, unidentified, Allen Freeman, Carroll Gideon Bull. Back row: unidentified students. (Courtesy of the Alan Mason Chesney Medical Archives of the Johns Hopkins Medical Institutions.)

immunization clinic to provide toxin-antitoxin treatments to susceptible children. In connection with this study, they discovered a rapid method for distinguishing between virulent and nonvirulent bacilli by injecting a small amount of culture into the skin of a guinea pig. The new method produced results in two days instead of ten, and used many fewer animals.

Roscoe R. Hyde directed his studies in the mid-1920s toward fundamental problems in immunology. He was especially interested in the heterophilic antigens. These substances, found in the tissues of many animals, could stimulate antibody production against unrelated substances even in widely different species. Hyde studied these antigens and the specificity of the antibodies produced. Antibodies, the mediators of acquired immunity, are unable in most cases to act alone, and require the cooperation of complement, a group of circulating plasma proteins with enzymatic functions.[53] Complement is activated by antigen-antibody reactions; when active, it can destroy bacteria and also cause tissue injury. Animals lacking in complement are thus especially important to investigators studying the activities and functions of heterophilic antigens, and Hyde was able to develop the first strain of complement-deficient guinea pigs for experimental purposes. He used these guinea pigs for a series of experiments, mainly published in the *American Journal of Hygiene*, which began the process of investigating and describing the effects of complement.[54]

Hyde also became interested in filterable viruses, and later taught courses on this subject. He conducted a variety of studies on influenza virus, infectious myxomatosis of rabbits, smallpox, and some of the tumor-inducing viruses. Under Hyde's direction, a small animal farm was established to breed rabbits, guinea pigs, and rats for experimental purposes. In addition to the complement-deficient guinea pigs, a highly homogenous strain of "Dutchbelt" rabbits was developed, and was widely used for research purposes.

Also in immunology, G. Howard Bailey became known for his work on the heterophilic antigens and the Forssman substance, which he and others tracked through a wide range of fauna and flora, from bacteria to man.[55] The presence of the Forssman antigen in infectious agents was especially enticing for immunologists interested in disease for it evoked such visions as possible cross-immunization by environmental agents (such as by foods containing the antigen) to protect against pathogenic organisms. Bailey and Sidney Raffel also worked on the problem of hypersensitivity to the horse serum used by pharmaceutical companies to produce antibodies for treatment of pneumonia, and they tried, unsuccessfully, to produce autoimmune disease in rabbits.

Teaching in the department centered on practical laboratory work: "The course for beginners consists of fixed exercises for which the student is given detailed outlines and protocols. The students prepare their own reagents. For example, they inject rabbits with red blood cells, bacteria—usually two varieties—heterologous proteins, bacterial toxins, etc., for the preparations of hemolytic, agglutinating, bacteriolytic, precipitating and opsonizing sera."[56]

Preparation of reagents could take a good deal of student time. Beef hearts were used to make antigen for the Wassermann tests, for example, so students had to buy these in the neighboring northeast market. Even more difficult was the process of catching sheep to take blood samples. The sheep were kept in a small pasture at the back of the school, now replaced by a parking lot. The sheep served several functions. They proved a cheap method of mowing the grass around the new building, they provided an endless source of interest and amusement for city children, and, most important, they were a convenient source of fresh blood for laboratory tests. An early student, Marie Koch, described the system: "We had to collect our sterile flasks and sterile syringes and everything and go down and try to lasso this darn sheep in the back yard. Finally, we'd get the sheep. Burt would shave its neck, and I had to stretch its neck and put in the syringe and that's how we collected our blood."[57]

Advanced students were provided with laboratory facilities for independent research. One such student, Herald R. Cox, became interested in the ricksettsia, a group of organisms that cause Rocky Mountain spotted fever and typhus. Cox became famous for his method of growing ricksettsia in fertile egg membranes, thus permitting the development of vaccines. Later, Cox was employed in the Lederle Laboratories and was engaged in developing one of the live polio vaccines. Several of the students went on to do fundamental research in immunology and others became practicing public health officers, directors of laboratories for state health departments, or workers in commercial companies involved in the development and production of vaccines.

There were few formal relationships between the departments in the School of Hygiene and other units of the university, but there were various informal connections. Hegner and Root had originally been members of the biology department at Homewood and continued to invite its members to share seminars and the luncheon meetings when mutual research interests were discussed. Ford had been a member of the medical school faculty and continued his relationships with friends and colleagues across the street. Medical staff at the hospital sometimes consulted members of the departments of "pathological hygiene" when patients arrived bearing unfamiliar parasitic or bacterial infections. The orientation of these departments toward biological research and the pathogenic organisms of disease thus helped diminish the distance between the School of Hygiene and other parts of the university.

Taken together, the departments of medical zoology (including protozoology, helminthology, entomology, and filterable viruses), bacteriology, and immunology provided research and teaching on the whole range of organisms known to cause diseases—the protozoa, worms, insects, viruses, and bacteria. Identification of these causal agents and the discovery of ways to control them or neutralize their effects had been central to the successes of scientific medicine and public health in the half century preceding the opening of the new school. Continued expansion of these areas of knowledge and their application to the health of populations had been confidently expected, and their research productivity more than repaid these expectations. However, both Welch and Howell were determined not to limit the scope of the school to investigation of pathological agents. They wanted an equally strong emphasis on healthy individuals and on the promotion of human health through environmental improvement, increased knowledge of nutrition, better sanitation, and more efficient planning and administration of health programs. These were the concerns of the departments of "physiological hygiene."

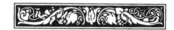

Creating New Disciplines, II:
The Physiology of Health

illiam Welch and William Howell, planning the new school, decided on two main divisions: the pathological and the physiological. They intended to emphasize their dual commitment to the study and control of the infectious diseases and also to the broader question of the study and protection of health itself. Welch wanted to break with the often narrow focus on specific diseases and to increase public health's range to include the social, environmental, industrial, and personal dimensions of health and illness. "Disease prevention and health promotion" were to be the dual concerns of the school.

In discussing the broader approach to public health, Welch frequently referred to the German hygienic institutes and particularly to Pettenkofer's Institute of Hygiene in Munich. The nineteenth-century German institutes had taken a "physiological" view of health and had analyzed the effects of environmental conditions on a population's health. Despite his own training and interest in bacteriology and admiration for the effectiveness of the germ theory of disease, Welch felt that many of the benefits of the environmental or physiological perspective were in danger of being lost in the rush to examine, identify, and describe the pathogenic organisms of disease.

Welch saw that the analysis of pathogenic organisms was only one set of approaches to health problems. The recognition of diseases as social as well as biological realities led to the understanding that their outbreak had much to do with social and sanitary conditions. Consequently, disease control required epidemiological, administrative, and sanitary expertise that went beyond the microscope or the laboratory bench.

The disciplines of pathological hygiene depended fundamentally on laboratory research, as has already been discussed. If one turned attention from the pathological organisms to the human host, however, laboratory research alone was not enough. The disciplines of physiological hygiene required the laboratory sciences but also, and often more important, field research and practice. Indeed, there was sometimes considerable tension between the disciplines concentrating on pure research in the laboratory and those emphasizing the practical application of existing knowledge. Some maintained that the school's mission was basic research, often considered synonymous with laboratory research, while others felt that research not directly applicable to real health problems should have no role in a school of public health. At the extreme end of the spectrum, a few people, especially those in public health administration, felt that the main point should be to apply already existing knowledge rather than devote resources to further research. (This last view was rare in the research-oriented Hopkins school, though common among public health officers in the field.)

The disciplines of physiological hygiene ranged across the spectrum: some focused on laboratory research, some on the geographical and statistical distribution of disease, some on the practicalities of administration and sanitary engineering. At times, those in different disciplines competed for funds and the "pure" versus "applied" debates became serious confrontations; usually, however, the battles were relatively mild ideological ones as faculty in the more applied fields defended their claim to be as legitimately "scientific" as those involved in basic research. Similarly, the departments concerned with understanding, maintaining, and enhancing the health of whole individuals had to defend the idea that their disciplines were as legitimately "scientific" as those focusing on pathogenic organisms.

Several disciplines had uncertain claims to scientific status within a school of public health. The fields of public health administration and vital statistics (or biometry) were well established in Britain but were little recognized as academic subjects in the United States, much less as fields for research. Physiology was a well-established discipline within medicine, but had to be adapted to the different needs of public health. Chemical hygiene, the forerunner of the field of nutrition, only existed in nascent form in agricultural colleges and experiment stations, its potential application to human health virtually ignored. Epidemiological studies in the United States were still in their early stages, the power of epidemiological methods still overshadowed by the more dramatic discoveries of the bacteriological laboratory. Sanitary engineering was a well-developed discipline, but was regarded by many as more practical than scientific, more engineering than hygiene.

The departments created for these disciplines in the School of Hygiene had few appropriate models on which to rely, and each had to stake out its own claim to practical significance and scientific importance.

The Rules of Right Living

Of the disciplines oriented to understanding the rules of maintaining and promoting the health of individuals, physiological hygiene was one of the most firmly devoted to "pure" laboratory research. The department of physiological hygiene, headed by William Howell, was central to Welch and Howell's vision of public health as a dual concept including both the prevention of disease and promotion of health. With the discrediting of older ideas about the environmental causes of disease, it was, however, necessary to reconceptualize the possible contribution of physiology to public health. As a leading American physiologist and professor of physiology at the Johns Hopkins Medical School, Howell was given the task of restoring physiology to a central place in public health and of redefining the relationship of good health to environmental conditions.

Howell decided his department should include several major areas: the study of the physical environment and its effect on health, working conditions and occupational hazards, diet and nutrition, and personal hygiene. Howell argued that the "external and internal environment" of man should be subject to scientific study and control in order to "realize the optimum conditions of health and to avoid the beginnings of constitutional and degenerative diseases."[1] Instead of simply controlling infectious diseases, the new science of physiological hygiene was to examine the means of "preservation of health" and the method of attaining maximum physical and physiological efficiency. Howell defined environmental health in the broadest possible fashion; his various discussions of environmental problems included the more familiar listing of specific living and working conditions, but also such issues as the complexity and speed of modern civilization, the dangers of the automobile, the threat of war and of famine, and the problems of population.

Howell gave personal hygiene an important, if subordinate, role in the protection and promotion of health: "We are as a matter of fact very ignorant in regard to what might be called the rules of right living, that is to say the kind of living that would maintain the functions of our body at the highest standard of efficiency. . . . Personal hygiene . . . calls for scientific study of the most exact kind."[2] Among the "rules of right living," Howell stressed the need for a calm approach to life, exercise, and fresh air. In popular radio broadcasts made for the Baltimore City

Health Department, he discussed "the evil influence that hurry and worry and excitement have on our digestive processes" and urged his audience to eat their meals in a leisurely fashion to prevent digestive disorders.[3] He also emphasized the need for more scientific studies of the chronic diseases:

The expectation of life at birth has been increased during the last fifty years by 10 years or more, largely through the control of the infectious diseases of early life. But most of us would place an equal or higher value upon the kind of knowledge that would enable us to avoid those disabling defects and illnesses that bring about chronic invalidism or impair our physical efficiency without killing us outright.[4]

Howell did, however, reject a suggestion from the National Research Council that he study the harmful effects of tobacco. A smoker himself, Howell said he thought such a study would be "not useful."[5]

Courses in the department of physiological hygiene dealt with occupational health, the physiological effects of environmental conditions, and personal hygiene. In his course on work, exercise, and fatigue, Reynold Spaeth described fatigue as "the most widely distributed of industrial hazards," causing injuries, absenteeism, physiological breakdown, and loss of productivity.[6] Spaeth's research centered on ways of improving industrial productivity and efficiency by reducing fatigue either through the improved design of tools or by introduction of rest periods.

Janet Howell Clark, Howell's daughter, taught a course on the physiological effects of radiation. Clark examined the implications of research on the biological effects of radiation for lighting schools, streets, factories, and offices.[7] Arthur Meyer taught about the physiological effects of other environmental factors: air quality, temperature, humidity, and ventilation. Meyer was primarily interested in the physiological effects of different mixtures of oxygen and carbon monoxide, and of dust particles in air.

Howell's lecture course on personal hygiene presented "the accumulated information from physiology, and from medicine in general, bearing upon the maintenance of the health of the individual, and upon those standards and rules of living which are conducive to the normal functioning of the body mechanism."[8] A course based on his *Textbook of Physiology* provided an introduction to physiological research for nonmedical students.[9] By all accounts, Howell was an excellent teacher. His lectures were clear and well organized, although he preferred, when possible, to teach small, informal classes. Alice Hamilton, a student of Howell at the University of Michigan, remembered his effect on a rowdy medical school class: "He would pause a moment, looking at the class, a small slight figure, then speak with his soft Southern accent, and at his first word the confusion would cease, the men would slip back to their seats and fumble for their pencils."[10]

In his papers and public lectures Howell made eloquent statements about the scope of public health and the possible contributions of physiology to health promotion. He provided at least a partial vision of a new science of the preservation of health and he inspired others with this ideal. In his research, however, Howell mainly continued his investigations on the mechanisms of the circulatory system and other basic physiological processes, extending researches started during his time at the medical school. While at the School of Hygiene, Howell discovered, isolated, and purified heparin, the blood anticoagulant, and he investigated many other factors involved in blood clotting. For his major research, he thus stayed with lines of investigation that had already proved productive and did not venture too far into uncharted territory. Howell's one excursion into environmental health research was comparatively trivial: a brief study of the relationship between humidity and comfort. For this, he installed an elaborate apparatus for regulating temperature, pressure, and humidity in student classrooms, intended to simulate both natural variations in weather and also the range of conditions to which industrial workers might be exposed.[11] He measured the effects of different temperatures and humidity levels on students' working efficiency and found that small changes in room temperature were much more important than humidity in determining student comfort.[12]

Howell was one of the earliest to struggle with the idea of creating a physiology and a philosophy of health, as distinct from the scientific study of disease. Moving from the world of medical research to public health, he tried to create a philosophy of public health, to articulate the relationships of environmental, occupational, and personal health, and to argue for the importance of environmental factors in the creation of optimum health. He provided the philosophical guidelines for the creation of a new field—the physiology of health—but he did not develop the field through his own research. The process of translating this philosophy into new research and practice was left largely to those who followed.[13]

The Diets of Rats and a Cure for Rickets

Elmer V. McCollum built the department of chemical hygiene into a world-famous center for nutrition research. McCollum probably did more than any other individual to improve the diet of the American people, through basic nutritional research, teaching, and popular lectures and articles. In 1951 *Time* magazine reported that "Dr. Vitamin has done more than any other man to put vitamins back in the nation's bread and milk, to put fruit on American breakfast tables, fresh vegetables and salad greens in the daily diet."[14] McCollum embodied Welch's ideal: a brilliant, dedicated, and original researcher, whose basic experimental work had profound importance for the public's health.

McCollum had not started his career with human nutrition, but with research on farm animals at the College of Agriculture of the University of Wisconsin, then the outstanding center of agricultural research. He had begun his research with the problem of determining why corn-fed cows were healthier than cows fed only on wheat or oats, a problem of obvious practical interest to farmers. Finding it difficult to reach any definite conclusions, he had decided it would be better to conduct nutritional experiments on rats, small, omnivorous animals that could easily be kept in large numbers, that grew quickly to maturity, and that reproduced rapidly.[15]

The dean of the state agricultural college was horrified when McCollum proposed using rats. The cow was an economically important animal; the rat was a pest. If it ever became known that the college was using tax dollars to feed rats, the public would be outraged. So McCollum began his rat experiments in secret, catching rats in an old horse barn. When wild rats proved too savage to maintain in the laboratory, he went to Chicago and bought albino rats from a petshop. When the little rats grew fat and healthy on a diet containing butter fat, but sickened on the same diet containing lard or olive oil, McCollum had the first clue leading to his discovery of vitamin A, and a convincing demonstration of the value of his research to the Wisconsin dairy farmers, who could now prove the superiority of butter over margarine.

Despite this discovery, McCollum's appointment as head of the department of chemical hygiene in 1918 was considered an adventurous one; he knew nothing of medicine, and was regarded as essentially an agricultural chemist. Physicians, pathologists, and even public health officials were remarkably uninterested in food, and most refused to believe that diet had any significance for the study of health and disease. Ernestine McCollum, who married McCollum during his retirement and was herself trained as a dietician, noted that it was practically impossible to get pathologists interested in the nutrition experiments: "The idea of food having anything to do with pathological conditions was incredible. . . . Curious attitudes people have towards food. It was something to be eaten and not important. If you had enough to eat, you were well fed."[16]

But McCollum quietly persevered, convinced that diet and nutrition were of immense importance to human health. In his laboratories at the School of Hygiene, he fed thousands of rats on hundreds of carefully controlled diets and was able to measure the effect of the presence or absence of many specific nutrients, including the vitamins, minerals, and amino acids. His research work was careful, patient, painstaking, and productive. In time, he was able to show a clear relationship between the deficiency of certain nutrients and clinical symptoms of specific diseases.

Some of McCollum's most important research explored the relationship of diet, sunshine, and rickets. At that time, children with deformed limbs caused by rickets were a common sight on city streets; the cure was unknown. McCollum had discovered that some of his rats fed only on

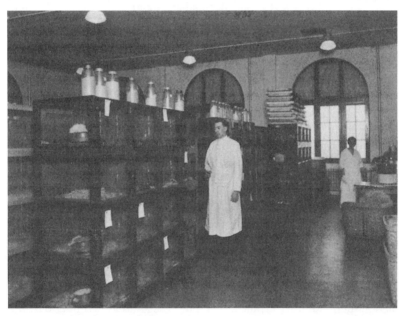

Figure 19. Rat colony, established by Elmer V. McCollum for the experimental study of nutrition, and used in the discovery of vitamins A and D. McCollum brought the first rats with him from the University of Wisconsin; the colony rapidly expanded in Baltimore, and some of their descendants still live in the School of Hygiene laboratories. Standing, Elmer V. McCollum, professor of chemical hygiene, (1917–44); in the background, his assistant, Nina Simmonds; circa 1920. (Courtesy of the Alan Mason Chesney Medical Archives of the Johns Hopkins Medical Institutions.)

cereal grains had developed a condition similar to rickets in children, but that the rats could be "cured" by small amounts of cod-liver oil. He then worked with John Howland, Edwards A. Park, and Paul Shipley from the School of Medicine to explore the clinical implications of these observations. McCollum and his co-workers tested the effects of over three hundred different experimental diets while the Howland group studied bone sections taken from the experimental rats.[17] They became convinced that an "organic factor" in the cod-liver oil was protecting the rats from rickets: rickets was thus a dietary disease caused by insufficiency of this unknown organic substance. When they presented this finding to the American Pediatric Society, one member of the audience, Dr. Chapin, objected:

I think there may be a deficiency in the food but it is the bad hygiene that supplements it. That has been called to my attention on the lower East Side where almost all Italians have rickets. They have come in and taken the rear tenements. . . . Now the Italian babies nearly all have rickets. . . . Rickets is very rare in Italy where the climate is mild and there is plenty of light and sunshine.[18]

McCollum decided to test the idea that rickets was related to sunlight. Every day, his co-workers carried little rats, fed on the deficient diets, into the sunshine. The rats got sunburned, and their ears peeled, but they did not develop any symptoms of rickets, while the control group, left behind in the dark laboratory, developed all the characteristic deformities of the disease.[19] McCollum's group concluded that the effects of sunlight and cod-liver oil were similar, if not identical, and that both could be used to prevent rickets.

From this point, McCollum and his co-workers concentrated on an effort to prove that the "anti-ricketic substance" was distinct from vitamin A. They were able to demonstrate that, after completely destroying the vitamin A in cod-liver oil through prolonged heating, it was still effective in preventing or curing rickets. They therefore announced the discovery of a "fourth vitamin, whose specific property, as far as we can tell at present, is to regulate the metabolism of the bones."[20] It would later be called vitamin D; its discovery led to a generation of children brought up on cod-liver oil, and the virtual elimination of rickets as a childhood disease.[21]

McCollum was convinced that many diseases of unknown origin were caused by nutritional deficiencies. Not only were rickets, scurvy, beriberi, and pellagra clearly related to diet, but, he thought, other more subtle conditions, including emotional states, could be traced to the presence or absence of certain trace elements in the diet. McCollum and his students studied the effects of the inorganic elements: calcium, phosphorus, fluorine, magnesium, manganese, iron, zinc, sodium, potassium, boron, and cobalt. Inferences from this research were reported by the newspapers in dramatic terms. The New York Times called manganese "the essence of mother love" (mother rats on a manganese-deficient diet neglected their babies), and magnesium was "the secret of philanthropy" because magnesium-deficient rats became extremely irritable and ill-tempered.[22]

McCollum and his associates called attention to the relationship between fluorides and healthy teeth. One of his students, Harry G. Day, later developed the fluoride toothpaste Crest.[23] McCollum also supported the fluoridation of water supplies, and energetically criticized excess sugar consumption as a cause of tooth decay.[24] Another associate, Donald K. Tressler, worked in McCollum's laboratory on improved methods for preserving fish; as the top researcher for Clarence Birdseye, he would later make important discoveries for the developing frozen food industry.[25]

Throughout his many years of productive research, McCollum had close relationships with his associates and graduate students. Describing his philosophy of teaching, he said:

I wanted my students to develop intellectual curiosity and the ability to satisfy it. The successful professor's horizons are broader than those of his students. It is his privilege and responsibility to help his students achieve maximum self-development. . . . His fitness for this role is determined by his ability to make his conversations and lectures more interesting than song, dance, drink, and fast driving.[26]

McCollum directed graduate students into his established research program in experimental nutrition. He disagreed with some faculty members who felt that students should be completely free to define their own problems for investigation. As a result of this philosophy, research in the department was closely integrated, and McCollum himself defined the problems worth investigating. The field of experimental nutrition was so new, and so rich in possibilities, that student researchers published a constant stream of scientific papers, and many of McCollum's students went on to become leading names in nutrition research.

The teaching in experimental nutrition was supplemented by introductory courses on subjects considered important for practicing health officers. A course on food production and distribution provided "lectures . . . followed by visits to manufacturing plants, warehouses and retail shops. The food and drugs act, the meat inspection acts, federal, state and municipal regulations, federal definitions and standards for foods, and labeling rules, are studied."[27] Olaf Rask offered a course in the chemical analysis of food and water, the detection of adulterants, and the exercise of government control over food products. Nina Simmonds, who assisted McCollum in his rat experiments, taught a course on experimental methods, and McCollum himself offered a course for discussion of the latest nutritional discoveries.

McCollum was happiest at work in his laboratory, but he was also deeply committed to popular health education. He surveyed the health conditions of children in the Baltimore schools, organized nutrition classes, and provided food supplements for undernourished children. He found that children living in the Negro Orphans' Home subsisted entirely on cereals, tubers, and roots, a diet that was inadequate for human nutrition. He arranged for half of the children to have a dietary supplement of milk powder for fifteen months. At the end of this period, it was obvious that although the children with the supplementary milk were healthy and of normal weight, the children fed on the institutional food were underweight and malnourished. McCollum then worked with charitable agencies in Baltimore to study the health status of 10,000 children in the public schools. Underweight children were organized into small classes of twelve to fifteen each and given regular instruction in hygiene and the selection of food. Teachers visited the children at home and tried to help parents improve their nutrition. Most of these children gained weight; the program showed the usefulness of even small changes in nutritional intake in improving child health, and provided a model of the kind of work that could be done by voluntary agencies in cooperation with public health authorities.

As a member of Herbert Hoover's Advisory Council on Nutrition, McCollum traveled around the country giving public lectures, urging mothers to serve milk, leafy vegetables, eggs, liver, and wheat bread. He summarized the results of his nutrition research in two books, *Food, Nutrition, and Health,* and *The Newer Knowledge of Nutrition,* both popular through many editions.[28] Between 1922 and 1946, McCollum and his associates wrote over 160 articles for *McCall's* magazine in a highly successful effort to educate housewives and mothers in the new understanding of nutrition. McCollum's articles had catchy titles meant to appeal to a popular audience: "Is Your Baby Running the Risk of Scurvy?" "Are There Such Things as Nerve Foods?" "Green Vegetables Are Unbottled Medicines," "My Husband Says I'm Hard to Live With," and "Eat to Keep Young."[29]

McCollum was also influential in national and international public health policy and in the politics of the agricultural and food industries.[30]

He served on the Permanent Committee on Nutrition of the League of Nations and gave advice on food and agricultural policies to developing countries. In the United States, he worked closely with the National Dairy Council to encourage the consumption of milk as a nutritionally valuable food. McCollum argued the advantages of what might today be called "natural foods." He criticized the milling industry for first removing nutrients from white flour, then adding back a few vitamins and calling the resulting bread "enriched" or "fortified." Instead, he stated that the industry should be decentralized so that bread would not have to be shipped and stored for such long periods, and less-refined flour could then be used. Barring that change, he recommended fortification with skim milk, brewer's yeast, and wheat or corn germ, rather than with synthetic vitamins.

McCollum did not win all his battles, but he was influential in convincing the American public to consume more milk, eggs, fruit, and vegetables, and fewer refined sugars and starches. His work on the vitamins, minerals, and trace elements provided much of the fundamental knowledge needed to produce not only healthy rats but healthy children.

In the last chapter of his *History of Nutrition*, McCollum asserted the importance of the scientific study of nutrition:

Before the emergence of the science of nutrition many millions of people in every generation, from ignorance, led lives blighted by malnutrition. . . . The new knowledge brought about improvement of health and its attendant elevation of the status of human life above the sordid, to a degree scarcely equalled by any other agency concerned with the prevention or cure of disease. [31]

The Causes and Distribution of Disease

While physiological hygiene and chemical hygiene were laboratory-based sciences, epidemiology introduced new methods of field research. Epidemiology involved the study of the actual distribution of disease among populations, and the gathering of statistical information in such a way as to discover the direct and contributing factors causing disease. The use of statistical information about large numbers of people allowed fresh, new ways of understanding diseases; it added powerful new research tools to the techniques of the laboratory. Since those in the biological sciences did not always perceive the potential of epidemiology, the discipline had to assert its central importance to the analysis and understanding of disease processes.

In 1919, when Wade Hampton Frost became head of the department of epidemiology, it was probably the first such department in the world. Epidemiology had not yet been constituted as a formal academic discipline, despite many classic epidemiological studies, most notably, perhaps, those to which Frost himself often referred: Snow on cholera, Budd on typhoid fever, and Panum on measles. The earliest generations of epidemiologists undertook what would later be known as "shoe leather epidemiology," going out into a community, visiting the homes of the sick, gathering information on water supplies, milk, and foods, looking for sources of infection, talking to public officials, observing local conditions, and gathering data on possible hazards to health.[32]

Frost's own early investigations of epidemic disease outbreaks—typhoid fever, septic sore throat, poliomyelitis, and influenza—had been models of "shoe leather epidemiology."[33] Even when he became professor of epidemiology, and began to analyze data gathered by others ("armchair epidemiology"), he remained firmly committed to field research and to recognizing the special value of direct personal observation of social and environmental conditions. In a period when laboratory research was widely regarded as providing the one route to fundamental scientific knowledge, Frost argued that epidemiology as "the method of experience" was essential in developing a practical knowledge relevant to the problems of disease prevention:

Any modification of the conditions of life as they exist in a community . . . requires something more than a knowledge of the specific organisms of disease, in terms of their reactions under the controlled conditions of the laboratory. It equally requires a knowledge of the community, of the psychology of the people, their social organization, the conditions and events of their everyday life. It requires that the knowledge of fundamental causes of disease be fitted together with the knowledge of people into a practical epidemiology, directly applicable to prevention.[34]

Frost also argued that epidemiology needed theoretical development, drawing on the theoretical understanding of disease derived from the biological sciences.[35] He was remembered for the painstaking way in which he searched for theoretical relationships in the disorderly accumulation of empirical facts about specific diseases. A friend and admirer, writing in the American Journal of Public Health, applauded this aspect of his personality:

We noted [in Dr. Frost] a restlessness whenever he confronted whatever presented the earmarks of an unattached fact. By "unattached" is meant some apparently sound observation without known relationships: a sort of toy balloon bumping against the ceiling, with its string dangling just out of reach. Faced with such a situation, Dr. Frost would pace the floor. . . . For him the problem could be settled only in one of two ways: the balloon must either be punctured or moored. If it arose because of hot air, then heaven help its launcher. If it floated merely because present knowledge was not tall enough to grasp the dangling string and tie it into basic facts, Dr. Frost reached for and usually grasped that string.[36]

Frost is widely recognized as having provided the analytic base and methodological principles for the subsequent development of epidemiology. Some have questioned whether his conception of the field included the chronic as well as the infectious diseases. In fact, his definition of epidemiology broadened over time as his work developed and expanded. In 1919, he defined epidemiology as "the natural history of the infectious diseases, with special reference to the circumstances and conditions which determine their occurrence in nature."[37] By 1927, he raised the question whether the term "epidemiology" should be applied to noninfectious diseases: "It is entirely in conformity with good usage to speak of the epidemiology of tuberculosis; and it seems customary also to apply the term to the mass-phenomena of such noninfectious diseases as scurvy, but not to those of the so-called constitutional diseases, such as arteriosclerosis and nephritis."[38]

In 1937, however, at the American Public Health Association meetings in New York, Frost declared that epidemiology included all diseases and hazards to health:

The health officer may well think of epidemiology as comprising the whole of the unremitting effort being made to clarify the relation between the diseases and disabilities which men suffer and their way of life. This view brings epidemiology into its proper relation to the health officer's administrative responsibilities . . . to modify the environment or alter the habits of people as to afford them protection against impairment of health.[39]

Frost saw epidemiology as a tool to be used by practicing public health officers and not simply as an academic specialty. Indeed, he urged health officers to conduct their own epidemiological investigations even if they had no specialized training: "The closer his [the health officer's] actual contact with people in their homes, in schools and in clinics, the better are his opportunities for observation, and if he lacks skill he need only confine himself at first to simple problems."[40]

During his time in Baltimore, Frost organized major research projects on the epidemiology of diphtheria, influenza, the common cold, and tuberculosis. The diphtheria study provided an analysis of the spread of infection in households and communities and highlighted the important role played by concealed infections.[41] The studies of influenza and the common cold were especially useful in developing statistical methods for following families over time to determine the frequency of respiratory infections.[42] The work on tuberculosis was important in initiating research on the chronic diseases. Frost argued that such studies required new methods of longitudinal analysis and he introduced methods of measuring the risk of developing disease over different periods of the life span.[43]

Frost had arrived at the School of Hygiene without teaching experience and with no models for developing a course of instruction. He cautiously introduced his first plans for the department: "The field of epidemiology as a separate department is not yet clearly defined . . . so that the scope and methods of instruction must be worked out gradually."[44] The "laboratory method" of teaching epidemiology that Frost subsequently developed became so successful that epidemiological departments throughout the country later copied it. He used real case studies to teach techniques of problem solving: he supplied original epidemiological data from ongoing investigations, suggested methods of analysis, and then let students debate possible approaches and solutions. Students were required to tabulate the crude data, state any pertinent facts known about the epidemiology of the disease in question, and present an interpretation of the whole set of data in written form.[45]

Lectures on epidemiological methods and the interpretation of field data supplemented laboratory classes. Students who loved the laboratory style of teaching sometimes found Frost's lectures dull; others realized "they were being treated to closely reasoned arguments and had better not miss a word."[46] If Frost discovered a flaw in his own argument, he became completely engrossed in the problem at hand, and often forgot his audience, apparently talking, debating, and muttering to himself at the blackboard. As one former student paraphrased Oscar Wilde's comment about Walter Pater: "Frost was not so much heard, as overheard." Working with individual students, Frost applied perfectionist standards. Many found this process exhausting, but also a superb training. As Ernest Stebbins, later dean of the school, explained, "If he tore your paper to pieces you knew it was good."[47]

Until 1929, Frost remained an active officer of the United States Public Health Service. He was frequently asked to consult on ongoing field investigations, and used these investigations to provide raw data for teaching and student research. He resisted pressure to take a high administrative position in the Public Health Service and, feeling torn between his dual commitment to the school and the service, eventually resigned the latter position in 1929. He continued, however, to be much in demand as a consultant to epidemiological investigations and gave freely of his time to those asking for his advice and assistance. Frost was also a scientific director of the International Health Board of the Rockefeller Foundation, where he successfully argued the position that practical programs of disease control must be aided by an ongoing process of epidemiological research.

In 1927, the International Health Board asked Frost to organize a conference on epidemiology at the School of Hygiene.[48] This conference, which brought together leading epidemiologists and state health officers, was influential in encouraging the development and institutionalization of epidemiology in health departments across the country. Fifteen years later, John A. Ferrell recalled the meeting:

In May 1927, about 60 scientists assembled in Baltimore to formulate plans for the development and enlargement of epidemiological services throughout the United States. At that time only a few state health departments had divisions of epidemiology which were supplying services of the caliber recommended by the conference. A recent review of the situation shows that the epidemiological services of these states have more than quadrupled in extent in the years since 1927.[49]

Through his research, teaching, and other professional activities, Frost played a major role in making epidemiology an analytic discipline, one that became central to public health theory and practice by relating the scientific knowledge and techniques of many disciplines to the practical problems of disease control.

Counting and Calculations

Epidemiology as a discipline later became firmly wedded to the mathematical methods of biostatistics. Not so at the beginning, when quantitative methods were often little understood or used in understaffed health departments that were overwhelmed with the practical problems of disease control. Biostatistics at Hopkins was first called biometry and vital statistics, so named by Raymond Pearl, a biologist who had studied "biometrics"—the quantitative analysis of biological processes—with Karl Pearson in London. Pearl became one of America's chief proponents of statistical biology. Welch's invitation to Pearl to become professor of vital statistics at the School of Hygiene in 1917 was an adventurous and imaginative move as it was extraordinary even to conceive of a professorship in vital statistics at that time. Statistics was usually assigned to clerks in public health departments—a routine recording of births, deaths, and infectious disease data. Welch wanted someone who could bring intellectual energy to this routine administrative task, who could provide a theoretical approach to quantitative methods as applied to human health and disease. In Pearl, Welch got all he wanted, and more.

Pearl felt that biostatistics opened up an exciting new field of biological investigation, one applicable to all manner of problems. He disliked the reductionist approach to biology, the analysis of the living organism into ever smaller component parts. Instead, he wanted to deal with large entities: the organism as a whole, the population as a functioning unit. Pearl wanted to address the great philosophical issues of biological existence by using mathematical methods. In his view, the mathematics of population groups offered a totally new approach to life, and to death.

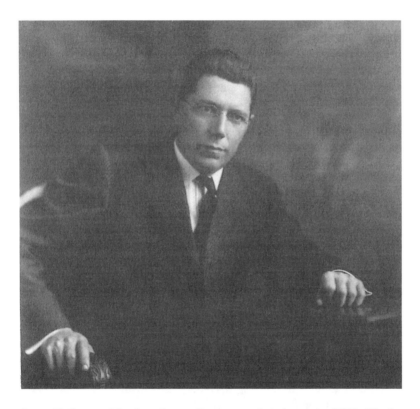

Figure 20. Raymond Pearl, professor of biometry and vital statistics (1918–25), director, Institute for Biological Research (1925–30), and research professor of biology (1925–40). Pearl wanted to address the great philosophical issues of biological existence by using mathematical methods; he studied the theories of population growth, longevity, alcoholism, tuberculosis, and cancer. (Courtesy of the Alan Mason Chesney Medical Archives of the Johns Hopkins Medical Institutions.)

Perhaps conscious that his own biological training was stronger than his knowledge of mathematical and statistical methods, Pearl brought with him to the school a young mathematician, Lowell Reed. Reed and Pearl had worked together at the University of Maine where Reed had become intrigued by Pearl's ideas about the possible applications of mathematics to biological problems. They continued to work together at the School of Hygiene with Reed as associate professor; when Pearl later established his own Institute of Biological Research, Reed replaced Pearl as head of the department.

Pearl and Reed had different and complementary skills; Pearl visualized a new kind of population biology and Reed contributed his knowledge of mathematics and statistical methods. The two also had very different personalities; Reed was known for his tact and discretion, Pearl for his aggressive and dogmatic style. Both men had great physical and intellectual energy. Pearl especially was impossible to ignore: a large, loud, ambitious man, with a totally original mind and a passionate dedication to his own vision of scientific truth. His interests ranged over many fields; his conversations and publications freely crossed the boundaries of biology, mathematics, philosophy, history, sociology, literature, and music. Pearl was egocentric and given to a high estimation of his own intellectual powers. He did not suffer fools gladly, and, in intellectual debate, was often all too ready to consider his critics as fools. Although he made more money than either Welch or Howell, Pearl always seemed to have felt himself shamefully underpaid, and he frequently threatened to leave the university for more lucrative positions.[50]

If Pearl could be overbearing, he could also be enormously stimulating. He had a wide circle of admirers and counted among his close friends many of the leading intellectuals of his time. One of his closest friends in Baltimore was H. L. Mencken, the author of acidic and often penetrating essays on the literary and social issues of the day. Pearl's own productivity, as measured by his hundreds of articles and books, was prodigious; his writings lucid and often fiercely controversial. Some thought Raymond Pearl the most brilliant scientific mind of his generation; others considered him a fraud and a charlatan. Few scientists had the self-confidence to question accepted conventions so relentlessly; few had the courage (or temerity) to follow their visions without regard for the warnings of the cautious.

Lowell Reed, by contrast, was a kindly, discreet, and tactful person, who tried to avoid any direct criticism of others' work. One of his students, Morton Kramer, described him as "a short, stocky man wearing a bow tie and a white lab coat—very outgoing, very warm, and very lucid in the way he explained things."[51] Reed was vital and energetic, but he never gave the impression of egocentricity or personal ambition; indeed, he was remembered for his remark that after a man retired, his imprint was about as lasting as that of a thumb pulled out of a bowl of water.[52] Reed published relatively few papers, these few carefully reasoned and argued. Generous in assisting others' work, his name appeared more frequently in footnotes and acknowledgments than on title pages. Margaret Merrell, student and later faculty member in the department, remembered: "A daily sight was Dr. Reed dropping by a student's office, chatting about what he was doing . . . putting into the student's mind some new idea in such a way that more often than not he thought it was his own."[53]

Reed was a superb teacher who could make a difficult subject perfectly clear. John Grant said of Pearl's teaching: "None of us in the class could understand his lectures, and we'd have to wait for Lowell Reed to come along and put in a few simple terms what Raymond Pearl had been telling us."[54]

In the teaching program, Reed taught statistical methods and Pearl taught the application of statistics to biological and medical problems. Reed supervised the "laboratory" part of the statistical courses, where students had the opportunity to practice methods of statistical analysis directly. Equipment assembled in the department included "modern computing and adding machines," "a complete Hollerith equipment for analyzing statistical data by use of punched cards," a photostat machine, a planimeter and integraph (used for drawing graphs), and a sampling machine, designed and built in the department, used for experimentally testing various sampling formulae.[55] In the laboratory classes, students learned how to apply these new pieces of technology to the problems of a health department. Lowell Reed and John R. Miner taught advanced classes on statistical theory, and William T. Howard, assistant commissioner of health for Baltimore City, taught a course on the statistical evaluation of public health programs.[56]

Pearl presided over a colloquium on the application of statistical methods to problems in biology, medicine, and hygiene, and also directed student research. His outline of research appropriate to the department included an astonishingly large array of subjects:

1. Theory of statistics, theory of correlation, life table construction, and probability.
2. The population problem, theory of population growth, growth of experimental populations, and vital index of populations.
3. Factors influencing the duration of life, experimental studies on drosophila, statistical studies in genealogical data, and deter-

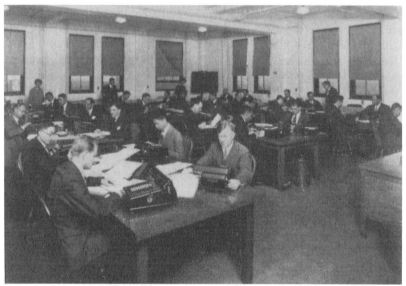

Figure 21. Lowell J. Reed teaching a class in the uses of computing machines, department of biometry and vital statistics, circa 1925. Reed (in bow tie) standing, back, far right. Margaret Merrell, his teaching assistant, standing, back, left, and Persis Putnam, back, center. (Courtesy of the Alan Mason Chesney Medical Archives of the Johns Hopkins Medical Institutions.)

mination of the relative influence of heredity and environment.

4. Constitutional, genetic, and environmental factors in disease and eugenic field studies.

5. Modification of the germ cells: experimental on drosophila, eugenic and statistical on man; the alcohol problem.

6. The natural history of disease, effectiveness of public health activities, biological classification of causes of death, and the influence of race on mortality.

7. Hospital statistics, studies in racial pathology, biometric analysis of clinical problems, and biometric studies in anatomy and physiology.[57]

Both Pearl and Reed were interested in the phenomenon of growth, and especially in mathematical methods for representing the growth of populations. In 1920, they published a paper applying a sigmoid curve to census figures for the growth of the United States population since 1790; they later called it the "logistic curve," demonstrating the growth and self-limitation of populations.[58] Pearl called this S-shaped curve the "law of population growth," and insisted that he had discovered "a new scientific law, comparable to Kepler's law of planetary motions or

Boyle's law."[59] Predictions of population size on the basis of this "law" deviated only 3.7 percent from figures later given in the 1940 census, but critics complained that Pearl's uses of the curve were vague and even mystical, and seized on the chance to question his statistical credentials.[60] Pearl, however, paid little attention to criticism, which he considered "the conservative resistance to any new idea," and he continued to promote the "law of population growth" in numerous publications.

Never to be accused of avoiding the big issues, Pearl decided to conduct research on the "duration of life," which he defined as follows: "Duration of life is an integration in the mathematical sense of the whole structural and functional constitution of the individual."[61] Once the determinants of "life duration" had been investigated, he declared, it should be possible to lengthen the span of human life.[62]

Pearl decided to start with lower organisms—fruit flies, rats, and mice—and to study their life duration under a variety of environmental conditions. He wanted to know whether duration of life was "a simple Mendelian character" and to investigate the extent to which inheritance determined an individual's biological future.[63] Engaged in a constant dialogue with the eugenics movement, Pearl believed strongly in the relative importance of heredity, but he also attacked many of the social and political ideas advanced by his eugenist friends. (For example, he said it was not necessarily a bad thing that the lower classes were reproducing at a higher rate than the upper classes, on the grounds that many of the most important social and intellectual advances came from people with lower-class backgrounds.)[64] Since he could not undertake experiments on human populations, Pearl proposed to study duration of human life by statistical studies of family histories.[65] He made an arrangement with the Johns Hopkins Hospital to use its autopsy records to investigate the biological aspects of senility and life duration, and the importance of hereditary factors in disease.[66] Pearl claimed to have discovered that "the duration of life is an inherited character of an individual, passed on from parent to offspring."[67] Of the relationship between heredity and environment in determining the length of an individual's life, Pearl added: "Heredity determines the amount of capital placed in the vital bank upon which we draw to continue life . . . while environment . . . determines the rate at which drafts are presented and cashed."[68]

Pearl asked the Rockefeller Foundation for more than $1 million to finance his research; after prolonged negotiations, he got $175,000 in 1925 to set up an Institute of Biological Research, with himself as director. Pearl promised "results of really revolutionary significance, perhaps of the same relative importance in the field of genetics that Bohr's work on the structure of the atom was in physics."[69] The institute gave Pearl a great deal of autonomy to pursue his own ideas. He had previously resisted the demands of teaching and even minimal bureaucratic controls, and complained: "To an investigator who is sensitive to the influences of the surrounding intellectual atmosphere, universities have a deadening and dulling tendency."[70]

Untrammeled by much association with colleagues, Pearl plunged ahead into an astonishing variety of research. He undertook studies of longevity, alcoholism, tuberculosis, and cancer, taking on, in rapid succession, the most recalcitrant problems in public health. Pearl found that the moderate use of alcohol was not dangerous and might even prolong life, a finding that has since been confirmed, but enraged temperance advocates in that era of Prohibition.[71] Curious about the point at which death occurs, Pearl found that the time of death could be different for different organs in the body. At the time, medical colleagues thought such studies ridiculous; now, they are of major importance to organ transplant surgery.[72] Even more outrageous was Pearl's firm support of birth control, and, with William Howell and others, he helped establish the first birth control clinic in Baltimore.[73] Pearl also founded and edited two journals, Human Biology and the Quarterly Review of Biology. As usual, these projects were ambitious ones: the former journal was to "serve as a medium for the publication of results of original research in all fields of human biology, including physical and general anthropology, anthropometry, vital statistics, human heredity and eugenics, prehistory, human anatomy, sociology, constitutional pathology, and psychobiology";[74] the latter journal was to provide "authoritative and comprehensive reviews of the present state of knowledge in the different fields of general biology" for an intelligent lay audience, and also to free the human mind "from the shackles imposed and maintained through the centuries by organized religion."[75]

Still looking for new fields to conquer, Pearl, as hospital statistician, continued to analyze the autopsy records of the Johns Hopkins Hospital. In the autopsy records, Pearl noticed a negative association between deaths from cancer and tuberculosis, actually a necessary negative relationship because a patient is unlikely to die of both diseases at once. Making a methodological blunder, Pearl suggested that perhaps tuberculosis protected against cancer, and he conceived the idea of treating cancer patients with tuberculin. After a few experimental studies on rats, he decided to extend the experiments to humans and arranged tuberculin treatments for some terminal cancer patients. After a year of apparently promising trials, Pearl believed that he had found

the cure to cancer, and risked his reputation by publishing his preliminary results in the *Lancet*.[76]

Meanwhile, Pearl had received an invitation to head the Bussey
Institute of Harvard. He publicly announced the offer, unaware that an
eminent Harvard statistician, Edwin B. Wilson, was campaigning
avidly behind the scenes against his appointment. The Harvard faculty
was divided on the issue, and finally the Board of Overseers narrowly
rejected Pearl's nomination. It was an embarrassing situation, and badly
damaged Pearl's reputation.

The Rockefeller Foundation now declined Pearl's suggestion that it
finance his Institute of Biological Research for another twenty years,
and instead gave the university a general grant for the biological
sciences, to be divided between the School of Hygiene and the School of
Arts and Sciences. Pearl's institute was closed in 1930, but Pearl stayed
on as head of a small department of biology, firmly under the administrative direction of the School of Hygiene.[77] Somewhat chastened,
Pearl continued his research, no longer with such complete freedom to
do as he wished. But Pearl's central ideal of applying statistical methods
to the holistic biology of life and death was never fully realized; biologists
moved toward molecular biology, and statisticians developed ever more
elegant solutions to mathematical problems. Pearl had nevertheless
done much to create the disciplines of biostatistics and population
dynamics. Whatever his mistakes and flaws, these fields owed much to
the intellectual energy of this passionate and original mind.

While Raymond Pearl had been trying to create a revolution in the
field of biology, Lowell Reed had been steadily developing the department of biometry and vital statistics, now renamed the department of
biostatistics. Under Reed, the department concentrated on the principles and methods for analyzing data about human health and disease.
Without Pearl's influence, the department focused less on the philosophy of biology and more on developing mathematical techniques of
analysis. Lowell Reed and Wade Hampton Frost became close friends,
and the departments of epidemiology and biostatistics often cooperated,
offering a joint seminar and pursuing mutual research interests. From
this period came the Reed-Frost epidemic curve and cooperative studies
on the epidemiology of influenza, the common cold, and tuberculosis.[78]
Margaret Merrell says of this collaboration: "As ideas were offered and
challenged, hats were frequently swapped, Frost as often as not wearing
the statistician's and Reed the epidemiologist's."[79]

The close collaboration between epidemiology and biostatistics
strengthened both disciplines. Initially, Reed had hesitated to take on
doctoral students because of doubts about their future professional

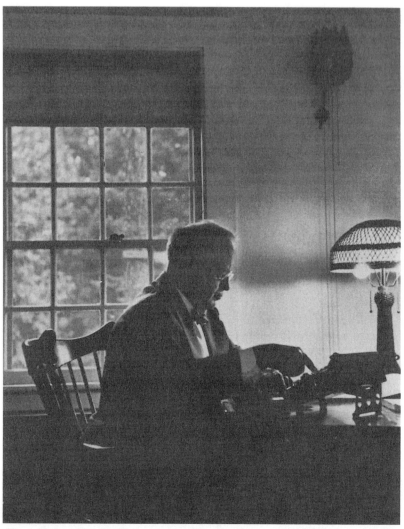

Figure 22. Lowell J. Reed at work (a) and at play (b). A mathematician, Reed was appointed associate in biometry and vital statistics (1919–20), associate professor (1920–25), professor of biostatistics (1925–46), dean of the School of Hygiene (1937–46), vice-president of the university and hospital, (1946–53), and president of the university, 1953–56. (Courtesy of Robert B. Reed, Boston, Massachusetts.)

opportunities; outside the department, statisticians were still expected to know "facts" rather than methods:

The emphasis on methodology and the failure to inculcate numerical data met with immediate outside criticism. . . . So ingrained was the idea that

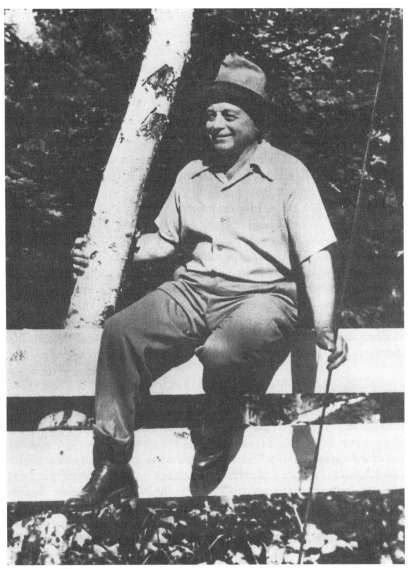

Figure 22 (b).

the statistician was a clerk with a status title, whose professional task was to compile those undigested figures, that Dr. Reed hesitated at the start to take on a doctoral candidate. . . . Opposition to a vital statistician engaging in statistical analysis died hard.[80]

Gradually, this situation changed until, by 1935, Reed could describe biostatistics as a "wide open field" for bright students with good training in mathematics and the sciences.[81] At the time, epidemiology was considered only an appropriate field for those with prior medical training; nonmedical men (and women) were often directed into biostatistics if their mathematical talents were considered promising. Gradually, Lowell Reed built the discipline of biostatistics until it was considered an essential tool for public health work, and the department at Hopkins was regarded as perhaps the strongest in the nation.

In addition to establishing statistical techniques for epidemiological analysis, Lowell Reed worked with members of the medical school faculty to develop statistical models in physiology and biochemistry. He collaborated more frequently on medical research projects than any other member of the School of Hygiene, consulting on research design and providing mathematical models and analysis.[82]

As Raymond Pearl's influence at Johns Hopkins declined, Lowell Reed's gradually increased. In 1937, he became dean of the School of Hygiene; in 1946, vice-president of the university; in 1949, vice-president of the hospital; and in 1953, president of the university. His calm and pleasant personality, his ability to pinpoint the essence of a problem, and his attention to detail were skills as useful to the administrator as to the teacher and statistician.

Putting Knowledge into Practice

The distance between the laboratory sciences and practical public health was at least partially bridged by the field researches of epidemiology, aided by the methodological tools of biostatistics. At the other end of the spectrum from "pure" research to its application came public health administration and sanitary engineering. These were the least academic and the most practical of the disciplines. To public health administration were consigned many elements of public health practice, from learning to organize and run a city health department to the methods of popular health education. Allen Freeman, who had been chosen to head the department after Sir Arthur Newsholme's initial two-year appointment, was a highly successful, experienced public health officer. Freeman had worked in public health projects in Virginia, Kansas, Iowa, and New York and had reorganized the entire public health service of Ohio before, as he put it, he moved "from a life of action to one of ideas."[83]

When Freeman arrived at the school in July 1921, wondering how best to organize the teaching program for the coming year, he found little trace of Sir Arthur's work: "There were some reports of British health departments and a splendid collection of books on the history of public health which Sir Arthur had bought for the school the year before. There were . . . no books on public health administration and no precedents for its teaching."[84] Freeman gave himself a month's vacation in Virginia, to try to distill his years of experience into a set of lectures for the incoming students. He later wrote about his own first efforts at teaching (he writes about himself in the third person):

He was forced to try many different methods before he could work out an effective schedule. Lectures he found to be of limited value. Through them he could give the students some idea of the history of public health and of the general principles of health organization. That was all. . . . In time . . . a modification of the seminar method was developed to meet the special conditions of the class and the subject. Each student was assigned a topic and was required to prepare an outline. . . . At the time a student's subject was discussed copies of the outline were distributed to the class and the student took his place on the platform beside the professor.[85]

Most of these students were practicing health officers, some with many years of experience. In seminars, they discussed actual administrative problems in public health based on their own experiences. They also observed field demonstrations of the various types of public health work being carried out in and around Baltimore. They spent their afternoons in the major divisions of the Baltimore City Health Department, the State Health Department, the Baltimore County Health Department, the Johns Hopkins Hospital, and the various volunteer organizations involved in local health and welfare work.[86] In addition to basic practical training in public health administration, promising students could participate in health surveys and research conducted for public health agencies.

Although Freeman wrote many articles and reports on various aspects of health department work, he never attempted to write a textbook. His autobiography is perhaps the best source for his ideas on administration. He followed no theoretical models of management technique; instead, he was extremely skilled at understanding the basis of political power in a community, identifying the most influential individuals, and persuading them of the need for effective public health programs. A friendly, hard-working, and almost self-effacing man, Freeman knew how to get people to take action by a combination of rational argument, tactful prompting, and appeal to self-interest. Avoiding identification with any extreme views, he liked to position himself in a central position as mediator in any argument. He disliked empty rhetoric and admired men who got things done. His practical orientation toward results could be seen, for example, in his bitter disappointment after attending a League of Nations conference in 1924: "It was concerned only with words: speeches, documents, conversations. Nothing might be expressed in such direct and simple terms as to be easily understood. For everything a formula must be found: an aggregation of words which would offend no one and commit no one. That the League was yet ready to bring about peace and justice between nations in this selfish, greedy, merciless world did not seem probable."[87]

Involved in a multitude of community health activities, Freeman was asked to serve on boards and committees, to conduct surveys, and to evaluate public health programs. As consultant to the Baltimore City Health Department, he evaluated their tuberculosis and venereal disease programs, and later helped the department adapt to the financial cutbacks of the depression years. As a member of the Maryland Occupational Disease Commission, he helped draft state legislation providing compensation for occupational diseases.

Although Freeman accepted the American division between curative and preventive medicine and the limitation that health departments should be concerned only with prevention, he was also interested in the organization of medical care. In 1928, he infuriated the College of Physicians in Philadelphia by arguing that medical services should be organized into group practices.[88] He participated in the medical care survey of Baltimore conducted by the Public Health Service in 1932, and also belonged to a local organization of businessmen set up to study the city government. Perhaps he did his most influential work for the Committee on Municipal Health Department Practice of the American Public Health Association. With the financial assistance of the Metropolitan Life Insurance Company, this group surveyed health department activities in all major metropolitan areas. Freeman wrote large sections of its final report, published in 1923, and providing by far the most complete account of public health practice in this period.[89]

In addition to his involvement in many local and national organizations, Freeman traveled extensively in Europe, sometimes in the company of Welch, and he studied the methods of public health administration in other countries. He especially admired the system of socialized medicine in Norway, but found the English health system "solid and substantial" with none of the "driving eagerness and urgent evangelism" of its American counterpart.[90] In 1926, Freeman went to São Paulo, Brazil, to assist in organizing the new Brazilian school of public health.

Freeman was always more a practical administrator and "man of action" than a scholar. His professional papers were careful, methodical, and often dull, in striking contrast to his lively and informal auto-biographical style. The department of public health administration lacked the glamour and excitement of pathbreaking scientific discoveries but gave the students their only direct experience of practical public health programs and thus better prepared them for future careers as practicing health officers.

Despite its somewhat pedestrian reputation in an institution devoted to scientific research, the department of public health administration later proved to be the major growing point of the school. It continually expanded in scope, spinning out new applied fields which later became programs and then departments in their own right: mental hygiene, maternal and child health, chronic diseases, behavioral sciences, medical care and hospitals, and international health. As the institution gradually became involved in more social and applied research programs in the 1930s, the department of public health administration became the focal point for these new kinds of activities. Befitting his organizational and administrative talents, Freeman became dean of the School of Hygiene in 1934, and directed its development into these newer areas of applied public health.

Of Sewers and Drains

The second important area of applied public health was sanitary engineering. Welch and Howell had wanted to include sanitary engineering in the school curriculum as part of their commitment to physiological hygiene, that is, to bring Pettenkofer's institute up to date by the emphasis on the prevention of disease through engineering methods. It was not, however, an easy matter to persuade physicians of the importance of sanitary engineering. Although sanitary engineering was taught at the School of Hygiene from the first year of instruction, the relationship of the discipline to the rest of the school remained complex and problematic for many years. Sanitary engineering was a professional specialty taught within the School of Engineering, and most engineers felt that it could hardly be properly studied, much less practiced, by nonengineers. At the same time, the existence of sanitary engineering within the public health curriculum offered an implicit challenge to the medical domination of public health. Most physicians and public health officers were more than happy to leave the technical details of sewage systems to the engineering profession. Because the provision of clean water and effective sewage disposal was a critical necessity for maintaining the public's health, sanitary engineering had to have a place in the curriculum, but teaching of sanitary engineering in the School of Hygiene was a source of tension for both physicians and engineers. The strains evident over sanitary engineering in the school were, of course, only one symptom of the professional competition between physicians and engineers over the proper direction of public health in the nation.

The early efforts to establish a close working relationship with the School of Engineering for teaching sanitary engineering had not been very successful. The professor of civil engineering, Charles Tilden, held a seat on the Advisory Board of the School of Hygiene but had appeared at few meetings. The actual teaching of sanitary engineering was done by Granville Reynard Jones, a practicing engineer. Jones took students for visits to local sanitary facilities, and delivered the address at the opening of the Baltimore City Filtration Plant in 1917 on "The Relation of Public Water Supplies to the Public Health." Jones was well qualified to teach sanitary engineering to public health students, but his career was abruptly terminated when he was commissioned a captain in the Sanitary Corps of the Public Health Service during World War I. While waiting for his discharge from the service, he contracted influenza and died at the end of 1918.

The curriculum of the engineering school, as described by Charles Tilden, was considerably less specialized than other engineering schools of the period. The Hopkins school followed an educational philosophy that might sound alarming to some of today's engineers:

The duty of the engineering school lies not so much in imparting certain items of knowledge to its students as in developing their intellects. The question of what to study is of far less importance than that of how it is studied. The engineer is essentially a creative animal, and the two qualities most necessary to the exercise of this function are imagination and faith. Imagination he must have to conceive and plan the things he must do, and faith to execute them—the faith that literally "removes mountains."[91]

Whatever this philosophy meant to the engineering students, it did guarantee that School of Hygiene students could take courses in the engineering school without being overwhelmed by technical information. They had an opportunity to interact with sanitary engineers and to get a practical sense of the "state of the art" in water purification and sewerage systems.

Associate professor John H. Gregory began teaching "Sanitary Engineering and Elementary Hydraulics" in the spring of 1919, and at the end of the year, when Charles Tilden resigned, Gregory was appointed professor of civil engineering. Gregory conducted joint inspection trips for engineering and public health students to visit a range of sanitary facilities: the water filtration plant at Baltimore Water and Electric Company, the water filtration system at Lake Montebello, the bridges over the Susquehanna River, the water purification, sewage screening and pumping station in Washington, D.C., the water purification and sewage disposal plant at Maryland State College of Agriculture, the sewage disposal unit at Baltimore Back River, the water filtration and sewage disposal system at Springfield State Hospital, and the sewage disposal unit of the Savage Manufacturing Company.[92]

Gregory had become interested in sanitary projects after contracting typhoid fever from the Hudson River; since that time, he had been "in the vanguard of those who argued for water reasonably free from microscopic inhabitants."[93] A successful consulting engineer, he had assisted with sanitary engineering projects in cities up and down the East Coast and in Columbus, Ohio. There, he had helped design the first large-scale plant for water softening; he had also drawn the plans for the huge Passaic Valley Sewerage system serving twenty municipalities. During the 1920s, Gregory seems to have withdrawn from his initial involvement with the School of Hygiene. Perhaps he was too busy with his consulting work but, in any case, Abel Wolman was asked to give most of the lectures at the school from 1921 to 1927 and again in 1936 and 1937. Wolman's energy, wit, and lively intellect delighted the students and immensely increased the popularity of the courses in sanitary engineering. Many reported his lectures as the best and most stimulating they had ever heard, on any subject.

Wolman did not limit himself to the traditional concerns of sanitary engineering: water and sewage. He held a broad and inclusive view of his field, including housing and working conditions, and he argued that "public health" as a social objective should include all approaches to improving people's environment for the protection of their health and comfort. He argued that efforts to improve living conditions in the cities need not wait until each specific reform was shown to be valid by statistical measures: "Fortunately in these fields, engineers have proceeded on the historically valid assumption that sometimes the instincts of man in his desire for these advantages are better guides to social action than are the failures of medical and statistical diagnoses to disclose their mathematical merit."[94]

At the time, Wolman was chief engineer at the Maryland State Department of Health, and he seemed to hold most of the unpaid jobs in the state; a kind of roving sanitary expert, he was also editor-in-chief of the *Journal of the American Water Works Association*, associate editor of the *American Journal of Public Health*, editor of the *Manual of Water Works Practice*, and editor-in-chief of *Municipal Sanitation*. Wolman considered himself first and foremost a practicing engineer, and he resisted the idea of full-time teaching although he was a frequent lecturer at Hopkins and Harvard, and gave occasional lectures at Southern California, Princeton, and Chicago.

In 1937, John Gregory died suddenly and unexpectedly. Wolman was immediately offered the job of professor of civil and sanitary engineering. He still resisted the idea of full-time teaching, feeling that if he stopped practicing as a sanitary engineer, he would soon find himself talking about the past, rather than current and future developments. To evade the insistent recruitment efforts of the university administration, Wolman submitted an unreasonable list of conditions for acceptance of the position: he would have to be the chairman of departments both in the School of Engineering and the School of Hygiene; he would need teaching and administrative assistants at both schools; and he would have to be free to continue all his outside activities. The university quickly accepted these conditions, although both faculties were upset by Wolman's insistence that engineers be admitted to the School of Hygiene and that sanitary engineers be required to take courses in physiology and biostatistics.[95]

Wolman had been much influenced by the work and ideas of William Thompson Sedgwick, who for thirty years had been chairman of the department of biology and public health at Massachusetts Institute of Technology. Sedgwick had vigorously opposed the monopolization of public health by doctors of medicine, and had argued for the importance of a new breed of people who combined engineering skills with public health concerns.[96] Wolman brought Sedgwick's ideas to Hopkins: he insisted that public health physicians understand the importance and basic concepts of sanitary engineering, and he also wanted engineering students to understand the concepts of epidemiology and the methods of biostatistics. The engineers preferred to take their own courses on structures and hydraulics; the School of Hygiene faculty preferred to teach physicians, but Wolman forced the reluctant engineers to attend classes in the School of Hygiene, and he forced the reluctant faculty to accept them. Perhaps to everyone's surprise, the combination worked extremely well; Wolman's students appeared at the top levels of public health administration and sanitary engineering posts around the world.

Although a master of the art of public speaking, Wolman disliked lecturing and ran his seminars with considerable informality. He did not attempt to fill his students with technical information but was more interested in their developing a critical capacity and analytical perspective: "I was reasonably convinced that what I was to try to do with a student was not to cram him with knowledge and information, but with

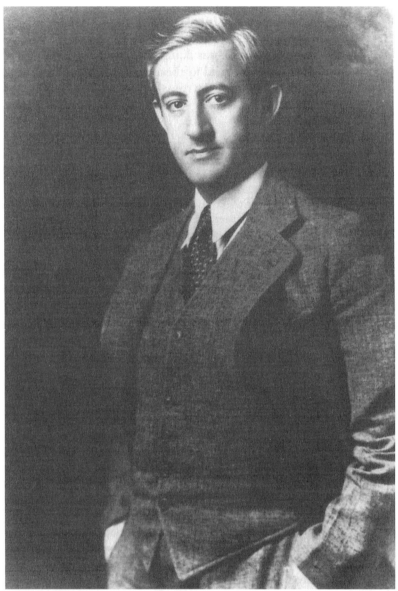

Figure 23. Abel Wolman, circa 1921. Wolman was assistant in sanitary engineering (1921), instructor (1923–27), and professor of sanitary engineering, both at Homewood and the School of Hygiene (1937–60). The architect of Maryland's water supply and sewage treatment facilities, Wolman became an international leader and consultant in sanitation and environmental health. (Courtesy of the Alan Mason Chesney Medical Archives of the Johns Hopkins Medical Institutions.)

The Physiology of Health / 153

a point of view, an attitude of inquiry, which ran all the way from the semantics with which he spoke or wrote to the actual quantitative aspects of whatever it was he was doing."[97]

Wolman emphasized the need to choose the most significant things to do, to avoid squandering time on trivial activities. He liked to tell the story of his meeting with the chief sanitary engineer of an (unnamed) South American country:

I said, "What do you do?" He said, "What I'm working on is swimming pool sanitation." I know the country pretty well; I looked at him, and I said, "Why are you working on swimming pools? Is that the central public health problem in your country?"—and I knew very well it wasn't. In the first place, they didn't need them, in the second place, they didn't have them. . . . The [sanitary engineer's] answer: "I'm working on swimming pools because I have a tremendous amount of material, stacked this high, on specifications for swimming pools from the United States."[98]

Wolman's students often remembered his pointed stories and common sense aphorisms for decades afterward. Wolman was indignant at the historical and cultural insensitivity he had often witnessed in his travels around the globe: "My criticism of the modern ignorant . . . is that you grab something you never heard of before and then you impose it, not only on the U.S., but on the rest of the world. It's nonsensical for us, and more nonsensical for the rest of the world."[99] Not surprisingly, Wolman was in great demand internationally as a sanitary consultant.

In Baltimore, Wolman was the architect of the city's expanded water supply and sewage treatment facilities built in the 1930s; his investigations in Maryland prompted the chlorination of the state's water supplies and later those of many cities in other states. He projected these cities' future water needs and arranged for dams and reservoirs; he figured out efficient and effective ways of dealing with sewage in a score of countries; and he cajoled and bullied the officers of the World Health Organization into making water and sanitation a top priority.[100] In a sense, his impact on the World Health Organization was similar to that on the School of Hygiene—by forcing public health experts, then mostly physicians, to recognize the basic importance of sanitary engineering and pure water supplies, he reintroduced a modern version of the environmentalist and engineering approach to public health that had characterized the great sanitary reforms of the late nineteenth century, but that had too often been forgotten in the intervening period.

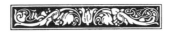

Surviving the Thirties

n its early years, the School of Hygiene passed rapidly through several important phases: the initial period of planning and organization of departments in the early twenties; a peaceful period of consolidation in the late twenties; a critical period of reevaluation and financial crisis in the early thirties; and another period of growth and recovery in the late thirties. During times of prosperity and growth, the underlying tensions between the pathological and physiological approaches to public health, the pure and applied sciences, laboratory and field research remained dormant. During periods of crisis, these tensions were intensified and played out in actual struggles over policy and funding.

When the school was launched in the 1920s, the laboratory sciences clearly occupied center stage. Almost all departments focused on laboratory research; even biometry and vital statistics was primarily oriented toward biological experimentation. Although epidemiology was strong under Frost, public health administration and health education had been almost afterthoughts in constructing the curriculum; disciplines with a directly practical orientation were not considered important from a scientific point of view.

By the 1930s, this attitude had changed. Now applied research had an increased respect and dignity; new funding supported projects in mental hygiene, child health, and venereal disease control. National and international visitors came to see the Hopkins experiment in public health administration in the Eastern Health District. Laboratory researchers now felt a need to explain the relevance of their work for public health practice.

This shift in focus, although real, should not be overstated. The School of Hygiene continued (and continues) to be primarily a research institution, based in the laboratory; it continued to emphasize the biological basis of health and disease rather than its social context. The pressures of the depression and the New Deal did, however, introduce a new balance in the thirties, and a new interest in community health services. This chapter concerns first the consolidation of the school in the 1920s during the relatively prosperous years of the Howell administration and then the crisis of the early thirties and the struggle and tensions provoked by limited budgets. The resolution of these tensions sets the stage for the development of community and applied research in the 1930s.

Peace and Prosperity: The Twenties

By 1926, the School of Hygiene seemed firmly established. The building on North Wolfe Street, if not elegant, was certainly solid and substantial. It was the visual equivalent of the endowment fund, guaranteeing the institution's permanence and future. The rotund figure of Welch, climbing the front steps for his Monday classes or greeting international visitors, provided reassurance and a certain glamour; in the administrative offices, the spare and dignified Howell ran the institution smoothly, calmly, and efficiently. The departments had been organized, and their offices and laboratories were producing a steady stream of research papers and publications. The teaching programs were also organized and running smoothly. There were now 146 students, 50 of them foreign physicians on Rockefeller fellowships, the rest North American scientists, doctors, and public health officers. The majority of the students took courses for one year or less, but about a third stayed for several years to complete doctorates.

During its first decade the school had thus been devoted to the primary task of establishing its program, departments, and disciplines, and setting the institution on a firm financial basis. In the second decade, it was subject to new internal and external pressures: the internal pressures created by the retirement of its founding fathers, Welch and Howell, and the external pressures created by the depression, the increased demand for public health programs and personnel, and the reduction of funding for research. Subjected to these new pressures, the school shifted its emphasis a little; although it lost some faculty and staff, most of the departments and teaching and research programs survived the depression intact, or even strengthened. The school as a whole was relatively insulated from the trauma of the depression by its endowment funds; tremors ran through the structure but most of it survived.

By 1926, William Henry Welch regarded his task of organizing the school as completed. By now, his position as director was largely honorary. He delighted in planning social occasions and splendid dinners for distinguished visitors. His influence with the Rockefeller Foundation, the Public Health Service, and other official bodies was enormously important in smoothing the way for the school's programs and activities; however, Welch's role was now mainly a ceremonial one, and he left the day-to-day running of the school to others. He usually appeared only on Mondays to give his course of lectures on the history of public health. Approaching his seventy-fifth birthday, Welch was still full of energy and enthusiasm, but he recognized that it was coming time for his retirement as director. He now handed over formal authority to Howell who already had the administrative responsibility, but not the title. Welch wrote to Howell: "You actually are doing the Director's work, and it is an immense satisfaction to me to feel that whatever honor goes with the position, will fall to you, who so richly deserve it."[1] Welch accepted a new position as professor of the history of medicine and honorary librarian of the Welch Medical Library, both the Institute of the History of Medicine and the medical library having been donated by the Rockefeller Foundation to offer Welch a "suitable resting place for his retirement."[2]

The School of Hygiene gave a farewell dinner in honor of Dr. Welch at the Maryland Club on December 20, 1926, with a menu that did justice to Welch's gastronomic reputation:

Maryland Oysters
Baltimore County Celery, Maryland Walnuts, Olives
Chesapeake Bay Diamond Back Terrapin
Maryland Beaten Biscuits
Baltimore County Cider
Roasted Susquehanna Ducks
Prince George's County Hominy Chafing Dish
Frederick County Ham and Lettuce
Carroll County Pumpkin Pie
Baltimore City Finger Rolls
Cigarettes, Coffee, Cigars.[3]

The *Baltimore Sun* noted that Welch was unperturbed by his birthdays, and took this one as an occasion to promise that the span of human life would be increased by proper attention to public health and preventive medicine. The press headlines announced: "Dr. Welch Declares Average Life Could Be Extended to 100 years: Urges as Much Care of Human Bodies as of Autos." Welch stated that the aim of living past one hundred was quite feasible but would require "learning the rules of health and applying them as assiduously as we apply ourselves to removing a rattle in our automobile engines."[4]

The Administration

During the 1920s, the school administration had been of the minimalist variety. Welch's approach was to give department heads virtually full control over the running of their departments and to leave routine academic policy decisions to the Advisory Board of the Faculty. He left to William Howell the daily administrative tasks of dealing with schoolwide operations, problems, and correspondence. As director of the school, and as a preeminent representative of scientific medicine in the United States, Welch received a flood of mail, much of which he simply ignored; it piled up on shelves, tables, and chairs unopened and unread. When his study table was completely covered with unanswered mail, he simply covered the piles with sheets of newspaper, and began new piles on top of the old. When a visitor found eight chairs full of unopened mail, Welch explained his system: "On that armchair there I have the letters that have come during the past week; I hope to read these in the near future. On that chair I have the letters that have come within the past month. On the other chairs are letters and magazines anywhere from six months to a year old which I hope to get to sometime."[5] Rockefeller Foundation officers and others who knew Welch well communicated with him by telegrams, which were generally opened and answered.

In contrast to Welch, William Howell dealt with correspondence in a disciplined and orderly manner. Fortunately, Howell had taken over the task of answering the mail, explaining that Welch was "not a very good correspondent."[6] Howell was aided by one secretary, the competent Louise Durham. Miss Durham seems at times to have kept the whole institution functioning; she arranged housing for foreign students, welcomed visitors, kept all the records, and did other essential tasks. Howell and Durham constituted the core administration; the other early staff members were Elizabeth Thies, the librarian, and Ethel Norris, an artist. W. Graham Boyce, the treasurer of the university, S. Page Nelson, the university's business manager, and William Howell managed the budgets and other financial affairs of the school.

The Advisory Board of the Faculty made all substantial decisions about academic policy. When first established, it was composed of the senior faculty.[7] As the faculty grew larger, the Advisory Board was restricted to the heads of the departments. The board discussed academic policy, and its members were "instructed to report to the Trustees from time to time their suggestions and to prepare and carry forward the proper arrangements for the instruction and graduation of students in the School."[8] The Advisory Board established committees as needed to deal with specific issues. Much of its business concerned relatively routine matters: the admission of students, the granting of degrees, and the appointment or promotion of staff.

The Executive Committee of the school prepared budgets, tried to make accounts balance, and, after discussions with the heads of departments, decided the salaries of each member of the faculty and staff. From 1918 to 1927, the Executive Committee was composed of the president of the university, the director and the assistant director of the school; after 1927, the university provost was added to the committee. These executive discussions were informal, and not until January 1929 were any records kept of the meetings.[9] After 1929, the process became increasingly formal, and the written budgets larger and more complicated.

The early administrative apparatus of the school was composed of three standing committees: on applications, publications, and the library. The committee on applications recommended student admissions to the Advisory Board; the committee on publications was responsible for the *American Journal of Hygiene*, the school catalog, and the *Collected Papers* of faculty research; the library committee ordered books and set library policy.

Research and Publications: The American Journal of Hygiene

Throughout the 1920s, six of the nine departments within the school were almost exclusively devoted to research in the laboratory sciences; even biometry and vital statistics was involved in animal experimentation. Epidemiology and public health administration were the only departments without a clear orientation to the laboratory sciences; these applied departments dealt with field research and public health practice. In its general orientation, the School of Hygiene more closely resembled the research-oriented ideal of an "institute of hygiene" than the practice-oriented ideal of a "school of public health." William Henry Welch had constructed the research institute he wanted.

The involvement with laboratory research and a concomitant focus on the biological basis of disease was evident in the research publications of the faculty and students. These were overwhelmingly oriented toward the "pathological" disciplines—the study of disease organisms. Helminthology, protozoology, and bacteriology tended to dominate by sheer volume of research papers and, therefore, to reinforce the impression that these fields constituted the central disciplines of a scientific approach to public health.

Welch decided, very soon after the school had been founded, that it should have its own research journal. At that time, the American Public Health Association produced the only American publication devoted to the field, the *American Journal of Public Health*. Here were published general articles on public health; in Welch's view, a specifically research-oriented publication was also essential. In 1920, Welch announced that he was forming the *American Journal of Hygiene*, with himself as general editor, to publish current research in hygiene.

Welch's decision created some consternation among the editors of other, possibly rival, publications. In July 1920, George Nuttall, editor of the English *Journal of Hygiene*, wrote to Welch suggesting that it would be "a pity to multiply journals" and that he should publish contributions from the School of Hygiene.[10] Welch wrote to Charles E. Simon:

You will be interested to know that I have a letter from Nuttall, who is evidently a little disturbed by our starting an American Journal of Hygiene. He suggests that there be added to his editorial board representatives from our School of Hygiene and that we send our contributions to his journal. This, of course, we cannot consider, and I have no doubt that I shall be able to make clear to him the need of an American Journal of Hygiene.[11]

Nuttall was apparently convinced, and he and Welch remained firm friends. But six months later, W. W. Hedrich, the secretary of the American Public Health Association, wrote to express his concern about possible competition between the *American Journal of Hygiene* and the *American Journal of Public Health*. Since Welch's publication was now inevitable, Hedrich asked Welch at least to consider changing its title so that the two journals could not so easily be confused. "There will probably be a good deal of confusion between your publication and the American Journal of Public Health. If your first issue has not yet appeared, may I suggest that you consider a change in title. A further source of confusion arises because of the fact that our Association once published an American Journal of Hygiene."[12]

Welch, however, stuck to his plans and managed to convince the editors of the other public health journals that his journal filled a different need and would not interfere with their circulations. Welch was also able to gain the cooperation and assistance of many of the leading public health men for his new journal. Besides the faculty of the School of Hygiene (Simon, Bull, Cort, Ford, Frost, Hegner, Howell, McCollum, and Pearl), Welch brought on, as assistant editors, such men as Hermann Biggs, Simon Flexner, Edwin Jordan, Graham Lusk,

W. H. Park, Milton Rosenau, Frederick Russell, Theobald Smith, E. R. Stitt, V. C. Vaughan, C-E. A. Winslow, and Hans Zinsser. Welch appointed Charles Simon as managing editor of the *American Journal of Hygiene*. Simon devoted great enthusiasm to the task and, with Welch's advice, essentially did all the work—soliciting papers, persuading reluctant authors, restraining the overly prolific, organizing, editing, and discussing manuscripts. The initial funding for the journal was $10,000 from the De Lamar Endowment, given to the Johns Hopkins University by Joseph De Lamar "to give to the people of the United States generally the benefits of increased knowledge concerning the prevention of sickness and disease and also concerning the conservation of health by proper food and diet."[13]

The first issue of the *American Journal of Hygiene* appeared in January 1921. Like the *Journal of Experimental Medicine* which Welch had started twenty-five years previously, the new journal would be devoted to publishing original research in a variety of scientific disciplines. Welch listed the specific disciplines expected to contribute to the *American Journal of Hygiene*: statistics, chemistry, physiology, pathology, bacteriology and immunology, medical zoology and its branches of protozoology, helminthology and entomology, epidemiology, and sanitary engineering. Although this list favored the laboratory sciences, the journal would also welcome field studies and research in the social and applied fields of public health.

It need hardly be said that scientific contributions to knowledge in the field covered by this *Journal* do not come solely from the laboratory, important as such contributions are. Of equal value are researches in the field, . . . investigations of the methods of administrative and other measures of prevention and of sanitation, studies of the influence of heredity, of acquired constitution, of diet, of social, environmental and other conditions upon health and disease, contributions to personal hygiene, to school hygiene, to industrial hygiene, to tropical hygiene, and other lines of research which it is unnecessary to specify.[14]

Despite these encouraging comments, the laboratory sciences heavily dominated the *American Journal of Hygiene* in its early years. The majority of papers were written by School of Hygiene faculty, and to a lesser extent by its students. The papers therefore represented the departmental and disciplinary organization of the school.[15] By far the largest number of papers came from helminthology, protozoology, bacteriology, and immunology. In 1925, for example, about 75 percent came from these fields with only a few scattered papers from epidemiology, biostatistics, chemical hygiene, and physiological hygiene. For several decades, the distribution of papers among disciplines followed this general pattern.[16]

A considerable number of papers were concerned with diphtheria and influenza, reflecting the research projects being jointly conducted in the departments of bacteriology, immunology, and epidemiology; a lesser number were devoted to malaria and measles. In general, these studies tended to focus on the pathogenic organisms rather than on the human host or the social context of disease.

In 1927, when Charles Simon died, Roscoe Hyde from the department of immunology was appointed managing editor in his place. General editorial control passed to an Editorial Board selected from the faculty of the School of Hygiene: Carroll Bull, William Cort, William Ford, Wade Hampton Frost, Elmer V. McCollum, and Lowell Reed, with William Welch as honorary chairman. Under Hyde's editorship the overall proportion of "basic" to "applied" research remained similar to that established by Simon. Only in the 1930s did the journal begin to pay much attention to field studies or epidemiology.

In May 1934, the journal published its first "epidemiological number" with articles on yellow fever, malaria, schistosomiasis, hookworm, ascariasis, diphtheria, and deafness. From this point, epidemiological studies started to appear somewhat more frequently than before. In 1938, the journal was divided into four sections: epidemiology, biostatistics, and general; bacteriology, immunology, and viruses; protozoology and malariology; and helminthology. The division by sections was dropped in 1941, and the proportion of epidemiological papers slowly increased in the postwar years; not until 1965, however, did the relative numbers of laboratory and epidemiological studies published shift sufficiently to justify renaming the journal the American Journal of Epidemiology.[17]

Though the American Journal of Hygiene was the single most important means of communicating faculty research, the papers published in other journals by the faculty and students were bound each year into volumes of Collected Papers, sold to individual purchasers, and sent free to institutions of hygiene, special laboratories, and libraries throughout the world. Within the school, there were also less formal methods for communicating research results and for discussing research findings before publication. Several departments held their own seminars, and the Society of Hygiene, originally formed by William Howell, had monthly meetings open to all members of the school and the general public. Society of Hygiene meetings kept people informed about research going on in the other departments. Lively discussions followed the papers and helped create intellectual exchanges among members of the different departments, students, and visitors.[18] Most of the papers presented at the Society of Hygiene, on topics ranging from African sleeping sickness to the etiology of rickets, later appeared in the *American Journal of Hygiene*.

While the Society of Hygiene mainly discussed original scientific research conducted within the school, the De Lamar lectures featured distinguished guests speaking to the public on general topics. In 1929–30, for example, the De Lamar lecture speakers included E. L. Bishop, the commissioner of public health of Tennessee, on "Tennessee's Child Health Program"; Stewart Paton, lecturer in psychiatry at the Johns Hopkins University, on "The Art of Living"; H. Gideon Wells, professor of pathology at the University of Chicago, on "The Relation of Heredity to Human Cancer"; M. E. Barnes, professor of hygiene and preventive medicine at the University of Iowa, on "The Problems of a County Health Officer"; Henry F. Helmholtz, professor of pediatrics at the Mayo Clinic, on "Preventive Pediatrics"; and George F. McCleary, deputy senior medical officer of the Ministry of Health, England, on "The Rise and Development of National Health Insurance in Europe."[19]

The Students

Many students coming to the School of Hygiene were, like the faculty, primarily interested in scientific research rather than in public health practice. Those without M.D. degrees were channeled into the Doctor of Science program, to be trained as scientific researchers in the different disciplines. These men and women were expected to become scientists and teachers of public health rather than practicing public health officers. Positions of administrative authority in public health departments were normally reserved for physicians. The profession of public health was thus caught in a contradiction: the leading positions were being kept for medical graduates, most of whom showed little interest in public health; the nonphysicians who displayed interest and enthusiasm for public health were not eligible for key professional jobs but worked in supporting roles in research and analysis.

Meanwhile, the faculty continued to worry that recent medical graduates were not attracted to schools of public health. In 1927, Victor Heiser of the Rockefeller Foundation interviewed members of the Hopkins faculty about their views of the relationship between public health and medicine and the reasons why young physicians were not drawn to the field. The problems seemed to be structural ones: in part economic, in part political, in part ideological. Most of the faculty agreed that small salaries and insecure positions made public health unattractive to physicians. Howell argued that the problem would not be solved until the whole structure of public health employment had changed:

Public health work . . . is attractive and important, and should appeal to the best of our medical graduates. The fact that it does not is accounted for by the unsatisfactory character of public health positions in this country at present. The leading positions . . . are regarded as political appointments, and are, therefore, subject to change with each change of administration. When a change in the status of our public health officers is effected, when the country at large adopts some such system as exists now in Great Britain, our schools of public health will enter upon their proper function.[20]

Quite apart from the insecurity of tenure were the relatively low salaries offered by even the more stable public health positions, much less than most physicians could make in private practice. The task was therefore one of attracting young physicians into public health against their own economic interests. In a conversation with Victor Heiser, Wade Hampton Frost expressed the belief that it could be accomplished. If only one percent of medical students entered public health work, it would be a sufficient number to provide the needed leadership. Frost mentioned Kenneth Maxcy as an example of a physician who willingly sacrificed a large income practicing pediatrics in favor of public health work. Frost was confident that other such physicians could be found.[21]

Kenneth Maxcy, the epidemiologist whose choices had inspired this optimism, was himself considerably more pessimistic. Maxcy succinctly summarized the concerns facing a medical graduate interested in public health:

Limited income. He must give up the hope of earning a large income and be content with a bare living for the rest of his life.
Insecurity of tenure. The feeling is current that in this field of work one is subject to the instability of political appointment.
Administrative duties. The graduating student, enthusiastic in his newly acquired power to diagnose and treat disease, sees little opportunity for its utilization in public health work.
Lack of prestige. Both the public and the profession are inclined to think of public health officials as largely recruited from the ranks of unsuccessful practitioners.[22]

Part of the problem of attracting medical graduates in public health was one of image and ideology. The image of the physician was a heroic one: the doctor struggled with life and death, while the fate of the patient hung in the balance. The relationship between doctor and patient was a personal and emotional one, a tie forged in dependence, trust, hope, and gratitude. By contrast, the public health officer was thought to lead an impersonal and unemotional life, dealing with the statistics of disease rather than individual lives. He had to demonstrate "statistical compassion": to find his personal gratification in lowering the population indicators of disease and disability. Public health practice was a success when events did not happen: although thousands of illnesses might be completely prevented, no one grateful patient was hauled back from the brink of death. The patients of the public health officer displayed no gratitude whatsoever.

The public health officer might also have to face antagonism from members of his own profession. Allen Freeman, a physician who had considerable experience as a public health official in Virginia and Ohio, argued that the interests of medicine and public health were in conflict since public health programs threatened the income of physicians, and the medical profession had increasingly come to resent public health efforts.[23] In Freeman's view, the problem had no solution.

The Rockefeller Foundation did try offering summer public health fellowships to medical students, in the hope of encouraging them to enter the field. The effort had little success; only three of ten 1925–26 fellowship students chose public health as a career; none of the eleven selected in 1934 entered public health on a permanent basis. The reasons they gave were the familiar ones: low compensation, insecurity of tenure, and political interference.[24]

The Rockefeller Foundation actually paid much less attention to the problem of developing public health in the United States than it did to the rest of the world. While the faculty of the School of Hygiene worried about attracting American physicians into public health, the International Health Board was actively recruiting and funding medical graduates from other countries. The International Health Board, in need of a continuous stream of professionals to staff health programs around the world, was offering generous fellowships and travel money to potential candidates. Its officers were able to select promising young physicians from a variety of countries and bring them to Baltimore for periods of public health training; then, help establish them in leadership positions within the health organizations in their home countries.

The mix of students at the School of Hygiene thus included two divergent groups: nonphysician graduates from the United States preparing for careers in scientific research and foreign physicians preparing for careers in international public health. The foreign students gave the School of Hygiene a thoroughly cosmopolitan air. Baltimore itself was a

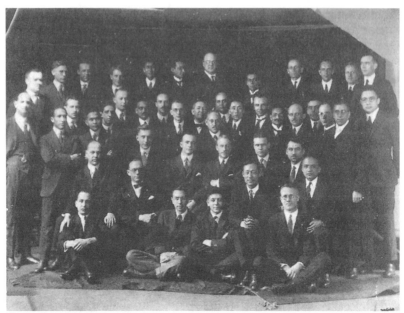

Figure 24. The Ubiquiteers, 1922–23. This student club was formed to promote friendly and informal cultural exchanges between students of different nationalities. From left, back row: Pinto, Dziuban, Cannon, Le Blanc, Baldwin, Chedt, Castro, Lambert, Fragoso, Kacprzok, Doering, Payne, Bishop. Middle row: Garcia, Battistini, Lara, Guernez, Rumreich, Mathur, Poch, Studeny, Haygood, Barbeau, Molloy, Kung, Van Dam, Edibam, Novakovic, Oliviera, Abadia, Hernando, Soper. Front row: Bermudez, Covington, King, Stoll, Greidanus, Larde, Sandground, Howell, Hu, Sweeney, Fear, Rozinek, Prommas. (Courtesy of the Rockefeller Archive Center, Tarrytown, New York.)

provincial city, a mixture of northern industrialism and southern social attitudes; the School of Hygiene was the one place in the city where people of many races and cultural backgrounds could meet on grounds of social and intellectual equality. The student club, the Ubiquiteers, had been formed specifically to promote friendly and informal cultural exchanges.[25] Baltimore itself could offer a chilly reception to foreigners. Ayodhya Das explained what it was like to arrive from India in 1932:

I had heard of the Mason-Dixon line. An ominous feeling crept into my mind, suggesting segregation and isolation. . . . The Rockefeller Foundation had very thoughtfully arranged for my accommodation at the Lord Baltimore Hotel for three days during which I was supposed to have found my digs. . . . A fellow worker from Lucknow had a bitter experience on getting hotel accommodation in Baltimore because he was rather dark in complexion. He ultimately went to a Negro hotel for the night. . . . An

Indian student rather dark in complexion used, while going to the School, his turban so that he may not be mistaken for a Negro. The street urchins used to hail him with shouts of "hi, buddy, let's have some magic."[26]

Both American and foreign students remembered with pleasure the close personal relationships between faculty and students at the School of Hygiene. The school, relatively small, allowed time for personal and intellectual discussions. Some departments organized regular lunches and "teas"; others had journal clubs for discussion of new articles and research. Especially interesting lunchtime discussions might last through the afternoon. Many faculty invited groups of students to their homes for dinner, where talk could continue late into the evening. The general impression given by alumni accounts is of an enthusiasm for research but a relaxed attitude toward time, with relatively few pressures.

Teaching could be challenging because it was difficult to arrange a course of instruction suited to students from a wide range of backgrounds, academic preparation, and practical experience. Whereas nonmedical students found the biomedical courses challenging, medical graduates found them repetitive; foreign students found some courses oriented toward North Americans irrelevant to their own needs. A report on the courses in 1922, for example, complained that the course on sanitary engineering was excellent for North Americans but that "the Latin students feel it will be impossible for them to apply any part of the subject as it is now taught and have requested that simpler means of water purification and sewage disposal be taught in greater detail."[27] The same report suggested that epidemiology deal with the control of malaria and yellow fever and that public health administration "include such phases of administration as have been found practicable in tropical countries."[28]

Despite such complaints, most students remembered the total experience of being at the school in positive, indeed, glowing terms. Leroy E. Burney's account, remembered at a distance of fifty years, was typical: "Every course I had was a new subject and a new experience to me. . . . I shall never forget the deep impression made by the small and devoted faculty and especially Drs. Frost, Reed and McCollum, three highly intelligent, scholarly, kindly men. . . . Exposure to them alone for nine months was a unique and unforgettable experience which helped to guide and shape my career."[29]

Speaking of her own student days, Margaret Merrell recalled: "I think that the School of Hygiene was an absolutely wonderful school in the whole spirit of the place."[30]

Two events provoked a crisis for the School of Hygiene in the early 1930s. The first was the retirement of William Howell in 1931. His retirement marked the end of the original leadership of the school and opened the way for changes in policy and curriculum. Howell had closely followed Welch's own direction of emphasizing the school's commitment to fundamental scientific research, but now the department heads who wanted more attention paid to public health applications had an opportunity to establish a new agenda.

The second crisis was a financial one. The school's endowment insulated it from the most devastating effects of the economic depression, but it was not completely immune. The income from the endowment fund was falling and continued to drop gradually over several years; for example, the interest on investments in 1930 was $250,000, and in 1933, $238,000.[31] The income from the endowment provided approximately 80 percent of the school's operating costs, so the cut in endowment income created increased competition among the departments for available funds.[32]

The simultaneous pressure of Howell's retirement and declining endowment income generated a reevaluation of the school's structure and purpose; suddenly, new committees proliferated to reconsider virtually all aspects of the school's activities and organization. Of these, the two most important were the committee on physiology and the committee on organization. Allen Freeman chaired the committee on physiology formed to discuss the future of the department of physiological hygiene. Wade Hampton Frost chaired the committee on organization formed to discuss the school's system of operation, administration, and future plans.[33]

The committee on organization met regularly for a year to evaluate the school's functioning and to assess its purpose.[34] The committee members started from the original Welch-Rose report of 1914 and agreed that its principles were sound, especially the emphasis placed on research, rather than training. They did not view as a problem the school's small number of students compared to the needs of the public health service. The committee particularly noted an appendix to the Welch-Rose report, written by Howell in June 1916, which concluded:

The benefits to be expected from the establishment of such an institute as that proposed are not to be measured solely by the number of students trained within its walls. The institute can supply only a relatively small number of those who desire to enter upon public health service. The far-reaching influence of the institute should be felt in the advancement of science and the improvement of the practice of public health, in establishing higher standards and better methods of professional education in this field, in stimulating the foundation of similar institutes in other parts of the country, in supplying teachers and in cooperating with schools of a simpler character designed for briefer technical training which should be established in each state in connection jointly with boards of health and medical schools.[35]

The faculty acknowledged the most common complaints about public health education at Hopkins. These included the school's failure to devote any significant attention to the social sciences or to the training of sanitary engineers, public health nurses, or health inspectors, and its failure to cultivate close relationships with the School of Medicine and with local health agencies. The issues demanding "more serious attention" were:

A definite policy of attracting physicians in fields other than public health to the School for graduate study; the building up of closer relationships to the School of Medicine, the Hospital and operating public health agencies, especially of this city and State; possibly more attention to the general field of the social sciences; and more extensive use of the facilities of the School in connection with the training of sanitary engineers.[36]

The committee declared that the failure to train public health nurses and inspectors had been due not to "inertia" but to "the growing conviction that training for these classes could best be provided elsewhere."[37]

Though the development of the school had closely followed its original plan, the growth of departments had been unplanned. The rule of only one full professor per department meant the newly promoted professors were given their own departments. The departments thus came to represent "fields marked out by the interests and special qualifications of individuals, rather than logically distinct subdivisions." This system could not continue indefinitely, so the committee suggested that appointments to full professor be made only when the school, as a matter of policy, intended to promote the independent development of a new field, and was furthermore willing to provide the appropriate salary and facilities; second, that when any existing chair fell vacant, the school should consider the redistribution of fields rather than the continuance of existing subdivisions.[38] Space for laboratories and offices was another problem. A "committee designated to survey space" in 1931, however, was able to do little more than suggest minor economies such as combining the use of laboratories for teaching purposes; competition for space would be an unending problem for the next fifty years.[39]

The committee on organization discussed the appointment of associate professors at some length and decided on three criteria for
promotion:

1. Such productiveness and initiative as justify the expectation that within
a few years, offers of appointment to higher position will come from outside
sources, or
2. Ability to fill a distinct and more or less permanent need in teaching,
and in either case,
3. Willingness and ability on the part of the University to provide a salary
appropriate to the grade, that is, generally not less than $4,000.[40]

The committee members agreed that the school did not want more
students but fewer, better students. They worried that some of the
students on International Health Division fellowships were "somewhat
ill-adapted because of inadequate preparation or attainments, or, in the
case of foreign students, because of unfamiliarity with our language."[41]
They applauded a "notable improvement in the quality of students
coming from the United States," but complained that "the total number
of students at the School is already quite large enough and probably too
large."[42] As before, too few recent medical graduates were being attracted into public health. Those who came tended to want the one-year
C.P.H. (Certificate of Public Health) rather than the longer period
required for the Dr.P.H. (Doctorate of Public Health) for perhaps
obvious reasons: the more advanced degree was not required for professional positions in public health. The committee recommended that
the degree of Master of Public Health (M.P.H.) be substituted for the
C.P.H., because a master's degree usually indicated more academic
weightiness than a "certificate."

The committee suggested reforms to make the curriculum more
flexible and also more compatible with that of the medical school.
Converting to a quarterly schedule met both of these objectives as it
made the School of Hygiene consistent with the School of Medicine and
shortened the required courses, so that students had more flexibility in
choosing electives.[43] The committee members also argued the need for a
local teaching and study unit in public health practice.

Upon Howell's retirement, the faculty decided to reduce the power of
the school's chief administrator and to make the position a rotating one.
The committee on organization suggested that the administrative head
of the school be a dean, elected by the Advisory Board for a period of
three years. The dean would be ineligible to succeed himself, so the
position would be held in succession by different members of the
Advisory Board.[44] This proposal, accepted by the university Board of

Trustees in February 1931, meant that the dean, having been elected by the other department heads, would be unlikely to act against their wishes; the short term of the deanship and the elective nature of the appointment thus curtailed the possibility of developing an independent base of administrative power. In 1931, the Advisory Board elected Wade Hampton Frost the first dean of the school under the new policy.

The committee on organization also restructured the standing committees of the faculty. After the Executive Committee, the most important single committee would be the committee on policy, with members "chosen by the Advisory Board without nomination from the Dean."[45] Initially, this committee would consist of two members of the Advisory Board appointed by the university president, and one directly elected by the faculty. The committee on policy would thus be essentially independent of the dean; it would consider all important matters of policy before these were presented to the Advisory Board for action.[46] Other school committees would be appointed by the president, on nomination by the dean. These were the committee on applications and curriculum; the committee on publications, responsible for the catalog and *Collected Papers*; and the editorial committee of the *American Journal of Hygiene*.

Invited by the committee on organization to discuss their views on the most important financial needs of the school, the faculty asked for more space, more research funding, more staff, and higher professional salaries. The committee decided that two needs were of sufficient urgency and importance to justify an appeal for special funds:

1. A farm for the breeding and special care of animals for experimental work
2. A field study and training area adjacent to the school and under its control, to be used for training nurses and for epidemiological research.[47]

The proposal for an organized field study and training area would have major consequences. The development of the Eastern Health District, established in 1932, is discussed in the next chapter. The proposal for an animal farm was referred to a special committee, and finally rejected for several reasons. Rats and mice were already being reared satisfactorily in the School of Hygiene, and rabbits and guinea pigs could easily be obtained. The breeding of dogs for experimental purposes was considered unwise as it "would soon become known to the antivivisectionists with undesirable results."[48] Research on large animals such as swine, sheep, horses, and cattle could be conducted better at agricultural experiment stations than at the school. The proposal for an animal farm, overwhelmed by various objections, including the budgetary crisis, was allowed to die a quiet death.

While the committee on organization was working out these various policies and proposals, the Executive Committee was dealing with the school's first projected budget deficit. The estimated expenses for academic year 1931–32 were $348,604; the estimated income, $333,500. The Executive Committee decided to meet the deficit by the following measures:

reduction in all increases asked for by the administration and departments of instruction

a reduction of 5 percent in the running expense accounts of the departments

a reduction of the appropriation for instruction in pathology, public health law and social hygiene

a reduction in salary for the Dean

suspension of appropriations for all research fellowships and graduate fellowships except for commitments made to students already in the school.[49]

In this first round of budget cuts, the largest single saving came from the reductions in proposed departmental budgets. The period of expansion was now over and the departments' plans were limited by the constraints of their gradually contracting budgets.

Physiological Hygiene

Because Howell's retirement as director of the school and as head of the department of physiological hygiene had come at a time of financial crisis, his department was in a weak position in the competition for limited funds. In addition, the committee formed to review the department was chaired by Allen Freeman, known to be critical of the department's orientation toward pure research and to believe that the school should emphasize more applied research and practical training. In October 1931, Freeman's committee decided that the budget of physiological hygiene should be reduced "to conform to the present financial situation of the School as a whole."[50] Arthur Meyer's appointment as associate professor in physiological hygiene was not renewed. The committee decided to defer the appointment of a new professor of physiology until determining "the place of physiology in future policy." It suggested that an effort be made to secure an acting head of the department to be appointed as associate professor or resident lecturer: "This candidate should be, in the opinion of the committee, a man in his early thirties who gives promise of development in research and who may in the future, on the basis of his accomplishments in the School, expect to be promoted to the professorship."[51]

This suggestion was remarkable for several reasons. In the first place, the report implied that the role of physiological hygiene in the school was somewhat doubtful; after one year, the committee had been unable to define its importance. Second, the committee had been unable to identify any suitable candidate for department head, thus reinforcing the idea that the department itself might be unnecessary. Third, if a younger person was to be sought, there were already two such candidates for the position. The problem was that both candidates were women: Howell's daughter, Janet Clark, was an associate professor and Anna Baetjer was an associate in the department. Both women were experienced in the field; both had been teaching major courses for several years and had published original research.[52] Both women certainly fulfilled one criterion for appointment as associate professor, giving "promise of development in research and teaching," but neither fulfilled the criterion of being "a man." In 1931, apparently, it was inconceivable that either be seriously considered as capable of heading a department. The committee on policy decided to continue, informally, making inquiries regarding "suitable and available men."[53]

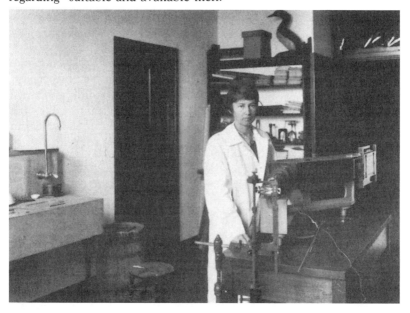

Figure 25. Janet Howell Clark, associate professor of physiological hygiene (1923–35), in her physiological laboratory, circa 1925. William H. Howell's daughter was trained in physics and studied the physiological effects of radiation on health. (Courtesy of the Alan Mason Chesney Medical Archives of the Johns Hopkins Medical Institutions.)

The financial status of the school continued to be problematic. In May 1932, the committee on policy stated that the budget for 1933–34 would have to be $20,000 less than that for 1932–33. The committee first considered and rejected as "inadvisable" a proposal to reduce all salaries by 10 percent.[54] It then considered and rejected a proposal to eliminate physiological hygiene as a separate department by combining it with McCollum's department of chemical hygiene. It recommended a third proposal to reduce all the administrative and departmental budgets, to limit the terms of appointment of associate professors to three years and to limit the salaries of new appointees to $3,000, and, as a matter of policy, to consolidate departments and resources whenever a professorship fell vacant "with more generous support for those that are continued."[55]

The first of the departmental consolidations had already occurred. When Charles Simon died in 1927, the departments of filterable viruses and immunology were merged. Roscoe Hyde was named professor and head of the new combined department of immunology.[56] This decision was not controversial; the department of filterable viruses was a small unit that had clearly been created by and for Simon. Without him, there was little justification for an independent department.

Physiological hygiene was more problematic, as it had been a founding department of the school. In January 1933, however, the committee on policy recommended that, as a temporary expedient, the departments of biochemistry and physiological hygiene be formally combined under the direction of Elmer McCollum.[57] The justification, that "the proposal is made as a means of developing the subject of physiological hygiene," was hardly convincing, for McCollum had little interest in physiological hygiene; the measure was strictly a holding action and a way of saving funds. The budget for physiological hygiene, already cut by half, was further reduced; Janet Clark and Anna Baetjer remained as the only full-time faculty.

In 1935, the committee on policy again considered the "future development of physiology in the school" and concluded that combining the departments of physiological hygiene and chemical hygiene, previously considered a temporary expedient, was not likely to be reversed "at any early date." They therefore recommended that Janet Clark and Anna Baetjer be formally transferred to McCollum's department; the budget for physiology would again be reduced, to "relieve the School from commitments of approximately five thousand dollars per annum."[58] Concerned that the school intended to abandon the department, Clark asked for a guarantee of her appointment and budget; when this was not forthcoming, she left to become headmistress of the Bryn

Mawr School, and later, professor of biology and dean of the Women's College at the University of Rochester. After her retirement, Clark returned to the School of Hygiene to continue her research on radiation and to lecture to students. She worked in her laboratory every day until the age of seventy-eight, and continued to publish papers almost until the day she died.[59]

Anna Baetjer remembered the period after Clark's resignation: "After that, being the youngest in the department at the bottom of the scale, I heard no more about abandoning the department. And then, I understand, what happened was that they decided to keep me on. I didn't cost them anything much to talk about. I was not expensive and yet I could keep the department going. . . . The man who was Dean at that moment really had no interest in the departments that were concerned primarily with basic research." Baetjer continued, "I was left entirely alone. I was put under Dr. McCollum. . . . Dr. McCollum said to me, 'I don't have any time, and as long as you stay in the budget, you can do anything you want.' "[60] It was a small budget; the departmental funds had been cut from approximately $25,000 to $5,000, the latter to cover the salaries and research expenses of Baetjer and one technician. William Howell, a calm and mild-mannered man, was moved to a formal protest:

One must conclude from these actions that the authorities in control of the School had decided that the Department of Physiological Hygiene had not justified its existence and was not of essential importance to the work of the School. The writer of this note greatly regrets this decision. What hygiene may be expected to accomplish in the long run is the establishment of standards of right living under optimal environmental conditions, seeking for a maximum of public health rather than a minimum of public disease. . . . It may be said, however, that the ideas embodied in the organization of this department have been adopted by other schools, so that the proper development of the subject, it is hoped, will not be unduly retarded by the unfavorable attitude of this School.[61]

Allen Freeman was now serving as dean, and in the perception of Howell, Clark, and Baetjer, he was trying to turn the school away from its original commitment to basic research by stressing only those aspects of the curriculum directly applicable in public health practice. The battle lines between "pure" and "applied" research had been drawn over the department of physiological hygiene. Budgetary constraints, Howell's retirement, and sexual discrimination had all worked against the department's interests.

Anna Baetjer was determined to keep the department, and Howell's ideas, intact. Ignoring the fact that she had only an associate appointment, and a miniscule salary, she single-handedly created a full teaching and research program for the students.

There wasn't anybody here. And I decided that if I wanted the department to continue . . . the only way to do that was to stop being a physiologist and see what the department had that I felt was of value to . . . our students at that time. . . . So I planned a course that would take all the things that we and everybody else had been teaching and rolled them all into one course . . . Industrial Hygiene and the Environment. Then I decided that the emphasis had to go on industrial hygiene as there was a great movement for the development of industrial hygiene in state health departments . . . and so I immediately began organizing more courses. . . . I quite enjoyed putting the emphasis on industrial hygiene but I had no choice anyway. This was it or there wasn't going to be a department at all. I so adored Dr. Howell that I wanted to keep his concepts and ideas alive in the school. I was alone, you see, for fifteen years.[62]

Anna Baetjer's previous research had been in "pure" physiology, but she now turned her attention to research in occupational health. For some years, she published little, but she then began a burst of productivity that established her name in occupational health circles and led to a raft of national and international honors. Somewhat to her embarrassment, as she refused to see herself as an expert, her book on women in industry became a classic in the field, while her other research established the connection between occupational chromate exposures and lung cancer.[63]

Until the war years, Anna Baetjer worked alone, with virtually no institutional recognition. Baetjer was aware that she received a low salary but reasoned that, as a single woman and member of a prominent Baltimore family, she did not really need money; she patiently waited for a promotion and was delighted when, after working for almost forty years, she was finally made full professor: "If you have a job you like and you're interested and people treat you properly, what difference does it make whether you're a man or a woman? If they don't look down at you, and they didn't, except salarywise. . . . But I loved doing what I wanted to do. . . . Nobody bossed me which was great."[64]

Despite the lack of institutional support, despite the budgetary massacre, despite the apparent disinterest of the school's administration, Anna Baetjer's strong will, independence, and boundless enthusiasm turned the most serious casualty of the depression era—the department of physiological hygiene—into an asset: a new, de facto, department of occupational health.

The crisis over the department of physiological hygiene was not the end of the financial problems of the depression era. In 1932–33, the school operated with a deficit; in 1933–34 the budgets were slashed again. All but the lowest paid faculty and staff took salary deductions.[65] These cuts were presented as "temporary deductions" rather than "reductions" in salary; when the financial status of the school improved, the money would be restored to individual salaries. To reduce operating costs further, the committee on policy recommended that the age of obligatory retirement be lowered from seventy to sixty-five years.[66]

Perhaps inevitably, the salary deductions raised the issue of the extent to which faculty members could supplement their salaries by working for other organizations. A committee on external relations was formed to consider issues of "conflict of interest." It asked all members of the staff to be "punctilious" in informing the president of "such of their activities as involve relations to other institutions of instruction or research, or to commercial or industrial agencies, where the relations in any way involve the interests of the University."[67] The committee unanimously agreed that the university should not own or control patents; its members disagreed whether individual faculty should do so. Reserving the right of final decision, the Advisory Board decided:

It is the policy of this School that, in general, it is undesirable for members of the faculty or others connected with the School to patent inventions and discoveries in the fields of medicine, hygiene, and public health. Should any member of the faculty or other person connected with the School consider it desirable, . . . it is expected that the question will be referred to the Advisory Board for consideration and recommendation.[68]

The committee on external relations declared that research grants from private firms and companies could be accepted on the condition that "the investigations are justified by virtue of their intrinsic scientific interest and that the results will be published without restriction."[69] Faculty were allowed to undertake work "of a commercial nature" in university laboratories during the summer months or at other times if such work did not interfere with academic programs, involved no expense to the university, and was approved by the president. Persons directly employed by commercial concerns were not to work in university laboratories on regular assignments except as approved by the president.[70]

These rules permitted faculty considerable freedom in their relationships to commercial enterprises. In actuality, several members of the faculty and student body already had such relationships. Two of the men working in the bacteriological laboratory, Veader Leonard and William Feirer, were employees of Sharp and Dohme, a somewhat dubious arrangement for an academic institution. When the issue was publicly discussed, Leonard and Feirer were formally invited to use the laboratory space as "guests" of the school, but both decided to withdraw.[71]

More commonly, corporations gave fellowships to an academic department to support graduate student research, often on a specific subject of commercial interest. Elmer McCollum was especially successful in obtaining this kind of student support. In 1925, E. R. Squibb and Sons gave McCollum's department a fellowship to study the "antirachitic factor" (vitamin D) in cod-liver oil, and they offered fellowships over several years for investigations of the fat-soluble vitamins.[72] Similarly, the Western Maryland–Fairfields Farms Dairy and the Certified Milk Producers Association, Inc., provided fellowships for research on milk and milk products, the Knox Gelatin Company for research on amino acid separation, and the Calumet Baking Company for studies of flour milling.[73] McCollum also obtained fellowship support from noncommercial agencies: the United States Bureau of Fisheries provided funds for research on the food value of fish; the National Dental Association provided a fellowship for research on the effects of faulty diet on tooth development; the American Dental Association and the dental staff of the Johns Hopkins Hospital gave a fellowship for the study of "dietary, pathological, and other dental problems"; and the Ella Sachs Plotz Foundation gave money for a study of dietary magnesium.[74] There was also funding in McCollum's department from the Mead Johnson Company, and from Lederle Laboratories.[75]

Several other department heads, especially Ford, Hyde, Hegner, Cort, and Pearl, were successful in obtaining outside funding from private sources. Sharp and Dohme gave the department of bacteriology generous support for research on disinfectants, and Wilson Laboratories provided funds for research on preventive dentistry.[76] The Eli Lilly Company gave the department of immunology fellowships for the study of respiratory immunity and for studies of viruses; the National Research Council provided support for Bailey's work on the heterophilic antigens.[77] Hegner obtained funding from the Committee on Scientific Research of the American Medical Association for his work on protozoal infections and from the International Health Board of the Rockefeller Foundation for his field studies in malaria control.[78] He was also given small amounts of funding by the National Research Council, the Gorgas Memorial Laboratory in Panama City, and the Bache Fund, and a much larger amount by the firm of Hynson, Westcott and

Dunning for "research on the value of mercurochrome in parasitic diseases."[79]

Cort's money came entirely from nonprofit organizations: the International Health Board of the Rockefeller Foundation, the American Child Health Association, and the American Association for the Advancement of Science.[80] Raymond Pearl had large grants from the Rockefeller Foundation, and also received funding from the Milbank Memorial Fund and the Josiah Macy, Jr., Foundation.[81]

The agencies providing other funds for research included the Carnegie Corporation, the Chemical Foundation for the Study of the Common Cold, the Commonwealth Fund, the Emergency Committee in Aid of Displaced Foreign Physicians, the Iddleson Foundation, the John and Mary Markle Foundation, Knox Gelatin Company, the National Cancer Institute, the National Committee on Maternal Health, the Research Corporation, the United States Public Health Service, and the Wander Company. Grants from corporations and nonprofit organizations provided "extra" funds for short-term projects. The income permitted additional research but was not basic to the financial structure of the school as it is today. From its foundation until 1939, the school's main source of income was the interest on its endowment, and second, tuition fees from the students. In this period, the school had no system of charging large "indirect costs" to research budgets. Since 1929, the school had set "overhead administrative charges" on external funding at 1 percent for grants not administered through university budgets, and 2 percent for grants with disbursements through the university. Thus, the school was supporting externally funded projects through the provision of space, equipment, and faculty time rather than using externally funded projects to help support the basic functions of the institution.[82]

With the budget at its lowest point, 1934 was probably the most difficult year for the School of Hygiene. As dean, Allen Freeman continued to make budget cuts throughout the school. The publication of the *Collected Papers* was discontinued in 1934, never to be resumed; support for the *American Journal of Hygiene* was cut; departments no longer had access to free services from the school mechanic and carpenter; the school draughtsman was laid off.[83] When department budgets were again cut, Pearl's department of biology was the only one exempted; his external funding insulated him from internal pressures. This distinction did not endear the biology department to the other faculty, nor did it guarantee its long-term survival; when Pearl died suddenly in 1940, the biology department was eliminated, with apparently little regret.

In April 1934, William Henry Welch died at the age of eighty-four. The members of the Advisory Board issued the following statement:

The passing of Dr. William Henry Welch on April 30, 1934, closed an epoch in the history of public health. The limitless future of that field of endeavor will forever bear the impress of his ideas and efforts. In the easy stride of his genius he created the School of Hygiene and Public Health of the Johns Hopkins University. Every element in the intellectual, the spiritual, and the material structure of that School is the product of his profound wisdom, far-seeing sagacity, and all-embracing humanity.[84]

The Recovery

For the School of Hygiene, the downward spiral of depression-era budgets began to reverse in 1935. The public funding of the New Deal had two major effects on the School of Hygiene: first, it shifted the school away from its earlier focus on the laboratory sciences and toward a new emphasis on applied research; second, it solved the problem of attracting medical graduates into public health through the provision of new fellowships and training funds.

The financial pressures of the early thirties had exacerbated underlying tensions between the basic and applied sciences. William Howell's department of physiological hygiene exemplified the basic science approach; this department produced basic research on blood physiology, but with little relevance to public health officers' daily work. Allen Freeman's department of public health administration represented the opposite pole. Freeman was a talented administrator who influenced public health practice in Baltimore by chairing committees, conducting surveys, and writing reports. His work was immediate and practical.

During the depression, when Howell retired and Freeman became dean, the focus of the school shifted from basic toward more applied research. The tension between these priorities was expressed in competition for funds, and the department of physiological hygiene was the main casualty. The department's budget was slashed and most of its faculty left. The teaching and research program only survived because of the persistence and indomitable will of one small lady who had been much underestimated, Anna Baetjer.

Two other departments were eliminated in the 1930s but at less cost; in combining the departments of immunology and filterable viruses under Roscoe Hyde, financial imperatives and academic coherence were well served. The department of biology, immune from budget cuts during the depression years, did not survive the recovery.

Individual faculty had also suffered. Only a few faculty members had left specifically because of salary deductions, but many of the associate professors had left at the conclusion of their limited three-year appointments. By the end of the thirties, the numbers of senior faculty had declined sharply and the faculty profile had shifted: now the school had two generations—one of older full professors, most of whom had been there since the early days, and one of young assistant professors.

By 1936, the School of Hygiene had an operating surplus for the first time in years. The amounts previously deducted from academic salaries were refunded; old apparatus and equipment were replaced; and funds were set aside to begin restoring lost services.[85] The economic depression continued into the war years and the departments still operated on restricted budgets, but the worst was over. Allen Freeman, who had presided over the school's financial crisis, stepped down, and Lowell Reed was elected as the new dean in June 1937.

Having survived the hardest years of the depression, the school was, in many ways, stronger than before. The most obvious benefit of the New Deal was the provision of public funding. The Social Security Act of 1935 expanded financing of the Public Health Service and provided federal grants-in-aid to the states to assist them in establishing and maintaining public health services.[86] Federal and state expenditures for public health actually doubled in the decade of the depression. For the first time, the federal government provided funds, administered through the states, for public health training. Federal regulations required states to establish minimum qualifications for the public health personnel employed through the new federal grants. Thus, it was no longer sufficient for state programs to employ any willing physician; some form of professional public health training was expected. The new availability of funds for public health education made it more attractive, and many physicians took the opportunity provided by fellowships to obtain one or more years of postgraduate training.

Funds for public health training came just at the point when many young physicians were finding themselves unable to begin private practices, as the underemployed or unemployed public could not afford medical care. The problem of attracting young medical graduates into public health seemed finally to have been solved through a combination of the carrot and the stick. The carrot, federal training grants, made additional years of schooling financially possible; the stick, the uncertainty of survival in private practice, provided a real incentive toward salaried employment. The new students and the new federal support for public health helped schools of public health survive and even expand during the later depression years.

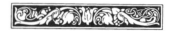

The Community as Public Health Laboratory

hroughout the 1920s, the idea of practical training for students in public health was more often discussed than implemented. The dual title of the School of Hygiene and Public Health suggested a combination of research and practice, but it had thus far been more an institute of hygiene than a school of public health. It offered an excellent education in the basic laboratory sciences but little practical training in administration or the kind of urgent field research expected of public health officers—immediate responses to immediate problems.

Perhaps the most important change in the school in the 1930s was a new orientation toward applied research. The most striking initiatives of the thirties occurred in applied public health programs: mental hygiene, child health, family planning, and venereal disease control. The locus of much of the school's research thus moved from the laboratory bench to the streets, especially the streets and houses immediately surrounding the School of Hygiene in East Baltimore. For the first time, the school developed a close working relationship with the City Health Department and was actively involved in the delivery of public health services.

In 1930, William Howell saw that, as more recent medical graduates were attracted into public health, the need for practical field training would become more urgent:

While our own School is well equipped for carrying on research work . . . we are deficient in facilities for practical field work. The lack of such facilities has not so far constituted an actual defect . . . since it has so happened that most of the students who have come to us for such courses have already had one or more years of practical field experience. But we must recognize the fact that in the future our students will more and more consist of recent graduates in medicine who have had no field work and who should have a certain amount of training of this kind.[1]

The Washington County Health Unit

The school had first tried to set up practical field training programs during the early 1920s. The most successful of these, the Washington County Health Unit, was a rural health district centered on the small city of Hagerstown. The school chose a rural area because the International Health Board wanted to develop a model rural health unit on the county level. The plan was "to make a complete epidemiological and sanitary survey of the conditions in a given county and to perfect an organization adequate to deal with these conditions."[2] Several counties had been eager to be chosen as the location for the new model health unit; after considerable discussion, Washington County was selected because it offered an opportunity to study both urban and rural health conditions and seemed to be within a reasonable traveling distance from the School of Hygiene in Baltimore.

Four agencies agreed to cooperate in the undertaking: the International Health Board, the Public Health Service, the School of Hygiene, and the Maryland State Board of Health. Among them, they supplied a staff of eight: a director from the Public Health Service, a sanitary inspector, a laboratory technician, a clerk, an attendant, and three public health nurses. The county was expected to furnish rooms for offices and a laboratory, and the outside agencies provided "a sufficient number of automobiles to enable the nurses, officers and attending students to make visits to houses in all parts of the county."[3] This level of staffing and funding provided the conditions for creating an ideal county health program; few counties at this time had even a single health officer, and most had no local health service at all.

The Washington County Health Unit had the following objectives:

a. To undertake intensive epidemiological and administrative study of important public health problems across the entire county.
b. To afford a field training base for students of the School of Hygiene and Public Health, and staff members of the State Board of Health, the United States Public Health Service and the International Health Board.
c. To demonstrate economical corrective measures for the problems and to stimulate the county and other political units to establish and maintain effective health services.[4]

The unit was only partially effective if evaluated by these objectives. The staff of the demonstration unit delivered a huge volume of services:

in the second year, for example, it provided 10,000 nursing visits, 4,300 clinic visits, and 5,700 laboratory examinations. The unit conducted school medical examinations and gave each child a "health score." The public health nurses made home visits, including pre- and postnatal visits to new mothers. They held clinics in Hagerstown for children and adults, and special clinics for the diagnosis and treatment of ear, nose, and throat problems, for dental problems, and for venereal diseases. The bacteriological laboratory examined smears and diagnosed patients for diphtheria, typhoid, tuberculosis, and gonorrhea.[5] The provision of these services did not, however, persuade the city or county to give any significant financial support to the unit's activities, which continued to be dependent on external funding.

The unit was also largely ineffective as a training area for the School of Hygiene. Because of the traveling distance between Baltimore and Hagerstown, students from the School of Hygiene were sent out to the demonstration unit for a week at a time to learn the operations of a model rural health unit. The students, however, missed regular classes for that period and many of them went to the countryside with reluctance.

In turn, the staff of the health unit was often unenthusiastic about teaching the students. The annual reports of the demonstration unit made little mention of teaching as it was not considered an important activity.[6] The faculty of the School of Hygiene rarely visited the demonstration unit, especially as the round trip to Hagerstown took at least six hours, given the automobiles and roads of the early 1920s.

The United States Public Health Service continued to conduct research in the unit, including the important Hagerstown Morbidity Studies by Edgar Sydenstricker, but the School of Hygiene gradually withdrew from using the unit for field training.[7] Washington County became an important base for community studies in the 1960s, but in the earlier period of the school's history, the faculty were more interested in developing a field training unit in a geographically convenient and easily accessible area. In 1923, Wade Hampton Frost began the lengthy series of discussions and negotiations that would result, some nine years later, in the establishment of the Eastern Health District of Baltimore.[8]

Strategies and Plans: Establishment of the Eastern Health District

Frost's initial plan for the Baltimore City field training area was ambitious. He wanted to develop a complete public health service "directly under the control of the School and integrated as closely as is possible with those health activities which legally can only be carried on by the City Health Department."⁹ Frost's plan included clinical work, practical training, and research opportunities for School of Hygiene students and public health nurses. Student nurses from the Johns Hopkins Hospital would work in the public health clinics; students from the School of Hygiene would participate in administering the clinics and "see all the procedures embraced in modern health service at first hand."¹⁰ The field unit could also be used for a special practical training program for public health nurses. The population of East Baltimore would be used for biostatistical and epidemiological studies of the "ordinary communicable diseases," including tuberculosis, and for studies of the problems of school health, nutritional status, maternal and infant welfare, and industrial hygiene. Frost suggested that the school would need an endowment for these activities, with an income of about $50,000 per year.¹¹

Frost explained his idea to Frederick F. Russell of the International Health Board "altogether unofficially and as a matter of personal information," and received an enthusiastic response.¹² Russell encouraged Frost to develop his plans for public health nursing, implying that the International Health Board would be interested in an expanded proposal: "I am sure that you will agree that it is best to look well into the future of the public health nursing situation in connection with the School at this time, so that the entire project may be considered as a unit, rather than to delay it to a later time."¹³

In response, Frost sketched out a plan for training graduate nurses in public health through a one-year course of lectures, laboratory work, and field training, warning, however, that the Advisory Board had not approved such a plan. The Advisory Board had considered public health nursing several times but had never yet accepted, even "in principle," the idea that the school should be directly involved in training public health nurses.¹⁴ The plans for a field training unit within the city met several major problems: the first was the apparent lack of enthusiasm of the Advisory Board toward any commitment to train public health nurses. The second problem was the opposition, overt or covert, from the commissioner of health of the City of Baltimore. The city health commissioner expressed formal interest, but actually acted to prevent the plan from being implemented. The commissioner, C. Hampson Jones, had personal and political reasons for opposing the plan. He was antagonistic toward the Rockefeller Foundation because his family's gas stations had been put out of business by the Rockefeller-controlled Standard Oil Company during the monopolization of the oil industry; he had therefore no intention of letting a Rockefeller-funded project "take over" any part of the city. He also considered the plan a possible threat to his authority and responsibility for public health services in the city.

Throughout the history of the Eastern Health District, the School of Hygiene faculty's desire to control the administration and organization of services, their need for freedom in developing research and teaching programs, and their critical attitude toward the city's public health programs were impediments to a happy and cooperative relationship. The commissioner of health had little interest in giving up administrative control over a part of the city, and even less interest in being shown "improved" methods of administration and management.

Discussions of the project thus continued throughout the 1920s with little result. While waiting for some more formal arrangement, Allen Freeman established a health center for infant and child welfare work in East Baltimore. Two McElderry Street houses belonging to the school were remodeled to provide facilities for voluntary organizations doing child welfare work, prenatal services run by the Johns Hopkins Hospital, tuberculosis nursing services provided by the City Health Department, and a dental clinic offered by the city for infants and preschool children. The School of Hygiene provided the space in return for "the privilege of keeping the records and of using the station for teaching and investigative studies."[15] From the point of view of the School of Hygiene, however, this arrangement was unsatisfactory because the faculty did not control the services offered; each organization conducted its own projects and simply allowed students to observe.

In 1930, a change in Baltimore City politics opened up new opportunities for cooperation with the City Health Department. A newly elected mayor, Howard Jackson, announced his intention to seek a new commissioner of health for the city. When he turned to Welch for suggestions of candidates for the job, Welch recommended Huntington Williams, one of the graduates of the first class at the School of Hygiene.

The selection of Huntington Williams as the new commissioner of health was typical of Welch's connections and influence. Williams's father, George H. Williams, the first professor of geology at the Johns Hopkins University, had been part of Welch's large, extended family network.[16] Although George Williams died at an early age of typhoid fever, his widow and Welch became close friends. They lived within a city block of each other and Welch often had lunch at the Williams's house on Cathedral Street. As a boy, Huntington Williams grew up listening to Welch talking about public health and medicine; on Welch's advice, he attended the Johns Hopkins Medical School and then transferred to the School of Hygiene in 1918. After graduation, he worked under Hermann Biggs (a former Welch student and friend), and perhaps the most powerful progressive public health reformer of the period. Williams became district state health officer in the New York State Health Department and worked there for ten years before being called back to Baltimore in 1931. Baltimore's commissioner of health, C. Hampson Jones, was still alive but elderly and in poor health, so the mayor created a new temporary position for Williams: assistant commissioner of health and director of health.[17]

In suggesting Williams for a health department post, Welch set the stage for future cooperation between the City Health Department and the School of Hygiene; Williams was the ideal man to create close relationships between the school and city health officials. Huntington Williams remembered that when he arrived in Baltimore "Dr. Frost and Dr. Freeman were camping on my doorstep."[18] A "committee" was immediately established to plan the Eastern Health District, but as Williams described it: "Well, it wasn't really a committee, it was a group of old friends just sitting around a table. . . . It was just as natural as running two rivers together."[19]

Within two months of Williams's arrival in Baltimore, Wade Hampton Frost was ready to travel to New York to discuss their plans with F. F. Russell, director of the International Health Division of the Rockefeller Foundation.[20] By early January 1932, Frost had Russell's preliminary agreement on a new proposal. The agencies initially participating in the planning, besides the City Health Department and the School of Hygiene, were the Babies' Milk Fund Association, the Instructive Visiting Nurse Association, the Johns Hopkins Hospital and Training School for Nurses, the Sinai Hospital, and the University of Maryland Hospital and Training School for Nurses.[21] The last two agencies later pulled out of the plan, making it essentially an agreement between the City Health Department and Johns Hopkins.

C. Hampson Jones died in April 1932; Huntington Williams was named the commissioner of health; and the plan for the Eastern Health District was formally submitted within a few weeks. The 1932 plan was, in fact, similar to the original proposal of 1923. It suggested the establishment of a special health district in which "all the lines of public health endeavor represented in the city will be developed to a maximum efficiency by selection of personnel, increased supervision, and better coordination of effort."[22] The area selected, immediately around the School of Hygiene, had a stable working-class population of about 60,000, of whom 80 percent were white, and 20 percent black. All existing services were consolidated into a single organizational unit under the direction of a full-time health officer who would represent the

City Health Department and also be appointed to the faculty of the School of Hygiene. Additional supervising nurses, a laboratory technician, and clerical personnel were to be hired. A field nursing staff of fourteen nurses, contributed by the participating agencies, would carry on a complete program of public health nursing and supervise student nurse training. Food and sanitary inspectors supplied by the City Health Department would help conduct a broad public health program; the School of Hygiene would provide the laboratory facilities. The Rockefeller Foundation was asked for $25,000 per year for five years to support the project. For the first time, the City Health Department warmly supported the proposal. Huntington Williams wrote to F. F. Russell:

From the point of view of the Baltimore City Health Department, and this is very strongly my own personal feeling, there could hardly be any development in Public Health Work in this city that would be of greater benefit than the establishment, and successful operation, of a Public Health District and Training Area such as is proposed. The two chief benefits which the City may hope to derive from the District are—The provision of opportunities for developing improved methods in City Health Administration; and the provision of facilities for training in public health of our Public Health Nurses.[23]

Williams was personally interested in the Eastern Health District because not only could he train his existing staff but the Rockefeller grant would also provide funding for highly trained new staff. This was the depression era, and Williams had already been asked to drop ninety-three people from the health department budget; the Eastern Health District would provide a much needed staffing supplement.[24]

Additional support for the Eastern Health District proposal came from the United States Public Health Service. When Williams was first invited to Baltimore, C. Hampson Jones, presumably with some urging from Mayor Jackson and William Welch, had requested a study of the health department's activities by the United States Public Health Service. In June 1932, this study was released. Written by Joseph W. Mountin, the study reflected the ideas of Welch, Frost, and Williams and strongly recommended an increase in the health department budget, increased coordination of the different health agencies, and administrative decentralization into health districts. The report might have been written by Welch or Frost, it so closely followed their ideas, even down to the plans for the Eastern Health District. The department was urged to develop closer links with local educational institutions: "Opportunity should be afforded students in public health, medicine, dentistry, nursing and social work either through observation or active participation. Ease and harmony in administration is usually promoted when certain clinics, hospitals, and areas of the city are selected for educational and study areas."[25] The final recommendations were quite specific, that "a special area of the city be set apart for the observation and instruction of new personnel and for the development and trial of public health procedures."[26] Without mentioning it by name, the Public Health Service report thus essentially recommended the Eastern Health District plan already formulated, and provided strong external authority for the idea. Four days later, the International Health Division awarded a grant to fund the first fifteen months of the Eastern Health District, beginning in September 1932.[27] In his letter of acceptance, Frost declared, "For the School of Hygiene, I believe that an active working connection with the district which is planned will mark a definite turning point, directing the interests of the School more and more toward the investigation of problems more directly related to actual public health."[28]

The summer of 1932 was devoted to meetings of participating agencies culminating in the selection of the district health officer. The position was accepted by Harry Stoll Mustard, formerly the assistant state commissioner of health for Tennessee, and later to be commissioner of health for New York City. Both Frost and Williams described Mustard as a master tactician, whose political skills were essential to the new job. Williams remembered Mustard's first meeting with the local physicians in September 1932:

The doctors in East Baltimore had a fit—almost unanimously they had a fit. Why? Because the public health nurses in the Health Department in years past felt that their day was successful if they could get Johnny Jones to have his tonsils out, and they were inclined to forget that each of these families . . . had a family doctor who had a personal relationship with that family and with that child. . . . We had a meeting in East Baltimore . . . so they would meet Dr. Mustard and see whether he was poison or not. Harry Mustard was an expert and had been doing this work for years down south, and he said to them, "Gentlemen, I know you're all apprehensive about me, I've made a lot of mistakes in the past, and I will probably go on making mistakes as long as I live, but one thing I can promise you, is that I won't do a thing to interfere with your private practice in these families. In other words, there will be no more yanking of Johnny's tonsils out regardless of the family doctor." So, the District got off to a very good start.[29]

Huntington Williams estimated that at that time there were perhaps one hundred physicians practicing in the Eastern Health District. In 1932, during the depression years, the physicians were especially concerned about possible threats to private practice and were thus alert to any potential interference from the health department. In an interview with the local press, Mustard emphasized that neither he nor his associates would give any medical treatment: they would encourage people to consult their own physicians and dentists about any health problems.[30]

Having reassured the physicians, Mustard and Williams also sought to reassure the local population that there would be "no invasion of homes," and that "residents of the two wards will not be made the subjects of experimentation in the public health field"; the people would, however, be offered an expanded range of services and information.[31]

The Eastern Health District organization started slowly, in part because of the need to reassure physicians and residents that their lives were not going to be dramatically disrupted. Martin Frobisher of the School of Hygiene took charge of the diagnostic laboratory, with Katherine Peirce and Mary Johnson as supervising nurses. The City Health Department physicians and nurses were gradually absorbed into the new organization. Training courses for public health nurses were started, and graduate students from the School of Hygiene began to gather data on the district for their thesis research. The work, begun in a building on Orleans Street, was soon moved to Monument Street to be closer to the School of Hygiene. The main achievement of the first year was completion of a health survey giving information on the morbidity, mortality, and social conditions of each family in the district. For this survey, twenty nurses worked for seven weeks gathering information door-to-door; the family files then organized provided a basis for many future statistical studies.[32] Sufficiently pleased with the first year's work, the International Health Board agreed to provide the remainder of the first five years' funding.

The initial administrative problems of the district were, said Frost, "rather discouraging" and it was "a tribute to Dr. Mustard's tact and patience" that they were successfully managed.[33] Wilson Smillie of Harvard, one of the district's critics, described its structural administrative problems:

We have the anomalous situation of the School of Public Health administering the health functions of a portion of the city without any direct responsibility to city government. It is true that the director of health work of the district, Dr. Mustard, is on the staff of the City Health Department and also on the staff of the School of Public Health, and it is probable that so long as the present personnel remain in office little administrative friction will occur. Nevertheless, the theoretical difficulty of divided responsibility exists.[34]

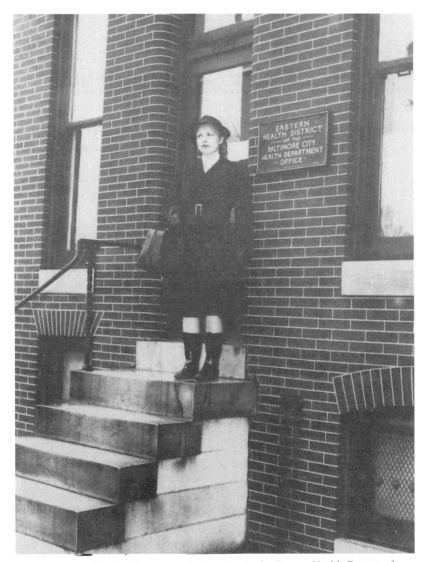

Figure 26. A public health nurse ready for visits in the Eastern Health District of Baltimore. The Baltimore City Health Department and the School of Hygiene and Public Health shared responsibility for research, training, and services provided in the Eastern Health District; public health nurses conducted house-to-house health interviews and provided a wide range of public health services. (Baltimore City Health Department photograph, courtesy of the Rockefeller Archive Center, Tarrytown, New York.)

Clearly, such an arrangement would work well only if the administrators were on amicable terms and shared similar goals. Mustard, Williams, Frost, and the faculty of the School of Hygiene worked well together in the early years, and the potential problems were thus minimized; later, these underlying structural problems became more evident and a source of much distress both to the health commissioner and to the School of Hygiene.

Studies in the Eastern Health District

The Eastern Health District was an area of approximately one square mile, bounded on the west by Caroline Street, on the north by Chase and Eager streets, on the east by East Avenue and Loney's Lane, and on the south by Baltimore Street. The area was made up of the row houses for which Baltimore is famous, with their white marble steps and rows of painted window screens. It was a settled, working-class neighborhood with a high proportion of homeowners. Many of the people were of German or Scandinavian origin; other residents included the Irish and the Italians, and the black population who were mostly migrants from the Maryland countryside, North Carolina, and Virginia. Sixty percent of the white population had been in America for three generations or more, the rest being more recent immigrants. Most of the whites were skilled workers and tradesmen: carpenters, mechanics, grocers, and electricians. Most of the black residents were semiskilled workers and laborers or members of what was still termed the "servant class." Wolfe Street marked the boundary between "white" and "colored" in an area clearly segregated by race. The black population lived to the west of this line, and the whites to the east. The boundary line was slowly moving east as whites moved out of the center city, but the racial mix of this settled neighborhood remained relatively stable until World War II.

The 15,000 families, or 60,000 people, living in this area were to be the "population laboratory" of the School of Hygiene. As Welch had conceived it, the population laboratory would be to public health training what the hospital was to medical training: the place where students could practice their professional activities under supervision, where scientific research could produce new knowledge, and where the population could also receive the best care and services available. The School of Hygiene emphasized the functions of research and training and the City Health Department focused on staff training and the delivery of services.

The people of the Eastern Health District were probably more extensively studied than any such population had ever been. The local newspaper explained: "Inquisitive visitors who ask very personal questions are no novelty to the people who live in Wards 5, 6, 7, 10 and the three borderline census tracts of Ward 8: They are, by all odds, the most interrogated, surveyed, examined, investigated and card-indexed citizens of Baltimore—and probably of the forty-eight states, Alaska, Hawaii, Puerto Rico and the Philippines."[35]

The baseline of the research was the district census survey carried out by the department of biostatistics in 1933, 1936, and 1939. Public health nurses and School of Hygiene students went house-to-house, noting all inhabitants, their occupations, illnesses, and medical care. They carefully recorded the number of rooms in each house, access to bathrooms, and the condition of the houses, as well as the presence of boarders and lodgers. Each census identified the families and individuals recorded in the previous surveys, to check population changes and identify a stable group for comparative studies.[36] As the newspaper graphically explained:

Biologists, pathologists and the like, when they work in laboratories, can lock their guinea pigs in cages and keep them under control until their studies are completed. But the director of the Eastern Health District can't build a fence around his bailiwick and keep his human specimens confined until precise conclusions are reached. In this land of the relatively free, our untrammeled citizens can pack bag and baggage and move at will, and they do. There is a steady flow of population into and out of the area, which means a constant changing of the statistical basis. The tuberculars, the syphilitics and the various others who were identified last year may be over the hills and far away this year.[37]

Residents who stayed in the area had "small chance of harboring diseases without knowing it. The most expert advice is theirs with or without the asking."[38] One of the most studied diseases was tuberculosis, and several students prepared doctoral theses on this subject under Frost's direction. These concerned such subjects as the morbidity and mortality of children exposed to household contacts with tuberculosis, evaluation of administrative changes in the city tuberculosis program, and studies of the medical care and preventive services received by tuberculosis patients.[39] The students charted the continuing decline in tuberculosis mortality and morbidity in the Eastern Health District, despite a continuing high rate of infection. Frost was able to argue in 1937: "We have already reached the stage at which the biological balance is against the survival of the tubercle bacillus. . . . This means that under present conditions of human resistance and environment the tubercle bacillus is losing ground, and that eventual eradication of tuberculosis requires only that the present balance against it be maintained."[40]

Students and faculty in the departments of immunology and epidemiology continued to study diphtheria, then one of the most prevalent and frightening of diseases, affecting especially young children. Under Martin Frobisher's direction, students gathered data on carrier incidence and immunity status at various age levels, and tested the relative success of different immunization procedures.[41] Three Schick test surveys of children in the Eastern Health District were carried out in 1922–24, 1933–34, and 1938–40, to measure the degree of both artificial and naturally acquired immunity to diphtheria. At the beginning of this period, almost no children had received artificial immunization; at the end of the period, about 90 percent of the children had been given artificial immunization, while the rate of natural immunity had remained unchanged. The studies documented public health progress in controlling the disease and showed what could be accomplished. At the beginning of the period, diphtheria had been a major cause of childhood deaths; in 1939, there were sixty-seven cases of diphtheria and only three deaths in the whole area.[42] Soon, diphtheria would vanish as a serious childhood threat.

Many of the research studies in the Eastern Health District concentrated on child health problems. These included major studies of measles, hearing impairment, and dental health.[43] The health services offered in the district also focused on child health. The district provided prenatal clinics and well-baby clinics, free smallpox vaccinations, diphtheria antitoxin, medical, dental, and eye examinations, instruction to mothers on child care, referrals to doctors and hospitals, and a constant stream of advice and information. Clinics were open every day with about fifty thousand examinations held each year, thus providing almost one examination for each inhabitant of the area. Beginning in 1938, all newborn children were followed with the aim of measuring the effects of prenatal and maternity care on morbidity and mortality in the first few years of a child's life.[44] As the Baltimore Sun reported, "Every child in the district, and a good share of adults, comes sooner or later into the grasp of a health officer or nurse. No child can escape. Some of them are under the benevolent dictation before they are born."[45]

In 1938, the United States Public Health Service in cooperation with the Milbank Memorial Fund and the School of Hygiene started an intensive study of illness and chronic disease among white families in the Eastern Health District. The Public Health Service pointed out that, while the major achievements of the previous fifty years had been the lowering of infant mortality and the control of infectious diseases,

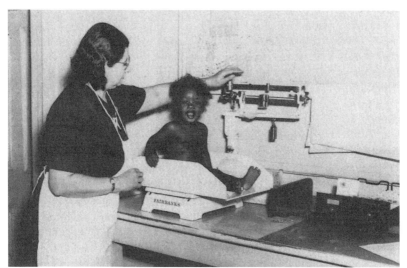

Figure 27. A nurse weighing a healthy baby in the Eastern Health District's well-baby clinic. All children were followed through the first few years of life and provided with comprehensive health examinations. (Courtesy of the Rockefeller Archive Center, Tarrytown, New York.)

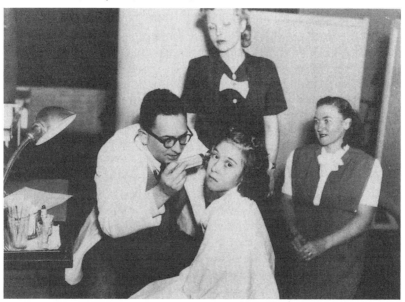

Figure 28. A child health examination, Eastern Health District clinic. Special research studies focused on child health problems such as hearing impairment, vision problems, and dental health as well as many common infectious diseases. (Courtesy of the Rockefeller Archive Center, Tarrytown, New York.)

future public health advances would have to be made in the preventive aspects of the chronic diseases such as cancer and heart disease. In 1938, there was still little information about the incidence of chronic disease in the population, or about the actual incidence of general illness and disability, including common but minor problems such as respiratory infections and digestive disorders. The survey of illness and chronic disease was intended to establish a data base for future public health studies and programs in these areas.[46] The illness and chronic disease researchers conducted monthly house-to-house surveys of all white families in selected city blocks of the Eastern Health District (about 1,500 families), asking them about all their experiences of illness in the preceding month. They carefully recorded all reports of minor and major illnesses and any medical care received, and these were supplemented by the records of sick benefit associations to determine sickness and death rates according to occupation.

The study found a rate of illness of slightly more than one illness per person reported over a twelve-month period, with about half of these being "disabling" (defined as causing loss of one or more days at work, school, or usual activities). The rate of hospitalization was about 5 percent of the total illness rate. The main causes of illness were minor respiratory diseases (almost half of the total), accidental injuries, "degenerative diseases" (including rheumatism, arthritis, and diseases of the heart and arteries), and minor digestive disorders. "Migrant families"—families that moved during the course of the study—were found to suffer a much higher rate of illness from all causes.

These studies served to highlight the importance of chronic diseases as the leading causes of death.[47] These diseases also generated by far the most use of hospital and medical care, and were the source of most time lost from work and other usual daily activities. The studies found that chronic diseases were present in 25 percent of the families and that "ambulatory cases" of chronic disease—18 percent of the population— were "a sickly group" that carried the main burden of illness, including infectious disorders and disability.[48] Specific studies of "the chronic disease family" noted that families with a case of chronic disease tended to show a higher illness rate for all members than did the general population, and at least one author suggested, following Sydenstricker, that this difference among families might be traced to diet.[49]

The most frequent chronic diseases reported in the population studied (in order of frequency) were hypertension, arthritis, heart disease, mental disease, neurasthenia, rheumatic fever, and diabetes. If cases of "mental disease," "mental deficiency," and "neurasthenia" were grouped together, they formed the largest single category of illness;

appropriately, therefore, much of the research developed in the Eastern Health District in the 1930s dealt with mental illness.

Mental Hygiene Studies

Perhaps the largest volume of work done in the Eastern Health District involved community-based mental hygiene studies. Until the establishment of the district, the School of Hygiene had offered little in the area of mental hygiene, although Welch himself had been involved in the national mental hygiene movement. William Welch and Adolf Meyer, the famous Hopkins psychiatrist, had been among the founding members of the National Committee for Mental Hygiene, a movement galvanized by the publication of A Mind That Found Itself in 1908.[50] This book, written by Clifford Beers, a former patient in a mental institution, was an eloquent plea for improvement in the conditions of people incarcerated in mental asylums, and for better understanding of mental illness. Welch had wanted to include mental hygiene in the early curriculum of the school and had asked Thomas W. Salmon, medical director of the National Committee, to become professor of mental hygiene in 1918.[51] But when Salmon was not interested in the position, the idea of creating a special department was indefinitely postponed. Esther Richards, the physician-in-chief of the Phipps Clinic of the Hopkins Medical School, offered two courses at the School of Hygiene, one on adult and one on child psychiatry. The Saturday sessions on child mental hygiene, open to Baltimore schoolteachers, were enthusiastically received. At the same time, Dr. Adolf Meyer, the director of the Phipps Clinic, was attempting to develop a scientific basis for the mental hygiene movement through a "socially oriented psychiatry" and a "biologically sound idealism."[52] In Meyer's view, mental hygiene was the social agent of psychiatry and a civic responsibility: psychiatrists should work with teachers, charity organizations, ministers, and physicians to promote mental health within communities, thus balancing their interest in the individual with a concern for family and social integration.

In 1932, the Rockefeller Foundation decided to begin a new funding program in mental hygiene, psychiatry, and the problems of human personality on the grounds that "while geneticists have minutely observed the fruit fly through hundreds of generations, and nutritionists and cancer researchers have life histories of the white rat and the mouse, the human individual—the presumed beneficiary of all this study—remains in large measure unknown."[53] The director of the International Health Division asked for suitable projects and invited Wade Hampton

Frost to stimulate suggestions from schools of public health. In 1934, Adolf Meyer's clinic was given a grant to develop pediatric psychiatry, and Frost was asked for "a modest project . . . [to] determine the steps which can be taken for dealing with the problem in a community."[54] Frost, Mustard, Meyer, and Williams discussed the possibility of a joint project and suggested "a thorough study of the records of the Phipps Clinic as pertaining to the population of the Eastern Health District . . . [to give] a fair idea of the gross magnitude of the mental health problem in a community."[55] Frost felt that such a project would require a well-trained psychiatrist working with a competent statistician and a social worker and that the records should first be studied to determine their epidemiological and statistical value.[56] Frost and Meyer, however, were far apart in their understanding of the project, and Meyer had little use for Frost's emphasis on epidemiological and statistical method. Frost wrote to John Ferrell at The Rockefeller Foundation:

As a result of repeated conversation with Dr. Meyer, I realize more keenly than at first how far apart are the viewpoints of the psychiatric institute and the School of Hygiene. The two groups think in such essentially different terms that at present neither really understands the other, and before any kind of effective collaboration can be established, it is necessary to build up some more solid basis of mutual understanding.[57]

In response, John Ferrell suggested the grant be made to the School of Hygiene rather than to the Phipps Institute, to strengthen Frost's hand "in an effort to have the community point of view emphasized in studies and plans."[58] Meyer, however, proposed a study unit "in which the School of Hygiene would have no part whatsoever except through a quite indefinite consulting relation."[59]

The problem was finally sorted out some months later when Allen Freeman, as the new dean of the School of Hygiene, engineered a compromise: the project would be a joint undertaking of the Phipps Clinic and the School of Hygiene.[60] In September 1934, the International Health Division provided $6,000 for a first exploratory study of mental hygiene problems in the Eastern Health District.

The difficulties of integrating psychiatry and epidemiology were not over; four years later, Freeman reported: "The problem is in its essence diffuse and difficult of exact definition in any of its stages. . . . There are no precedents. . . . The clinical psychiatrist is in general both ignorant and scornful of statistical procedures. The epidemiologist is in general both ignorant and scornful of psychiatry."[61] The mental hygiene study struggled through this unpromising beginning, to produce a considerable volume of work that helped open up the new field of community mental health.

The first step was to find out how much mental disease and disorder actually prevailed in the population of the Eastern Health District. Records were collected for all people who had been seen at a mental hygiene clinic, admitted to a mental hospital, or recorded by any agency as "exhibiting behavior indicating the probability of some mental defect or disorder."[62] This initial census produced the names of 2,500 individuals, or about 4½ percent of the population; another 1,300 names were collected from police files of "adult delinquents" who had been arrested for some type of offense.[63]

At that time, there was little concern about the individual's right to privacy or the confidentiality of information; it was not considered problematic for the police, the courts, welfare agencies, and other public and private agencies to share information about their clients. The names of individuals being treated for psychiatric problems were simply added to those who had been in trouble with the police or those who had appeared on the files of social service agencies as "showing difficulty in adjusting to their . . . environments."[64]

All individual files were then examined and classified by the psychiatric staff into "reaction types": psychotics, psychoneurotics, psychopathic personalities, postpsychotics, mental deficients, epileptics, and the "maladjusted."[65] The staff then attempted to calculate the prevalence rate of the various disorders so defined: a notable finding was that 25 percent of psychotics were receiving no treatment, but apparently were being successfully managed in their own homes.[66] This was one of the first efforts to measure the prevalence of mental disorders in a community (as distinct from studies limited to those under treatment) and it suggested that such community-based studies could offer a broader perspective on the prevalence and management of mental illness. The problem with such studies was the inadequacy of the classification of mental illness and the inability of psychiatrists or statisticians clearly to distinguish symptoms, diseases, and social judgments.[67] Adolph Meyer had been a leading opponent of the effort to provide a classification system for statistical purposes, believing as he did that the life history of the individual was the most significant element in the etiology of psychiatric illness. From this point of view, the very attempt to provide a psychiatric nosology was misguided.[68] The interests of the statistician and the practicing psychiatrist seemed fundamentally opposed.

Undaunted by such caveats, the mental hygiene researchers attempted to measure the prevalence of "personality disorders," defined as major failures of personal and social adjustment. They found an "unmistakable" association between personality problems and low economic status, with the lowest income groups having about six times the number of problems as the highest income groups. "Housekeeping status," whether the home was clean and well kept or dirty and neglected, was also measured and found to be strongly associated with personality problems.[69] Males had a higher rate of personality difficulties than females, blacks than whites, and Jews than non-Jewish whites. In general, the highest rates of personality disorders were found among the largest families, among adolescents, and among those about forty years of age. Whites living in areas with significant numbers of blacks also had higher rates than those in all-white areas, and the researchers suggested that the former were the least stable and settled neighborhoods.[70]

The mental hygiene researchers usually did not attempt to interpret the meaning of their statistics; obviously, the choice of variables for measurement—race, religion, level of cleanliness—disclosed the underlying hypotheses of the study, but there was little explicit discussion of their meaning. At a meeting in 1937 to celebrate the twenty-fifth anniversary of the Phipps Clinic, Ruth Fairbank, the mental hygiene study psychiatrist, presented a series of charts providing a summary of the "epidemiological" facts.[71] (The habit of putting "epidemiological" in quotation marks was Fairbank's own.) The first five charts mapped the residences of psychotic and postpsychotic cases, those with educational and social problems (including mental deficiency), juvenile delinquents, adult delinquents (from the police records), and maladjusted individuals. The last and largest group, the "maladjusted," included alcoholics, those with family difficulties, and "the individuals who find it practically impossible to get along without guidance and who often need financial aid as well."[72] A final chart showed the "social factors considered to be favorable and unfavorable to the youth." This chart, prepared by the Baltimore Criminal Justice Commission, mapped the schools, churches, houses of prostitution, saloons, gang hangouts, and "saloons known to be hangouts." From a glance at the maps, the audience could see that the maladjusted and the juvenile and adult delinquents tended to be clustered in the western and southern parts of the district, which also had more saloons, gang hangouts, and houses of prostitution.

The psychotics, adult delinquents, and the maladjusted were marked on the first three maps by red and black pins. On the fourth map, the pins represented juvenile delinquents. Newspaper reporters expounded on the moral of the maps for the public: "Each pin represents a child. Unless something is done for them, they will become red or black pins on the other maps—criminals, psychotics, public charges. They are not pretty—these maps, if you know what they mean." What was to be done about the juvenile pins?

In the Eastern district of the Health Department, an experiment is being tried. If successful, it may build a wall between young lives and the night outside; between pins that mean children and pins that mean wasted lives . . . . Science believes that if children are given proper training during the first six months of their lives they may be saved from many environmental maladjustments. So, in the Eastern District, mothers are being taught, and being directly helped, to mould tiny, inarticulate lives in the hope of reducing the number of red and black pins of 1950.[73]

The messages about social problems from the pin charts had thus abruptly been reduced to a question of early childhood training. If the mothers could but raise their children in the best possible manner, the social environment—the saloons, gang hangouts, and houses of prostitution—would become irrelevant; the associations between poverty and "maladjustment" found in the statistics could be transcended by the maternal-child relationship. A social problem had been transmuted into an emotional problem, located within the family, and made the subject of advice to mothers.

This move, from a social to an emotional problem, was a staple of the child guidance and mental hygiene literature.[74] The Baltimore Mental Hygiene Study thus shared the theoretical ideas and assumptions current in the mental hygiene movement. Having concluded that social maladjustment stemmed from emotional maladjustment (and therefore poor childhood training), the next step was to offer a practical solution, namely, an educational program for parents. According to Ruth Fairbank, the study had found many behavior problems in children and adolescents stemming from oversolicitous parents and a lack of discipline: "Common sense must grant that the period of growth is the ideal time to develop and foster such habits as emotional control, self-reliance, self-dependence, and the ability to get on with one's fellows." The solution was to show mothers how to train their children in "very simple rules of habit training, discipline, and the principles of self-control and self-reliance."[75] The texts used for training in self-discipline and self-control were Thom's *Everyday Problems of the Everyday Child* (1927), Blatz, Millichamp, and Fletcher, *Nursery Education* (1935), and Richards, *Behavior Aspects of Child Conduct* (1934).[76]

In 1935, therefore, the Mental Hygiene Study group opened a Mothers' Advisory Service. Mothers visiting the existing clinics were invited to discuss any problems in child behavior with the psychiatric staff: "An effort is made to get facts which convey an estimate of the intelligence and emotional stability of the parents. Facts are sought which indicate the degree of family harmony or lack of it, which show the attitude of the parents toward the child and with which to evaluate the responsiveness of the mother in terms of her interest and capacity to carry out a plan for her child."[77]

While the mother was being interviewed, the child stayed in a playroom and was observed by a social worker. The child's behavior was noted and compared to scales of "normal" development.[78] The problems described by the mother or observed in the child's behavior were plotted on charts, with black boxes for "good" behavior and red boxes for "problems."[79] Each time the child returned to the clinic, his or her progress could be measured by the number of objectionable red boxes and positive black ones.

Marcia Cooper, a student in the School of Hygiene, wrote her doctoral dissertation on the Mothers' Advisory Service, and offered a series of case studies. John, for example, was the third child of a young Irish-Italian couple; the father was a grocery clerk. The parents had a limited income but a "keen determination to do well by their children and a comfortable warmth in family relationships."[80] At one year and eight months, John had a series of problems, each measured by the little

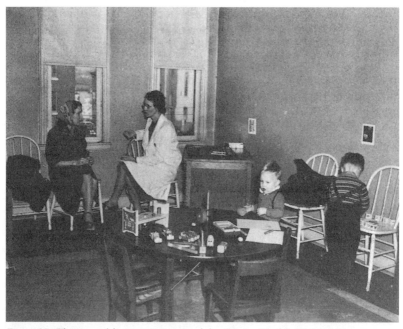

Figure 29. The mental hygiene program of the Eastern Health District. The Mothers' Advisory Service was intended to prevent mental health problems in adults by attention to early childhood development. Here the psychiatrist interviews a mother while her children are playing. (Courtesy of the Rockefeller Archive Center, Tarrytown, New York.)

red boxes: he was not weaned (one red box), had temper tantrums (two red boxes), was left-handed, and his mother was trying to correct it (one red box), and he had retarded speech development (one red box). Four months later most of the problems had gone: he was weaned, had fewer tantrums, had a fair vocabulary, and understood both English and Italian. He was still left-handed, but his mother had decided not to worry about it. Another four months later, he had no tantrums and was talking well, but was jealous of a new baby and refusing to give up his crib. In another four months this problem seemed to be over, but John now refused to keep his clothes on—a new red box. He was three years and two months by the time this final problem had been solved: potentially, a model citizen, and "a demonstration of what can be accomplished with what might be considered unpromising material."[81]

In general, the mothers seemed grateful for this advice and many, like John's mother, returned regularly to the Advisory Service to report their progress. As the psychiatrist explained, they were "not apt to be reached by modern theories in regard to child training made available through the literature."[82] The public health nurses acted as popular translators of the latest theories and as experienced advisers to worried mothers. When a mother seemed to have psychiatric problems herself, she could have an appointment in a public clinic.

By available accounts, the service was a popular one, and it was gradually expanded, offering a psychiatric consultation service to all physicians and medical clinics in the district. As a clinical service, however, the Mothers' Advisory Service did little research and could not demonstrate that it actually helped the children, much less that it had any effect on the problem of juvenile delinquency. From the School of Hygiene's perspective, the service was unsatisfactory in generating research results about the promotion of mental hygiene and the prevention of mental disorders. When Paul Lemkau came to the school in 1939, initially to analyze and publish some of the Mental Hygiene Study data, the service was holding group sessions for mothers to discuss their problems with child rearing. Lemkau noted: "This was conceived to be a preventive activity. Nobody has every shown that it was, but it was conceived to be. Certainly, it was obvious that it made people feel better. . . . I find myself increasingly skeptical about the long-term effect of these things."[83]

The idea that a Mothers' Advisory Service could prevent the social and psychiatric problems of adulthood was naive, if well intentioned; part of the evangelical thrust of the mental hygiene movement, it was at least reassuring to mothers worried about their children's behavior. As Allen Freeman concluded, "The prevention of mental disease rests on no such simple and well understood principles as those which underlie the prevention of communicable disease or the promotion of maternal and infant hygiene. It has as yet developed no simple and effective administrative technic."[84]

The mental hygiene study continued for a number of years, through World War II. Christopher Tietze, an Austrian refugee who joined the project as statistician, became acting director; later, Paul Lemkau was appointed psychiatrist and director of the project, and Marcia Cooper was appointed psychologist. They reanalyzed much of the data from the 1933 and 1936 surveys and published a series of papers on the prevalence of different kinds of problems in the community.[85] Lemkau started teaching in the School of Hygiene, and organized a course using family case study conferences in the Eastern Health District. He later explained his conception of community-based mental hygiene in a text for public health students, *Mental Hygiene in Public Health* (1949).[86] At the time, mental hygiene programs were developing more rapidly than there were trained psychiatric staff to run them, giving rise to professional disputes between the representatives of the mental hygiene movement and psychiatrists who felt that they alone could offer responsible therapy. Paul Lemkau did much to argue for the important role of public health nurses in mental hygiene programs and helped overcome some of the resistance shown by psychiatrists to the idea that nurses could be competent to deal with psychiatric problems in the community.[87] By World War II, the Hopkins Mental Hygiene Study had contributed to bringing public health and psychiatry into somewhat closer alignment, and thus helped provide a basis for the enormous expansion of mental hygiene in the postwar period.

The Bureau for Contraceptive Advice

A very different initiative, but with a similar goal of improving the physical and mental health of Baltimore families, occupied the attention of several other Hopkins faculty members. Though this effort, the Bureau for Contraceptive Advice, was considered too controversial for official Hopkins sponsorship, faculty members initiated and sustained it. It represented a voluntary, cooperative effort by several faculty members of the School of Hygiene and the School of Medicine working in association with some of Baltimore's more progressive physicians and concerned citizens. Four leaders on the original Committee on Contraceptive Information were J. Whitridge Williams, professor of obstetrics in the School of Medicine, William H. Howell, then director of the School of Hygiene, Raymond Pearl, then the School of Hygiene's professor of biometry, and Adolph Meyer, the Hopkins psychiatrist who was working with other faculty members on community health efforts.

As head of obstetrics in the Johns Hopkins Hospital, Williams had worried about the effects of frequent childbearing on women already weakened by serious medical conditions such as cardiac disease, tuberculosis, severe anemia, and gynecological disorders. Howell and Pearl were both concerned about health at a population level and had tangled with and criticized the eugenics movement; interested in Margaret Sanger's efforts to open birth control clinics for women, they also wanted to avoid the public and political accusation of social radicalism associated with Sanger's tactics. All three men thought it should be possible to offer birth control services "on conservative and scientific lines" and to open a clinic both socially and medically respectable.[88]

On March 22, 1926, sixteen of Baltimore's more prominent civic and medical leaders (eight women, eight men) met in the School of Hygiene to organize the Committee on Contraceptive Information. Concerned about the possible legal implications of their actions—Sanger and her supporters had repeatedly been jailed—they elected Judge Jacob Moses as chairman and asked him to explore quietly the attitude of the state's attorney and local judges, should they decide to open a birth control clinic.[89] The committee elected William Howell as first vice-chairman, Raymond Pearl as second vice-chairman, and Donald Hooker, who had been associate professor of physiology under Howell at the School of Medicine, as treasurer.

Judge Moses reported back that neither State's Attorney O'Connor nor Judge O'Dunne would interfere with their plans, and Whitridge Williams was then asked to prepare a policy statement for the proposed clinic. Williams suggested that only women referred by their physicians should be accepted; each referring physician would be asked to sign a statement that, in his or her opinion, the mental or physical condition of the woman would be aggravated by further childbearing.[90] An advisory group of doctors would make certain that no advice was given to "unsuitable cases." Dr. Bessie Moses, who had graduated from the Johns Hopkins Medical School and had worked with Williams in the department of obstetrics, offered to serve as medical director of the clinic at the nominal salary of $500 per year. She then traveled to New York to observe the clinics being run by the Birth Control League and the Committee on Maternal Health, and reported back that an assistant would be needed to follow up cases, that fees should be implemented based on the patient's ability to pay, and that it would be preferable to have separate clinic days for "colored" and white patients.[91]

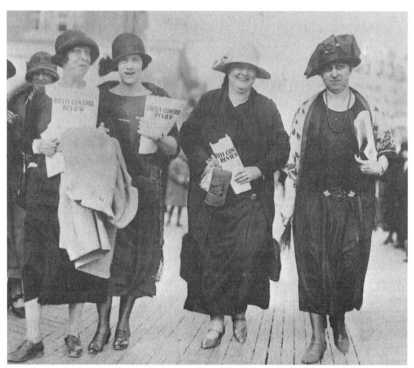

Figure 30. Volunteers selling copies of Margaret Sanger's *Birth Control Review*, circa 1917–25. In 1926–27, William H. Howell and Raymond Pearl helped create the Bureau for Contraceptive Advice and opened one of the earliest family planning clinics in the country. (Courtesy of the Sophia Smith Collection, Smith College, Northampton, Massachusetts.)

Within six months of their first meeting, the members of the committee felt ready to open their new clinic. They decided, however, to postpone their plans until after the sessions of the state legislature for fear that legislation might be passed to suppress their work. Meanwhile, they formed a finance committee to solicit funds quietly from people thought to be sympathetic; the treasurer, Donald Hooker, personally guaranteed the funds needed to purchase a building on North Broadway.[92]

Williams, Pearl, and Hooker formed a Maryland subcommittee to cooperate with Margaret Sanger's National Committee on Federal Legislation. They sent out a letter to all members of the Maryland State Medical Society, all hospital superintendents, and all social agencies informing them that the Bureau of Contraceptive Advice, "conducted along the most ethical lines" and "limited entirely to those who really need its services," was ready to see patients referred by "reputable physicians."[93] The bureau would evaluate "the efficacy of the advice given" and "determine the relative value of the various methods which may from time to time be recommended." Only patients referred for reasons of mental or physical health were to be accepted.

The bureau was formally opened and the first patient seen on November 2, 1927. By May 1928, the Bureau for Contraceptive Advice had been incorporated, a Board of Directors selected, and Bessie Moses had already seen 74 patients.[94] At this time, contraception was only beginning to be considered as a medical problem; no mention was made of contraception in medical textbooks, and medical schools usually ignored the subject. Few physicians were prepared to advise their patients on contraceptive methods, even in cases in which pregnancy was admitted to be medically dangerous.[95] In Baltimore, most physicians were apparently relieved to have a respectable clinic to which they could refer patients; within the first year, 86 physicians had referred 168 patients to the bureau.[96]

Moses herself saw most of the patients coming to the clinic. She elicited a careful medical, social, and sexual history from each patient, then provided a pelvic examination. Most patients were fitted with vaginal diaphragms and advised to use spermicidal jelly, followed by a soapy warm-water douche from six to twelve hours after intercourse. They were asked to return to the clinic after one week. Given the fact that physicians so rarely gave contraceptive advice, it is especially interesting to note that approximately 85 percent of the clinic patients (including 80 percent of the Catholic women) had already practiced some form of contraception, either intermittently or regularly throughout their married lives. Usually, patients had tried several different methods with little success; the most frequently reported methods were condoms, douches, coitus interruptus, suppositories (tablets, jelly, sponges, etc.), and the so-called safe period. Unfortunately, women using the "safe period" were avoiding intercourse for five days before and after their menstrual periods on the mistaken information that these were their most fertile times. Usually, patients had tried combinations of methods in a desperate attempt to avoid conception.

An enormously high proportion of the women reported having had illegal or self-induced abortions. Of the 1,152 patients seen in the first five years of the clinic's operation, 1,008 abortions were reported, a figure that Bessie Moses noted was a minimum estimate since many women would have been reluctant to admit to a criminal activity. Indeed, about half of the women reported having had abortions. Some had had only one, but others had had as many as ten or fifteen and one woman had had twenty-five, the first "criminally induced" by a physician and the other twenty-four self-induced after she had learned the technique.[97]

Virtually all of these women reported multiple prior pregnancies and many had serious medical problems. Whitridge Williams categorized the first year's 168 patients into four groups for purposes of analysis. The first group of 70 patients had been sent to the clinic for "purely medical indications" such as tuberculosis, diseases of the kidneys, nervous disorders, or organic heart disease. The second group of 23 patients had a history of multiple pregnancies resulting in undernourishment, anemia, and general debility. The third group of 60 women Williams considered "more debatable." They had had excessive numbers of pregnancies in a relatively short period of time (9 children in 9 years, 12 children in 14 years, and so on) and were economically unable to support their existing families. There was insufficient information to categorize the final group of 15 patients, but Williams concluded: "In general, I have no hesitation in stating that the material has been carefully sifted, and that great discretion has been exercised in selecting the patients to whom advice has been given."[98]

In his statistical analysis of patient records, Raymond Pearl noted that all patients were married, and the average length of marriage was twelve years; half had borne more than five children and some as many as twenty-six children. Pearl refuted the usual criticisms of birth control, that only young, single, irresponsible, and/or wealthy women would try to avoid conception. The evidence, he said, contradicted the frequent claim that "the economically less fortunate and less foresighted elements of the population would not avail themselves of contraceptive advice."[99] From a survey of the occupations of the women's husbands, Pearl concluded that 94 percent "cannot justly be accused of belonging to the 'upper classes,' though they may include a great many desirable citizens."[100]

In the first five years of operation, more than one thousand women visited the clinic. The Milbank Memorial Fund financed a study of the 1,152 patients and the efficacy of the contraceptive advice given. One thousand and sixty-nine women had been given contraceptive advice; 95 percent of these had been fitted with diaphragms. Of these, about 20 percent had never returned to the clinic. Follow-up studies found that many women had moved and could not be located, some were separated or divorced, some had been unable to use the method, some had given in to their husbands' objections, and some lacked carfare or shoes to attend the clinic.[101] Moses reported that many used the diaphragms without telling their husbands. "In one case a patient's husband refused to allow her to use the diaphragm whereupon she was given another which she used without his knowledge for four years."[102] Only 45 percent of the women had successfully avoided pregnancy, and of the patients with undesired pregnancies, three had died following induced abortions.[103] Eleven of the women had died from other conditions. In general, the clinic's 45 percent success rate in controlling fertility was a marked improvement on the 15 percent success rate calculated from the reports of the women's own efforts at birth control.

When the clinic had been in operation for five years, the Board of Directors met to consider its future. Pearl commented on the difficulties of attempting to combine research studies with pure birth control activities; the initial studies of the first 1,000 cases were almost complete, and the question was whether to discontinue the work of the bureau or reorganize to conduct a birth control clinic "in the usual sense of the term."[104] Bessie Moses argued that discontinuing the clinic would have serious social consequences for the women being helped. The Board of Directors thus decided to close the research project (and the bureau) but to continue the clinic "for the benefit of the women of Baltimore." A new organization, headed by Mrs. Richard Jackson, would be responsible for fund-raising; the clinic would now be prepared to treat any patient "whether referred by a physician or by a social or charitable agency, for medical, economic or other reasons."[105]

The new Baltimore Birth Control Clinic was run almost exclusively by women. There were fourteen women on the Board of Directors and, by 1937, five women physicians at work in the clinic. Men, however, served on the Medical Advisory Board and contributed financially to the effort. The clinic was now completely independent of Hopkins (in fact as well as on paper) although several members of the faculty, including William Howell and Abel Wolman, were listed as sponsors. The clinic no longer had the objective of scientific studies but intended "to assure wives the right of voluntary motherhood" and "to promote economic independence and a decent standard of living."[106] In September 1937, a second clinic was opened in Hagerstown, Maryland; in October, the Howard County Maternal Health Center was organized in Ellicott City for "the wives of neighboring farmers and millhands"; and in November, the Northwest Maternal Health Center, sponsored "by the best conservative element among the colored citizens" was opened.[107]

The Baltimore Birth Control Clinic provided funds for several of these clinics and provided training in contraceptive methods to physicians organizing and working in similar clinics throughout the state. The main Baltimore clinic reported 3,265 patient visits in 1937 and a constantly increasing demand for further services. Their annual report included some of the letters received from mothers; presumably these were found helpful in fund-raising efforts. The following letter was typical:

Dear Doctor:

I am a mother of seven children and I am writing you as to my condition about having children. When my first child was borne I had a midwife, and my family doctor told me when the fifth child was borned I was in no condition to have children, this child was a bridge birth, and then the sixth came along and this baby was almost strangled and the seventh I suffered all the time I carried her, and this baby was borned in the University Hospital.

My husband hasn't been working steady and I can't pay much, but will do my best. We have seven children and the oldest is only 13 years and my husband is not making anything. . . . I hope you will please examine me, as I have all that I can do to take care of seven children without any more. . . . I will thank you from the bottom of my heart for all your trouble and do my best to pay as I am not able to pay much.

So please let me know what to do.[108]

In 1938, the Baltimore Birth Control Clinic became a member of the national Birth Control Federation. When several birth control groups merged to form Planned Parenthood in 1942, Bessie Moses became director of the Maryland Association. The small local effort started with considerable daring by a few Hopkins doctors and their influential friends in 1926 had become part of a major national and international movement which was dramatically to transform women's abilities to plan and control their reproductive lives.

The Syphilis Study

In addition to providing a home for services such as the Mothers' Advisory Service and the Baltimore Birth Control Clinic, the Eastern Health District provided a research base for many epidemiological studies on the infectious and chronic diseases. One of the most important infectious disease projects was a study of syphilis initiated with a Maryland State Health Department grant in 1936. Thomas Parran had just become head of the United States Public Health Service and was committed to a major national campaign against syphilis; as head of the division of venereal diseases, he had been involved in the Tuskegee experiment and had written books and popular articles on syphilis control.[109] A forceful and dynamic man, he wanted to break through the wall of silence and force the public to confront the scope and magnitude of the syphilis problem. In 1936, he placed the problem of syphilis on the national agenda with a massive publicity campaign.

The School of Hygiene obtained a grant of $10,000 from the State Health Department to train public health specialists in venereal disease control. The International Health Division of the Rockefeller Foundation agreed to "loan" one of their staff members, Thomas B. Turner, on the condition that he organize a community program for syphilis control, using the facilities of the Eastern Health District and the School of Medicine.[110] "Tommy" Turner had trained in medicine at the University of Maryland and Johns Hopkins before moving into biomedical research. A skilled bench scientist, he had also gained public health experience in Jamaica as head of the International Health Division's program against the tropical disease yaws. He then worked at the Rockefeller Institute in New York before returning to Hopkins to conduct laboratory research on syphilis in the School of Medicine.[111] Turner now agreed to work in the department of bacteriology in the School of Hygiene and conduct basic epidemiological studies of the incidence and prevalence of syphilis in the local community. These studies were intended to provide a baseline against which the relative success of syphilis control programs could be measured.

In the 1930s, public health clinics for the diagnosis and treatment of syphilis were clearly inadequate. The recommended schedule consisted of at least forty weekly treatments, with alternating courses of injections of arsenicals and heavy metals; in 1933, because of budget cuts during the depression, the Baltimore clinics had cut back to four treatments with arsphenamine, enough to render the patient noninfectious, but not enough for a cure.[112] Those suffering from syphilis were often considered immoral and undesirable persons and syphilis itself could not easily be discussed in public, factors that only compounded the problems of venereal disease control.

In the Eastern Health District, Turner and his staff undertook extensive community surveys and collected data from clinics, hospitals, and health department records. They identified a "discovery rate" of syphilis in whites of approximately two cases per thousand and in blacks, of approximately thirty per thousand.[113] Hospitals and private practitioners were encouraged to conduct Wassermann tests on all patients; attempts were made to find, examine, and treat the sexual contacts of those infected.[114] In studying the incidence of syphilis, Turner and his staff attempted to separate new cases of syphilis from those previously known, and to separate early and late infections; they tried various methods of estimating the prevalence of the disease and the trends of syphilis rates over time. The results of these studies were published in an extensive series of papers that gave an epidemiological picture of the extent of syphilis in a representative urban community and provided the methodological tools for conducting similar studies elsewhere.[115] Turner became a national consultant and adviser on syphilis control; his students went on to staff venereal disease control programs across the country. With the entry of the United States into World War II in 1941, Turner volunteered for service and was assigned as director of the army's venereal disease unit working from the surgeon general's office for the duration of the war.[116] The syphilis studies in the Eastern Health District continued through the war years, and in 1945, researchers helped evaluate the new and successful treatment of syphilis by the "miracle drug" penicillin.

The Future of the Eastern Health District

The Eastern Health District continued to be a site of community-based health studies during and after the war years. A survey of the prevalence of illness in families and of their medical care needs was started in 1938 and continued for five years. It laid the basis for the Baltimore Medical Care Program for the recipients of public assistance inaugurated in 1948 after much discussion and planning. The "rodent ecology" project started during the war explored methods of controlling the rat infestation of inner city neighborhoods; the study eventually concluded that rehabilitation of old and delapidated housing was the only effective method of keeping the rat population under control.[117] Child and maternal health services, prenatal care and well-baby clinics helped to keep the mortality rates in the Eastern Health District well below those for the city as a whole.

In 1938, the Eastern Health District was expanded to include several more city wards, almost doubling its population size. The rest of the city's health department programs were now reorganized on a district basis. The organization of the Eastern Health District provided a model for the decentralization of health department programs in other city units.[118] This reorganization, however, also emphasized the anomalous status of the Eastern Health District in being partially under the jurisdiction of the School of Hygiene and partially under the authority of the city health commissioner, a structural problem that had been there from the beginning. When Harry Mustard left the district in 1937, and Ernest Stebbins was offered the job of director, he declined, and explained: "In talking with Dr. Reed and Dr. Frost in the school, I got the impression that I would be an employee of the school, a regular faculty member, while from Dr. Williams I got the impression that I would be under his direct supervision and that he would have to approve all the activities in the District."[119]

Howe Eller did accept the job and, as an astute diplomat, managed to wear both hats as a member of the City Health Department and the School of Hygiene faculty. Later administrators, Harry Chant and George Silver, had to deal with the problems of a deteriorating relationship between the City Health Department and the school.[120] From the point of view of the faculty, the health commissioner too often tried to interfere in the conduct of their research and training programs; from the point of view of the commissioner, such interference was his duty and responsibility in protecting the population from overzealous and sometimes insensitive researchers. Huntington Williams, in defending his position, told the story of a research project on the prevalence of venereal disease among high school students:

There was a Roman Catholic secondary school, and you know high school students have a way of getting together in a manner that isn't quite elegant, if you know what I mean. They sent for me because the headmistress of this school in the Eastern Health District was in tears. They were starting this from the school on Good Friday. Now the School of Hygiene does not keep a religious calendar in front of it, but they couldn't have chosen a worse subject, or a worse day to start than Good Friday, so I was asked to go to the school and call off the dogs, you know?[121]

Williams eventually insisted on approving all research plans and all field interviewers, steps that, from the School of Hygiene perspective, simply slowed up their research program. Again, in Williams's words:

We [the health department men] would go out all unsuspecting and be told: "Dr. Jones was in here yesterday and he asked the most fantastic questions we ever heard. Who in the hell is Dr. Jones? Is he one of your men?" We'd reply, "Oh no—he must be from the School of Hygiene" and then we'd run home and call Dr. Jones and ask what he was doing out in the district without getting any clearance. We finally worked out a scheme with the School of Hygiene where they practically promised me that they wouldn't send out any Dr. Joneses without my having had him in my office and talking to him to find out what kind of guy he was.[122]

Some of the School of Hygiene faculty and district health officers were irritated by Williams's insistence that they spend a lot of time cultivating good relationships with local medical practitioners; Williams was convinced that this was the secret to accomplishing public health reforms.

In Williams's view, these disagreements were mainly squabbles "within the family," although they were sometimes only resolved with the expenditure of much "blood, sweat, and tears."[123] One of the most serious disagreements came over the location of a new building for the Eastern Health District; the School of Hygiene had bought land next to their main building, intending to build new offices and laboratories there, but Williams adamantly refused to place the building anywhere within four blocks of the school. He felt that some geographical distance was necessary to guarantee the autonomy of district health activities. In this instance, Williams won the struggle and, after protracted negotiations, the building was finally placed on Caroline Street, just outside the forbidden four-block radius.[124]

Despite these problems and struggles over the authority (and credit) for the Eastern Health District, the district was an undeniable success. In the 1930s it received a steady stream of national and international visitors interested in the research and training programs. In 1938, the International Health Division described the district as "an outstanding success in providing practical field training for students in public health; in providing a population group, exceeding 100,000, unequaled anywhere in the country for study purposes because of the complete family records now available; and in elevating public health standards and practices in the City of Baltimore, as well as serving as a model and stimulus for comparable developments in other schools of public health."[125]

VIII

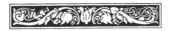

Extending the Hopkins Model

he School of Hygiene and Public Health at Johns Hopkins had been the central hub of the Welch-Rose organizational plan for public health education. As previously discussed, this plan proposed the creation of one or more research institutes at the center of a network of schools spread out across the country. The central institutes, the focal points for the production of knowledge, would be linked to a web of smaller schools responsible for educating local health officers to implement the results of research. Rose had hoped that schools of public health could be built in every state, and following the model of agriculture, provide extension courses and practical training programs to reach out to local health officers in small towns and rural counties. According to this plan, full-time trained public health officers in every county health department would eventually put this knowledge into practice. Knowledge would flow in both directions: epidemiological investigations at the county level would be used for teaching and research in the state and central schools of public health, and the conclusions reached in the research institutions would, in turn, be fed to local communities for action.

When William Henry Welch won the competition to start the first of the central research and training institutes supported by Rockefeller Foundation dollars, he gained the responsibility of defining public health education and thus much of the future content of public health. As we have seen in the definition of public health unfolding at Hopkins, the conceptual frameworks and methodologies of public health were aligned with those of scientific medicine, and research predominated over practice in producing new knowledge. Twenty-five years later Welch's research institute was thriving. As measured by any criteria of scientific productivity, it was a resounding success. A small number of faculty were churning out research results and publications at a rapid

215

rate. They were training a small and select group of students conversant with the latest research methods, and many of these students were becoming leading teachers and researchers in public health.

New Schools of Public Health

Once the Hopkins school had defined its model of public health, other schools tended to pattern themselves in that image. Even the pioneering Harvard-MIT School for Health Officers, which had preceded the Hopkins school, was restructured to resemble the one at Hopkins. The choice of Baltimore as the location for the school of hygiene had infuriated President Charles Eliot of Harvard but he then changed the name of his School for Health Officers to the "School of Public Health of Harvard University and the Massachusetts Institute of Technology."[1] In 1920, William Thompson Sedgwick, professor of biology and public health at MIT and founder of the school, agreed that, in order to offer degrees and attract outside funding, the school should be legally affiliated only with Harvard, maintaining simply a loose cooperative relationship to MIT, since neither school's legal charter allowed the granting of joint degrees.[2]

In agreeing to this plan, Sedgwick was essentially abandoning his conception of public health training as equally related to sanitary engineering and medicine. As a biologist, Sedgwick had never accepted the idea that an M.D. was a necessary qualification for public health practice; as a professor at MIT, he had argued for the important contributions of sanitary engineering as well as the biomedical sciences to the new profession of public health.[3] Sedgwick's ideas, however, had been unpopular with the medical profession and had not received financial or institutional support; by 1920, with Welch's school thriving in Baltimore, Sedgwick knew that public health had become essentially a medical specialty, that the M.D. degree was required for the higher-level positions, and that, therefore, the influence of sanitary engineers, biologists, and other nonmedical specialists would be severely limited.

With Sedgwick's blessing, Harvard established a new School of Public Health, located beside the Harvard Medical School. In an important symbolic move, the school cut its ties with engineering and moved over into the medical environment. In 1921, the Rockefeller Foundation approved the undertaking and gave Harvard $1,160,000 in endowment, $500,000 for a building and $25,000 a year for five years to support the new Harvard School of Public Health. The school opened its doors to students in 1922.

The organization of the Harvard school differed from that at Johns

Hopkins in having a much closer relationship to the medical school, a relationship so close that the School of Public Health would have difficulty maintaining its financial and organizational independence. The dean of the School of Medicine, David L. Edsall, was also made dean of the School of Public Health. The existing university departments of preventive medicine and hygiene, industrial medicine, tropical medicine, comparative physiology, and sanitary engineering were placed in the new school, and additional Rockefeller funding was used to finance new departments of bacteriology and immunology, vital statistics, and child hygiene.[4]

In its early years, the School of Public Health developed in the shadow of the Harvard Medical School. The budgets of the two schools were closely intertwined, an arrangement that did not encourage the independent development of the School of Public Health. The argument for an intimate relationship between the medical and public health schools was that the School of Medicine would thus be imbued with the spirit of public health. This argument turned out to be a naive hope: Harvard Medical School continued, as did Johns Hopkins Medical School, to demonstrate a distinct lack of interest in public health. The perspective of medicine was not, after all, determined by administrative arrangements, but was the synthesis of more fundamental political and economic forces. Bringing medical and public health education together was rather like merging a large corporation with a small one; public health tended to become submerged in the powerful interests of academic medicine and clinical research. Lengthy financial negotiations between Harvard and the Rockefeller Foundation partially resolved these questions in 1946 when the School of Public Health was placed on an entirely separate budgetary basis from the School of Medicine.[5]

Jean Alonzo Curran has fully described the history of the Harvard school in his *Founders of the Harvard School of Public Health* (1970).[6] Here it is sufficient to note a few similarities and differences between the Hopkins and Harvard schools. Both were identified with strong medical schools and with the "medical model" of public health; both were clearly oriented toward research, with a relatively small and elite postgraduate student body, and both were similarly organized into departments and disciplines. There were differences in emphasis. In its early years, the Harvard school made its most distinctive contributions in areas in which the Hopkins school was weakest. For example, in industrial hygiene, Cecil and Philip Drinker developed a pioneering program, and in child hygiene, Harold Stuart undertook long-term studies of child growth and development. Hopkins was especially noted for epidemiology and nutrition research, while Harvard was stronger in industrial and child hygiene. Organizationally, the Hopkins school was an independent institution, and the Harvard school had a complex administrative and financial relationship to the medical school. The Hopkins school, the larger of the two, tended to attract more foreign students, especially to its programs in medical zoology. Both schools trained a small number of United States students (especially relative to the demand for public health officers) and tended to offer an elite route into high-level public health positions.

With the founding of the Hopkins and Harvard schools, several other universities in the United States established public health programs. In 1915, Yale University had developed a department of public health within the School of Medicine, led by Charles-Edward A. Winslow; Columbia University then established the De Lamar Institute of Public Health, and the University of Michigan created a division of hygiene and public health. Several of these programs were divisions or departments of medical schools and were smaller or less well endowed than Hopkins or Harvard, but all tended to follow a similar basic model as to the content and methods of public health.

Public health education developed rapidly in the 1930s when many schools expanded their facilities as increased funding to train and employ qualified public health officers became available. In 1935, the Social Security Act provided the first federal funds for public health training. By 1936, the American Public Health Association reported that ten schools offered public health degrees or certificates requiring at least one year of residence; of these, the largest were Johns Hopkins, Harvard, Columbia, and Michigan.[7] By 1938, more than four thousand individuals, including about one thousand doctors, had received some public health training with funds provided by the federal government through the states. In 1939, the federal government allocated over eight million dollars for maternal and child health services, over nine million for general public health work, and over four million earmarked for venereal disease control.[8] Federal laws required states to establish minimum qualifications for health personnel employed through federal assistance; they recommended at least one year of postgraduate education in an approved school of public health in addition to basic educational qualifications. By 1938, the states budgeted for over 1,500 public health trainees, including doctors, nurses, engineers, and research workers.[9] The existing training programs were filled to capacity. In 1938, Lowell Reed, then dean of the Hopkins School of Hygiene, could tell the medical school: "The School of Hygiene doesn't need medical school recruits. Plenty of recruits are now coming from the

Social Security program, and the quality has come up abruptly in the last five years."[10] In less than twenty years, public health became institutionalized as a distinct field of knowledge requiring specialized training.

One consequence of the rapid development of public health education was that doctors, nurses, and engineers were being separately trained. Sanitary engineers were usually trained independently in schools of engineering; public health nurses were being trained in nursing schools; and physicians were trained in schools of public health.[11] The separate public health training programs for the three groups meant that they were not used to working together on research projects or practical programs. The physicians were usually trained in research institutes, while the sanitary engineers and public health nurses were given a more practical or vocational education. Thus, the three groups retained separate professional identities, even as employees of the same public health departments and programs.

International Expansion

Wickliffe Rose, made director general of the International Health Board of the Rockefeller Foundation in 1913, was in a position to expand his conception of public health training and implementation from a plan for the United States to a plan for world public health. He decided his first task should be the extension of hookworm control programs, begun in the southern states, to other countries, and "so far as practicable to follow up the treatment and cure of this disease with the establishment of agencies for the promotion of public sanitation and the spread of the knowledge of scientific medicine."[12] Rose spent much of his time traveling: in the first year, to England, the British West Indies, Egypt, Ceylon, and Malaya. Joseph White traveled for the board to Panama, Costa Rica, Guatemala, and Nicaragua. As a result of these preliminary investigations and contacts, hookworm control programs were started in British Guiana, Trinidad, Grenada, St. Vincent, St. Lucia, Antigua, Panama, Costa Rica, Guatemala, and Egypt. In the next few years, the International Health Board expanded its focus to include malaria and yellow fever as well as hookworm, and developed major programs in China, Latin America, and Central America.

International Health Board officers from the United States started these programs in cooperation with national governments, but their goal was to train local public health officers to carry on the projects when the Rockefeller Foundation withdrew. To this end, they gave Rockefeller Foundation fellowships to selected health officers and medical graduates in countries where their programs were operating; the Fellows came to the United States for public health training and then usually returned home to participate in the International Health Board programs. Eventually, the board intended to establish national schools of public health in these countries with faculty selected from the countries concerned and trained in the United States. In other words, the original "Rose plan" for public health training would be implemented on an international level rather than only within the United States.

Despite the complexities of national and international politics, a remarkable number of international health programs were established. The Rockefeller Foundation helped establish schools of public health in Brazil, Bulgaria, Canada, Czechoslovakia, England, Hungary, India, Italy, Japan, Norway, the Philippines, Poland, Rumania, Sweden, Turkey, and Yugoslavia.

The project of developing international schools of public health relied heavily on what the Rockefeller Foundation referred to as the "West Points of Public Health." For the United States and, to a large extent, for all countries under its influence, these were the Johns Hopkins School of Hygiene and Public Health and the Harvard School of Public Health. For almost all the British colonies and Commonwealth countries, this role would be filled by the London School of Hygiene and Tropical Medicine, which the Rockefeller Foundation funded in 1922; for Canada and the British West Indies, the University of Toronto School of Hygiene was funded in 1924. In China, the Peking Union Medical College, opened in 1919, provided an elite form of medical and public health training in a country somewhat isolated from United States influence. Later, schools in India, Japan, and the Philippines provided centers for professional health training on the western model. Thus, a network of training centers was established in Europe, Latin America, and Asia, with faculty and students rotating among these centers on Rockefeller fellowships, teaching exchanges, and research projects. The Rockefeller Foundation had a goal to reduce provincialism and nationalism, to expand international cooperation in public health, and to create a "world commerce in ideas": "The search for truth and its application to human need is a vast, worldwide cooperative task which demands constant interchange of ideas and more intelligent team-work among workers. Every country should seek entangling alliances in a league for scientific progress."[13]

Wickliffe Rose based much of his international health program on a study of the British experience in the colonies; the British had the most extensive knowledge then available of tropical medicine and public health administration. Rose first traveled to London to consult with the British government and the Colonial Office; after meeting with Lord Crewe, the secretary of state for India, and the Right Honorable Lewis Harcourt, the secretary of state for the colonies, he obtained official invitations to visit the colonies and begin work in Egypt, Ceylon, Malaya, and the British West Indies. As George Vincent explained:

From London and the British Isles as the center of a common culture, political control, financial and commercial activity, educational ideas, social prestige, and family ties, go influences to every quarter of the globe. . . . The progress of medical education and public health in the British Isles and in strategic parts of the Commonwealth is of moment to vast areas of the world, to millions of human beings both within and without the borders of the Commonwealth. The Rockefeller Foundation in carrying out a policy of international cooperation has found particularly valuable opportunities to aid British undertakings all the way from London and Edinburgh to Hong Kong and Sidney.[14]

Rose regarded the London School of Tropical Medicine, founded in 1899, as the "nucleus" for a future international school of hygiene and public health; working with the Ministry of Health, the University of London, and the Colonial Office, he negotiated the establishment of a new school of hygiene. The school was endowed by the Rockefeller Foundation in 1922 with $2 million and incorporated under a royal charter in 1924 as the London School of Hygiene and Tropical Medicine.[15] Men being sent to the British colonies as public health officers were trained in London. The British Empire was the London "sphere of influence," and the majority of students worked in colonial health programs. The London school also acted as a research and training center for several European countries, and physicians interested in tropical diseases could obtain advanced training in London. Thus, Rose's vision and Rockefeller funds helped to transform the London school into a central hub for the British Empire analogous to the Hopkins and Harvard schools in the United States.

The School of Hygiene at Toronto, formally established in 1924, acted as the main research and training center for Canada. Compared to Hopkins and Harvard, the Toronto school paid more attention to practical training for public health work: academic training in the laboratory sciences was supplemented by strong practical programs provided by members of the Toronto City Health Department.[16] The school provided postgraduate training in public health engineering as well as diplomas for public health nurses and physicians. Most of the students trained at Toronto became public health officers and public health nurses in the provincial and local health services of Canada; some became teachers of preventive medicine in Canadian medical schools.

By this time, the Rockefeller Foundation had withdrawn from most of its public health activities in the United States and focused almost exclusively on promoting international health programs. The Rockefeller fellowship program proved to be an effective method of recruiting for international public health. Thus, international students comprised a high proportion of the student body in the three "central" schools—London, Hopkins, and Harvard. The conscious plan of the foundation was to use the fellowships to train promising people in the central schools so they would return home and, with foundation help, develop programs and schools in their home countries. As Raymond Fosdick described it:

Rose and his successors as head of the International Health Board undertook the implementation of a bold and creative plan literally to girdle the globe with schools and institutes of public health, including public health nursing. . . . The schools and institutes were located in Prague, Warsaw, London, Toronto, Copenhagen, Budapest, Oslo, Belgrade, Zagreb, Madrid, Cluj, Ankara, Sofia, Rome, Tokyo, Athens, Bucharest, Stockholm, Calcutta, Manila, São Paulo, and the University of Michigan. . . . A migration of public health personnel back and forth across national boundary lines would be an enriching experience by which the new ideas and techniques of one area could become the common property of all.[17]

Evaluation of Schools of Public Health

During the 1930s, schools of public health in the United States were requesting funds for expansion from the International Health Division. To identify where "limited sums of money might have the most far-reaching influence," the Rockefeller Foundation decided to assess the status of public health training compared with the future need for trained workers.[18] The evaluations of the public health schools revealed continuing problems and tensions in public health education; the issues identified in John A. Ferrell's initial evaluation and the subsequent in-depth study were similar to those that had proved problematic for the Hopkins school. Recurrent themes included conflicts between the emphases on research or on practice; problematic relationships between public health and medicine; and conflicts between emphases on health or on disease.

In 1938, John A. Ferrell consulted Thomas Parran, surgeon general of the United States Public Health Service, and Martha Eliot, assistant chief of the United States Children's Bureau, for advice on how to evaluate the schools. He then gathered information about the degrees granted and numbers of students graduated each year from each school.[19] Seeking to compare the numbers trained with the numbers needed, Ferrell used information from the United States Public Health Service and the American Public Health Association to suggest that 1,500 physicians, 6,000 nurses, 750 sanitary engineers, and 500 "others" (statisticians, chemists, bacteriologists, etc.) should be trained over the next ten years. Looking at public health graduates for the previous two years, Ferrell found a shortage of physicians and nurses, and a slight "oversupply" of engineers and "others."[20] He concluded that considerable foundation aid for public health training would be required.

Ferrell went on to criticize existing programs in public health education. The segregated training of physicians, nurses, and engineers caused "needless difficulty" when these groups tried to work together in public health organizations. Furthermore, most physicians in medical schools and hospitals still lacked any understanding of public health, again causing "needless difficulty" for all concerned. Ferrell recommended that all public health schools offer training programs in which the different professions would work together, and develop field study areas "comparable to the Eastern Health District which the Hopkins School of Hygiene and Public Health has developed."[21]

After reading Ferrell's report, the scientific directors of the International Health Division authorized a critical study of the accomplishments of the schools and institutes of public health in the United States, Canada, and Europe. They selected Thomas Parran, the surgeon general, and Livingston Farrand, recently retired as president of Cornell University, to study the United States and Canada.[22] Kenneth F. Maxcy of Johns Hopkins was asked to survey the European schools, but when war conditions in Europe made such a visit impossible, A. J. Warren, the International Health Division representative in Europe, was asked for a brief "confidential report" on the European schools.

Warren reported that, though some of the European institutes of hygiene were successful, London was the only school that "might be compared with the Schools in the United States."[23] Most of the European institutes were administrative units of national health services responsible for technical and administrative work; few were actively engaged in research. They offered training courses for public health officers varying in length from four months in Turkey to twelve months in London and Athens. The schools were expected to need occasional external support; even the successful London school was not adequately supported by the Ministry of Health.

In late 1939, Thomas Parran and Livingston Farrand presented a thorough report on schools in the United States and Canada. The Parran-Farrand report provided an intelligent review of existing programs, a fairly trenchant critique of their limitations, and selective praise for their accomplishments. This report justified decisions to increase support for public health at the schools classified as "national and international"—Hopkins, Harvard, and Toronto—and to offer new funding to schools then classified as "regional"—at the University of California, the University of Michigan, and Vanderbilt University.

Parran and Farrand discussed the growing acceptance of professional public health training, most recently in federal requirements for specialized training of public health personnel. The need for public health training was, however, better established as an ideal than as a reality. The Public Health Service surveyed health department personnel and found that one-half of the physicians, one-third of the nurses, and two-thirds of the sanitary officers had no public health training whatsoever: they were scandalously undereducated by the newly created contemporary standards.

Parran and Farrand noted that public health services were expanding rapidly with increased public funding. Their forecast was made "as the business analysis which guides a manufacturer in the development of plant and working force."[24] To estimate training facility requirements, they considered the need to educate existing public health department personnel, to replace retirees and part-time workers, and to staff the programs authorized by recent legislation. They suggested a minimum of 289 public health physicians and between 2,000 and 4,000 public health nurses each year. The need for other kinds of public health personnel—sanitary engineers, statisticians, and so on—would also increase dramatically.

What of the existing facilities for public health education? Twenty-four schools and universities in the United States offered postgraduate courses in public health. However, their graduates would not be sufficient to meet the projected need for trained personnel.

Johns Hopkins was the only school at which the applicants for admission significantly exceeded available capacity. At Hopkins, the administration complained that large student enrollments were taxing the facilities "to the utmost." The Parran-Farrand report noted that the School of Hygiene had "resisted all attempts to make it more of a vocational school" and "practical methods" had been subordinated to "the teaching of principles" (p. 33). They declared the departments of biostatistics, biochemistry (nutrition), and epidemiology especially good, with epidemiology giving "inspiration and cohesiveness to the work of the whole school" (p. 32). They accorded the Eastern Health District great importance, and urged that it be funded permanently. They recommended the appointment of additional professors in bacteriology, biostatistics, epidemiology, and especially public health administration, the departments with the heaviest teaching loads. Their major criticism involved "a certain isolation" from the medical school and other university departments (p. 27). They commended the recently created syphilis training program as "the first occasion upon which the School of Hygiene, the Medical School, and the Johns Hopkins Hospital have cooperated so actively on any project" (p. 65).

At the Harvard School of Public Health, Parran and Farrand rated industrial hygiene as "outstanding" and sanitary engineering as "economical and effective." They commended the child hygiene program and the teaching of epidemiology and preventive medicine. However, they considered the communicable diseases facilities inadequate, and criticized the school for "the lack of proper arrangements for practical teaching and field work in health administration and epidemiology" (p. 45). They felt Harvard lacked "an integrating force comparable with the laboratory influence at Toronto and the epidemiological influence at Johns Hopkins": and noted a recurrent problem with "the fair division of funds between the Medical and Public Health Schools" (pp. 46, 48).

At Toronto, Parran and Farrand were favorably impressed by the research in physiology, immunology, and nutrition, by the integration of practical and theoretical training, and by the facilities for public health nursing:

Our general impression of the Toronto School is extremely favorable. It has directed itself to the particular problem of training medical officers of health and seems to have done an excellent job. The spirit of research permeates the institution, yet emphasis upon research has not resulted in courses too theoretical for practical administrative purposes. Clearly associated with the medical school, it has not been dominated by it. Functionally, its relation to the public health nursing school seems ideal (p. 60).

Parran and Farrand considered the relationships of the public health schools to departments of social science and to medical schools. They found consistent neglect of the social sciences in all three schools.[25] Relations with the medical schools varied among the three: Hopkins had failed to develop any close relationship; Harvard was dominated by the medical school; only at Toronto was there a "close coordination" without "domination."[26] Nonetheless, all of the schools were declared a good investment of foundation funds and all wanted additional support.

Even with the expansion of programs following passage of the Social

Security Act, the national need for public health training went far beyond the capacity of existing schools. Federal training funds now averaged $1,320,000 annually; $103,000 had been allotted to the universities of California, Michigan, Minnesota, Vanderbilt, and North Carolina to develop short courses. These short courses were recognized as a first emergency measure to be followed by development of more adequate postgraduate training at the new regional schools. With Social Security Act funding, the University of Michigan expanded its "division" of hygiene and public health to a "school," offering graduate training in public health to over three hundred students. The University of Minnesota's department of preventive medicine and public health now offered graduate training and boasted excellent facilities and expanding student numbers despite a small budget. Columbia University's department of public health was headed by Haven Emerson and comprised a major department of the medical school and an important center for public health training in New York City. At Yale University, public health was also organized as a part of the medical school, directed by Charles-Edward A. Winslow, "one of the leading philosophers of the public health movement in the United States and perhaps its foremost interpreter" (p. 75). At Yale, integration with the clinical departments was "unusually good," although the public health program was "less weighted in the fundamental sciences than seems desirable" (p. 76). At Vanderbilt University, the schools of Engineering, Nursing, and Medicine were each offering courses in public health. These were "short courses" of three months' duration, supplying practical training for southern public health officers. Both Vanderbilt and the University of California, which had also been offering short courses, were planning to expand.

In their final recommendations, Parran and Farrand suggested increased support for Hopkins, Harvard, and Toronto. This funding would sustain research in public health disciplines, but would not solve the national needs for public health training. For the latter purpose, the report recommended that regional training schools be supported in the Far West, the Midwest, and the South. Berkeley, Michigan, and Vanderbilt seemed likely locations to provide a second tier of public health education: schools oriented to practical training more than to research. Support for such regional schools could come from ten-year grants, "sufficient only to achieve reasonably good training courses for public health personnel" with research projects to be considered separately, and on their merits, so as not to divert support from the primary teaching functions (p. 89).

The relationship of the principles of public health to those of medicine was a continuing preoccupation of those organizing and implementing the expansion of public health education, just as were the institutional relationships between medical and public health schools. The fond hope that schools of public health allied to medical schools would serve to permeate those medical institutions with the spirit of preventive medicine had proved illusory. Johns Hopkins and Harvard had had little impact in changing the basic orientation of medical education. Reformers constantly advocated improved teaching of preventive medicine in medical schools so that "practicing physicians, upon graduation, understand something of the methods and approaches of public health and . . . develop a social conscience as to the unmet needs of the people in the mass" (p. 90). After twenty years of public health teaching, however, public health and medicine still seemed far apart and often moving in opposite directions. The situation in 1939 suggested a thriving and expanding public health movement, supported by new federal and state health programs, but developing in general isolation from the medical profession as a whole.

The officers of the Rockefeller Foundation, who were pouring money into medical education as well as into public health, continued to be optimistic that eventually the two would form a closer and more harmonious relationship. Indeed, they often asserted that, with the increasing success of medical science in curing disease, the emphasis within medicine would gradually shift from cure to prevention. The industrial and mechanical metaphors in which they conceptualized medicine transformed this dream into good business sense:

A railway spends more money on train and track inspection than on wreck crews. The average automobile owner is on the watch for signs of motor trouble and does not wait until there is trouble. The factory manager looks solicitously after his machines and does not wait until there is a breakdown. The human body, which is vastly more complex than any machine, is in need of vigilant care and frequent examination. Yet for the most part it is neglected until pain and disability sound an unmistakable alarm. Then the doctor is called in and too often expected to do the impossible. He is thought of as a wreck crew rather than as a train and track inspector.[27]

Deciding that a shift in emphasis from curative to preventive medicine needed some encouragement, the foundation funded projects in medical schools to "permeate the curriculum with the preventive idea." At the Harvard Medical School, for example, it provided funds to "assist every teacher in the medical school to include in his courses the preventive aspects of his subject."[28] Now shifting to a new set of metaphors, it urged doctors to use the "telescope" to view the distribution of disease throughout a community as well as the "microscope" to perceive the effects of disease within an individual body. The same observer could alternately use a telescope or a microscope, and medical students ought to learn to use both.

In most medical schools, however, the teaching of preventive medicine was poor or nonexistent. In 1931, Waller S. Leathers, dean of the School of Medicine at Vanderbilt University, had surveyed United States medical schools and concluded that in most schools, the teaching of preventive medicine was "of a desultory, uninteresting, and poorly organized type."[29] In 1933, the recently reorganized division of medical sciences of the Rockefeller Foundation thus made the teaching of preventive medicine and hygiene in medical schools a funding priority.[30] Teachers of public health and hygiene used Rockefeller funding to travel to other universities and medical schools and observe methods of teaching and curriculum organization.[31] John Fitzgerald, from the University of Toronto, and Charles Smith, from Stanford University, undertook an intensive survey of the teaching of preventive medicine, public health, and hygiene in North American and Western European medical schools.[32]

This survey produced few constructive ideas. No one seemed ready to provide dynamic leadership to the scattered forces trying to change the orientation of medical education. In part, at least, it was a political problem: preventive medicine, to the extent that it was equated in many physicians' minds with "socialized medicine," represented a potential economic threat; medical schools were, in general, more willing to express vague support for the concept of preventive medicine than to provide active advocacy or financial commitment to the idea. As far as most physicians were concerned, public health continued to be the weak sister of clinical medicine.

Public health and medicine remained quite distinct: the one oriented toward the analysis of health and disease on a population basis, the other oriented toward individual patients. The economic support of each was fundamentally different: one dependent on government-funded salaried positions, the other on the entrepreneurial basis of private practice. Efforts to merge public health and medical education were hardly likely to be successful so long as the organization and economic foundations of preventive and curative services were thus strikingly opposed.

In the United States, reformers tended to approach this structural problem as though it could be solved by joint educational programs.

These, however, were mainly remarkable for the recurrent enthusiasm of the efforts and the consistent failure of the results. Reviewing the organizational relationships and cooperative efforts between schools of public health and schools of medicine, Russell Nelson, president of the Johns Hopkins Hospital, later noted: "It is a sad story of unfulfilled expectations, numerous failures, frequent tensions, and some bad feelings."[33] Rejecting the idea that schools of medicine and public health should be combined or that medical schools should "take over" public health, Nelson added: "Medical schools are already too large and complex to manage their present, and future, responsibilities, let alone take on others. . . . In short, medical schools don't want to take over public health; the idea, it seems to me, appeals only to some administrators and armchair critics."[34]

John Hume, dean of the School of Hygiene and Public Health, agreed that the independence of schools of medicine and public health was necessary: "Examples do exist of single schools that provide faculty for both medical and public health students. In general, however, insofar as the public health element is concerned, when the schools are separate the programs are stronger, have a broader spectrum of training and research programs, as well as expertise, and greater overall resources."[35]

Although the separation between medical and public health education seemed necessary in the United States context, it was often a barrier to those attempting to organize health services in developing countries. Luis Fernando Duque of Colombia (South America) bitterly attacked the rigid separation in the early development of schools of public health and medical education in Latin America:

The health professionals shut themselves up in their schools of public health, and the physicians stayed within the walls of the medical schools and hospitals. The latter felt that public health specialists "were no longer doctors," while the health people believed themselves to be crusaders in a cause they had to win, imposing it if necessary on the community as well as on other physicians who did not understand them.[36]

Guillermo Arbona, the secretary of health of Puerto Rico, agreed that developing countries could not afford to separate responsibility for preventive and curative health services; for rationality and economy, they needed integrated health systems.[37] In the same vein, John B. Grant of the Rockefeller Foundation repeatedly argued the idea that health services could be more efficiently and effectively provided if based on the concepts of regionalization, integration of preventive and curative services, and community health centers.[38] Grant insisted that medical education in developing nations should be oriented toward prevention, with training in administration, epidemiology, and the social sciences. Indeed, he believed that such changes would transform medical education in the United States as well as in the rest of the world: "This trend, it seems to us, will occur as much in the richer and more highly developed countries as in the developing areas of the world. It will leave no justification for the existence of separate schools of public health, as such."[39]

The concepts of regionalization and the integration of curative and preventive services were, however, more often honored in rhetoric than in practice. The relationship between schools of medicine and schools of public health (or departments of preventive medicine) would continue to be marked by tensions and distance, with sporadic efforts to create cooperative programs of teaching and research. In summarizing the pragmatic case for the independence of schools of public health, Milton Roemer concluded that the academic environment of patient-oriented clinical medicine was simply not conducive to the growth of the community-oriented public health discipline.[40]

If public health and medicine were to be brought closer together, the integration would have to happen in practice and not simply by creating joint educational programs. By the 1930s, many progressives in public health were suggesting just such an integration. They did not intend simply to introduce an epidemiological perspective into schools of medicine; they wanted to reorganize medical care. In his presidential address to the American Public Health Association in 1926, C.-E. A. Winslow had first suggested that public health was at a "crossroads," and posed a challenge to public health officers to become involved in planning the organized community medical services which, he said, would come "as surely as the sun will rise tomorrow."[41] Between 1927 and 1932, the Committee on the Costs of Medical Care issued a stream of reports calling for the extension of basic public health services and the group organization of medical care.[42] Henry Sigerist at Johns Hopkins became the leader of an influential group of socially committed physicians and public health specialists who promoted the idea of a national health program combining both preventive and curative health services.[43] Edgar Sydenstricker elaborated the argument for a greatly expanded view of public health including the provision of medical care, improved housing, control of environmental hazards, and economic security for the whole population:

Society has a basic responsibility for assuring, to all of its members, healthful conditions of housing and living, a reasonable degree of economic security, proper facilities for curative and preventive medicine and adequate medical care—in fact the control, so far as means are known to science, of all of the environmental factors that affect physical and mental well-being.[44]

Arthur Viseltear and others have analyzed the subsequent struggles within the American Public Health Association over the proper scope of public health.[45] When the National Health Conference, convened in 1938 by President Roosevelt, recommended a national health program to promote both expanded public health and medical care services, an APHA Committee, chaired by Abel Wolman, applauded the proposal and suggested that state health departments carry out the task of planning, integrating, and coordinating services. The Wagner Bill, submitted to Congress in 1939, was to provide enabling legislation to allow states to expand the provision of health and medical services.

Within the APHA, however, opinion was sharply divided. The more conservative public health officers, led by Haven Emerson, then professor of public health administration at Columbia University, opposed the proposed involvement of the federal government in medical care or any blurring of the traditional division between preventive and curative services. Abel Wolman, as president of the American Public Health Association, supported the Wagner Act, while also stressing the importance of the states' role in implementing the proposed national health program. The debate continued within the APHA between "progressives" who wanted public health and medical care services to be provided in a single, unified system and "conservatives" who wanted to leave well enough alone: to confine public health to its traditional preventive activities and categorical programs, while leaving medical care to the clinicians.[46]

These debates reflected divergent political philosophies and different attitudes toward the whole economic and political principles of the New Deal. Increasingly, the progressives in public health looked to the federal government for public health legislation and a broader scope of activity, while those favoring traditional practice looked to state and local health departments. An inability at the national level to implement the proposed national health program resulted in a continuing division between these two approaches. When federal programs were finally implemented to provide medical care for specific populations, they bypassed state health departments and created new administrative structures at the local level. The failure to create a national health program was thus also the missed opportunity to integrate preventive and curative services, to close the gap between public health and medicine. As Wilson G. Smillie and many others have noted, preventive services could not effectively be incorporated into medical practice unless there was some change in the system of payment for medical services in the United States.[47]

Internationally, primary care programs tried to integrate preventive and curative services, but the medical model of curative care continued to dominate.[48] In the United States, public health and medicine continued to take separate paths. Schools of public health increasingly oriented themselves toward the new federal initiatives and became more involved in national and international health policy, paying less attention to the activities and problems of local health departments. The medical schools remained largely unruffled by these debates and divisions; they continued to develop ever more sophisticated scientific research, to provide the basis for more effective diagnostic and therapeutic tools, and to give lip service to the need for prevention.

Public health education and medical education thus continued on largely separate tracks. In theory, public health and medical education could well be provided together; in practice, the two thrived best apart. Public health took pride in its separate identity by noting the deficiencies of individual private practice and the limitations of the medical gaze on the individual body; it cultivated a broader (and possibly subversive) view of whole populations. Patterns of health and disease were mapped onto whole communities, not limited to individual tissue cultures. The new and different kind of knowledge thus produced was now gaining some social recognition, and even financial support from the new federal health research establishment. Public health was distinctly separate from medicine and at times aggressively independent. At Johns Hopkins, the single street separating the School of Hygiene and the School of Medicine still marked a great divide: Wolfe Street was often called "the widest street in Baltimore," and only a few brave souls crossed this boundary on a regular basis.

Yet, even as public health remained separate from medicine, they were also irrevocably, inescapably linked. As we have seen, public health education had been conceived on the medical model, and leadership positions were still largely reserved for physicians. The Hopkins school was oriented toward the education of physicians: the M.D. degree was required for admission to the Dr.P.H. and M.P.H. programs, and these degrees in turn guaranteed access to significant public health positions. The core of the curriculum was also heavily weighted toward basic biomedical knowledge, with some extension to applied fields.

The concept that professionals other than physicians could specialize in public health was only slowly accepted. Until Abel Wolman arrived to challenge this medical chauvinism, few engineers could be seen at the School of Hygiene; sanitary engineering classes were treated as dull but necessary obligations, requiring excursions to the foreign territory of the School of Engineering on the other side of town. Public health nurses were virtually ignored. Vaguely regarded as a form of vocational training not deserving of serious intellectual effort, public health nursing was left to others. The doctors were thought of as the leaders, researchers, and teachers of public health; the nurses as their patient and faithful assistants. Nurses were thus only slowly and reluctantly admitted to the M.P.H. and Dr.P.H. programs. Gradually, the engineers and nurses were followed by others, and the doors of public health were opened wider to admit lawyers, economists, sociologists, and even the occasional anthropologist or historian.

Besides a similarity in their primary orientation to physicians, the School of Hygiene also shared many fundamental values with the School of Medicine. Perhaps most important was their shared emphasis on research. Critics complained that the School of Hygiene was too exclusively focused on research and paid too little attention to practical education and community service, just as critics of the School of Medicine complained that it favored medical research over medical care.[49] L. E. Burney summarized the complaints about public health education: "If it's any consolation, they are similar to those of medical and other graduate schools. You are becoming institutes of research—teaching is subordinate to research."[50] As was the School of Medicine, the School of Hygiene was unapologetic about its research orientation; both believed scientific research to be their central purpose and felt that critics had simply failed to understand the nature of the enterprise. Much of the research conducted at the School of Hygiene was also compatible with medical school interests: it tended to focus on the study of biological organisms rather than the social context of disease. Despite the dual vision of public health, incorporating both biological and social determinants of health and disease, the school was heavily weighted toward the investigation of the biological components of this equation. These components were investigated often in the laboratories on both sides of Wolfe Street, and less often, in the surrounding streets and neighborhoods.

Although the focus of research at the School of Hygiene and other schools of public health continued to broaden in later years, their foundations in biological and biomedical research continued to exert a strong influence. Advocates of a more social orientation to public health education continued to argue the importance of the social and political sciences, law, economics, and popular health education:

The basic sciences of public health are not anatomy, etc., but statistics, sociology, economics, political science, nutrition, sanitary engineering, management, ecology, etc. . . . Their major places of learning are not at laboratory benches or bedsides, but in communities, urban and rural, and at local, intermediate, and at central levels. Of course, there are also certain biological aspects to public health but its central goals and its daily tasks are social.[51]

After World War II, the School of Hygiene moved into new and expanded areas of public health concern including the social sciences, engineering, and environmental health sciences, chronic diseases, and the organization of medical care. This, however, was a new and different period of expansion, to be discussed in a subsequent volume. By 1939, these issues were only on the horizon, and had not yet had any significant impact on the curriculum.

In 1916, when the plan of public health education was originally outlined, as we have seen, there were three possible approaches to public health: the social, the engineering, and the biomedical. Public health education could have been organized around any of these; at Hopkins, at least in its early years, the biomedical orientation overwhelmed the engineering or environmental approach, and the social and political sciences were almost completely ignored. Welch and Howell's original plan for the school had suggested a balance between the pathological and physiological divisions. To organize the curriculum in this fashion meant a break with the dominant conception of public health as concerned only with the control of infectious diseases; it meant a reaching out into largely unknown and unexplored territory—the physiology of health. As we have seen, this exploration was partially successful.

The study of health, as opposed to the study of disease, had a long struggle to find a firm intellectual and institutional basis. As previously discussed, the department of physiological hygiene under Howell was oriented toward studies of health rather than disease. Although it tried to take a broad, environmental view of public health, it could not immediately articulate a comprehensive research program based on this alternative conception. By the depression era, although Anna Baetjer was able to organize and maintain a program on occupational health, the department had become a casualty of restricted funds.

McCollum's experimental studies of nutrition constituted a much more immediately successful route toward developing a physiology of health. Here, research in the laboratory constituted a direct link between the larger social, economic, and environmental issues and the improvement of the public's health. In McCollum's case, the difficulty of introducing a new approach to public health may be measured by the fact that local health departments and the medical profession paid little attention to the new knowledge of nutrition. Instead, it reached the country as a whole through the medium of popular education, domestic science departments, and mass circulation women's magazines.

In general, the Hopkins School of Hygiene had an ambivalent relationship toward the practice of public health on a local level, and this ambivalence tended to be well justified. The school's problems with local health departments could be illustrated by its relations with the Baltimore City Health Department: strained and rather distant in the 1920s, and coming closer only in the 1930s, thanks to a Hopkins-trained commissioner of health and a generous Rockefeller grant to facilitate their cooperation. The Eastern Health District, whatever its problems, was successful in bringing together the research-oriented School of Hygiene with the City Health Department's interest in the direct organization and provision of services on the local level. The departments of epidemiology, biostatistics, and public health administration were thus directly connected to local community health problems, especially in the 1930s and 1940s. Later, the interests of the school and the city again became more distant. Population health surveys using statistical methods developed techniques for sampling large populations rather than comprehensive studies of a single community. Telephone surveys replaced the door-to-door calls of the visiting nurse, and graduate students spent their time developing questionnaires and computing statistical correlations rather than flooding the neighborhood to ask questions about venereal disease, tuberculosis, or mental hygiene. The City Health Department, on the whole, was relieved: the task of running their services could sometimes be much easier without the constant questions, even interference, of faculty and students. Here, too, the School of Hygiene followed a trend to increased involvement in national and international programs rather than in local city activities.

Although the focus and form of public health education continually changed, we can freeze this process in time and say that by 1939 the "Hopkins model" of public health education meant a concentration on the biomedical sciences, supplemented by sophisticated attention to statistical and epidemiological methods. The School of Hygiene produced highly trained health officers and prepared researchers and teachers to staff other schools of public health; its influence was spread around the globe by the training of international students from many nations. It provided a powerful focus on the epidemiology and control of specific diseases: in the early years, especially the infectious and parasitic diseases; in later years, the chronic diseases.

The economic and political crisis of the depression and the New Deal had helped to institutionalize public health both on a local and national scale. New interests and new funding had stimulated the development of "applied" public health into such areas as the creation of child health, mental hygiene, and venereal disease programs. Later, as these fields developed, public health expanded its efforts into environmental and industrial health, maternal and child health, mental health, population dynamics and family planning, international health services, the organization of medical care, the economics and management of medical institutions, and the control of medical costs. The social sciences and health education eventually found a role in the curriculum, and overall, the basic sciences were balanced by more emphasis on the social application of services. These developments, however, were built on the basic foundation established from 1916 to 1939; these were modifications rather than transformations of the original plan of Wickliffe Rose and William Henry Welch.

In general, the emphasis of the original Welch-Rose report on research actually helped the schools of public health to expand their focus beyond the boundaries of public health departments, thereby adding new areas to the curriculum. Public health education outgrew the traditional definitions of public health and prepared students for a wide variety of careers in federal and state governments, international agencies, academia, and health and social welfare institutions. The initial insistence of the Welch-Rose report on creating an independent status for schools of public health also meant that these schools need not remain closely wedded to the medical model or subordinated to the demands of the medical curriculum. Instead, schools of public health could be free to continue defining and redefining their purpose and activities in response to political and economic pressures and newly perceived health needs.

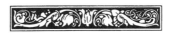

Notes

The main manuscript sources used for this study are the Alan Mason Chesney Medical Archives of the Johns Hopkins Medical Institutions, Baltimore, Maryland (hereafter AMCMA) and the Rockefeller Foundation Archives of the Rockefeller Archive Center, Pocantico Hills, North Tarrytown, New York (hereafter RFA).

Chapter 1   Toward a New Profession of Public Health

1. Charles E. Rosenberg, *The Cholera Years: The United States in 1832, 1849, and 1866* (Chicago: University of Chicago Press, 1962).
2. Robert H. Wiebe, *The Search for Order, 1877–1920* (New York: Hill & Wang, 1967).
3. J. H. Powell, *Bring Out Your Dead: The Great Plague of Yellow Fever in Philadelphia in 1793* (Philadelphia: University of Pennsylvania Press, 1949).
4. See, for example, Erwin Ackerknecht, "Anticontagionism between 1821 and 1867," *Bulletin of the History of Medicine* 22 (1948): 562–93.
5. Baltimore City Ordinance 11, approved April 7, 1797, as cited in William T. Howard, *Public Health Administration and the Natural History of Disease in Baltimore, Maryland, 1797–1920* (Washington, D.C.: Carnegie Institution, 1924), p. 50.
6. During epidemics, the clergy led days of fasting and prayer. In Baltimore, in 1819, they claimed success in turning the wind to a northwesterly direction, thus saving much of the city from a threatened epidemic of yellow fever. See Howard, *Public Health Administration*, p. 87.
7. G. W. Adams, *Doctors in Blue* (New York: Henry Schuman, 1952). According to contemporary accounts, the main causes of death were "typho-malaria" (perhaps a combination of typhoid fever and malaria), camp diarrhea, and "camp measles"; scurvy, acute respiratory diseases, venereal diseases, rheumatism, and epidemic jaundice were also widespread in army encampments. See, J. J. Woodward, *Chief Camp Diseases of the United States Armies* (Philadelphia: J. B. Lippincott Co., 1863).
8. *Proceedings and Debates of the Third National Quarantine and Sanitary Conference* (New York: Edward Jones, 1859), pp. 179–80.
9. R. G. Patterson, *Historical Directory of State Health Departments in the United States of America* (Ohio Public Health Association, 1939).

10. S. W. Abbott, *The Past and Present Conditions of Public Hygiene and State Medicine in the United States* (Boston: Wright & Potter, 1900).

11. For a complete history of the founding of the National Institute of Health from its beginnings in this one-room bacteriological laboratory, see Victoria A. Harden, *Inventing the NIH: Federal Biomedical Research Policy, 1887–1937* (Baltimore: Johns Hopkins University Press, 1986).

12. John Blake, *Public Health in the Town of Boston, 1630–1822* (Cambridge: Harvard University Press, 1959); Barbara Rosenkrantz, *Public Health and the State: Changing Views in Massachusetts, 1842–1936* (Cambridge: Harvard University Press, 1972); John Duffy, *A History of Public Health in New York City, 1625–1866* (New York: Russell Sage Foundation, 1968); John Duffy, *A History of Public Health in New York City, 1866–1966* (New York: Russell Sage Foundation, 1974); Stuart Galishoff, *Safeguarding the Public Health: Newark, 1895–1918* (Westport, Conn.: Greenwood Press, 1975); Judith Walzer Leavitt, *The Healthiest City: Milwaukee and the Politics of Health Reform* (Princeton: Princeton University Press, 1982).

13. Charles-E. A. Winslow, *The Life of Hermann M. Biggs: Physician and Statesman of the Public Health* (Philadelphia: Lea & Febiger, 1929); E. O. Jordan, G. C. Whipple, C.-E. A. Winslow, *A Pioneer of Public Health: William Thompson Sedgwick* (New Haven: Yale University Press, 1924); James H. Cassedy, *Charles V. Chapin and the Public Health Movement* (Cambridge: Harvard University Press, 1962); Rosenkrantz, *Public Health and the State.*

14. Charles E. Rosenberg and Carroll S. Rosenberg, "Pietism and the Origins of the American Public Health Movement," *Journal of the History of Medicine and Allied Sciences* 23 (1968): 16–35; Richard H. Shryock, "The Early American Public Health Movement," *American Journal of Public Health* 27 (1937): 965–71.

15. Barbara Rosenkrantz, "Cart before Horse: Theory, Practice, and Professional Image in American Public Health," *Journal of the History of Medicine and Allied Sciences* 29 (1974): 57.

16. Stephen Smith, "The History of Public Health, 1871–1921," in Mazyck P. Ravenel, ed., *A Half Century of Public Health* (New York: American Public Health Association, 1921), pp. 1–12; Mazyck P. Ravenel, "The American Public Health Association: Past, Present, Future," in ibid., pp. 13–55.

17. See Mary P. Ryan, *Womanhood in America: From Colonial Times to the Present* (New York: Franklin Watts, 1975), pp. 225–34.

18. The American Red Cross had been formed in 1882, the National Tuberculosis Association in 1904, the American Social Hygiene Association in 1905, the National Committee for Mental Hygiene in 1909, and the American Society for the Control of Cancer in 1919. See Wilson G. Smillie, *Public Health: Its Promise for the Future* (New York: Macmillan Co., 1955), pp. 450–58.

19. Robert H. Wiebe, *The Search for Order, 1877–1920* (New York: Hill & Wang, 1967); Samuel P. Hays, "The Politics of Reform in Municipal Government in the Progressive Era," in Samuel P. Hays, *American Political History as Social Analysis* (Knoxville: University of Tennessee Press, 1980), pp. 205–32; Samuel P. Hays, *Conservation and the Gospel of Efficiency: The Progressive Conservation Movement, 1890–1918* (Boston: Beacon Press, 1968); Daniel T. Rogers, "In Search of Progressivism," *Reviews in American History* 10 (1982): 115–32.

20. William Henry Welch, "Sanitation in Relation to the Poor," an address to the Sanitation Organization Society of Baltimore, November 1892, in *Papers and Addresses by William Henry Welch*, vol. 3 (Baltimore: Johns Hopkins Press, 1920), p. 598.

21. For a classic statement of this argument, see Max von Pettenkofer, *The Value of Health to a City*, translated with an introduction by Henry E. Sigerist (Baltimore: Johns Hopkins Press, 1941), pp. 15–52.

22. Welch, "Sanitation in Relation to the Poor," p. 596.

23. Charles Chapin, "Pleasures and Hopes of the Health Officer," in Clarence L. Scamman, ed., *Papers of Charles V. Chapin, M.D.: Review of Public Health Realities* (New York: Commonwealth Fund, 1934), p. 11.

24. Thomas M. Rotch, "The Position and Work of the American Pediatric Society toward Public Questions," *Transactions of the American Pediatric Society* 21 (1909): 12.

25. Charles Chapin, "How Shall We Spend the Health Appropriation?" in *Papers of Charles V. Chapin, M.D.*, pp. 28–35.

26. Martin J. Schiesl, *The Politics of Efficiency: Municipal Administration and Reform in America, 1880–1920* (Berkeley and Los Angeles: University of California Press, 1980).

27. William T. Sedgwick, "Scientists and Technicians in the Public Service," as cited in Jordan, Whipple, Winslow, *A Pioneer of Public Health*, pp. 133–34.

28. George M. Sternberg, "Sanitary Lessons of the War," in George M. Sternberg, *Sanitary Lessons of the War and Other Papers* (Washington, D.C.: Byron S. Adams, 1912), p. 2; see also, Graham A. Cosmas, *An Army for Empire: The United States Army in the Spanish-American War* (Columbia: University of Missouri Press, 1971).

29. Howard A. Kelly, *Walter Reed and Yellow Fever* (Baltimore: Medical Standard Book Co., 1906).

30. Sternberg, "Sanitary Problems Connected with the Construction of the Isthmian Canal," in *Sanitary Lessons of the War and Other Papers*, pp. 39–40.

31. Raymond B. Fosdick, *Adventure in Giving: The Story of the General Education Board* (New York: Harper & Row, 1962), pp. 57–58.

32. For the Rockefeller Sanitary Commission, see John Ettling, *The Germ of Laziness: Rockefeller Philanthropy and Public Health in the New South* (Cambridge: Harvard University Press, 1981).

33. Wickliffe Rose, *First Annual Report of the Administrative Secretary of the Rockefeller Sanitary Commission* (1910), p. 4, as cited in Raymond B. Fosdick, *The Story of the Rockefeller Foundation* (New York: Harper & Brothers, 1952), p. 33.

34. Ettling, *The Germ of Laziness*, pp. 220–21.

35. George Rosen, "The Committee of One Hundred on National Health and the Campaign for a National Health Department, 1906–1912," *American Journal of Public Health* 62 (1972): 261–63; Alan I. Marcus, "Disease Prevention in America: From a Local to a National Outlook, 1880–1910," *Bulletin of the History of Medicine* 53 (1979): 184–203.

36. Irving Fisher, *A Report on National Vitality, Its Wastes and Conservation*, Bulletin 30, Committee of One Hundred on National Health (Washington, D.C.: Government Printing Office, 1909).

37. For a detailed history of the Public Health Service, see Ralph C.

Williams, *The United States Public Health Service, 1798–1950* (Washington, D.C.: Government Printing Office, 1951).

38. For Sedgwick's rather lyrical view of bacteriology, see William T. Sedgwick, "The Origin, Scope, and Significance of Bacteriology," *Science* 13 (1901): 121–28.

39. As cited in Jordan, Whipple, Winslow, *A Pioneer of Public Health*, p. 57.

40. Charles V. Chapin, *Municipal Sanitation in the United States* (Providence, R.I.: Snow & Farnham, 1901).

41. Charles V. Chapin, *The Sources and Modes of Infection* (New York: John Wiley & Sons, 1910).

42. Hibbert Winslow Hill, *The New Public Health* (New York: Macmillan Co., 1916).

43. Ibid., p. 69.

44. Ibid., pp. 19–20.

45. Ibid., pp. 134–35.

46. J. Scott MacNutt, *A Manual for Health Officers* (New York: John Wiley & Sons, 1915), p. 85.

47. Charles-Edward A. Winslow, "The Untilled Fields of Public Health," *Science* 51 (1920): 23; see also, C.-E. A. Winslow, *The Evolution and Significance of the Modern Public Health Campaign* (New Haven: Yale University Press, 1923).

48. See Barbara Sicherman, *Alice Hamilton: A Life in Letters* (Cambridge: Harvard University Press, 1984), pp. 153–83.

49. Milton Terris, ed., *Goldberger on Pellagra* (Baton Rouge: Louisiana State University Press, 1964). See esp. Joseph Goldberger and Edgar Sydenstricker, "Pellagra in the Mississippi Flood Area," pp. 271–91.

50. For a detailed examination of this point in the case of tuberculosis, see Bonnie Kantor, "The New Scientific Public Health Movement: A Case Study of Tuberculosis in Baltimore, Maryland, 1900–1910" (D.Sc. diss., School of Hygiene and Public Health, Johns Hopkins University, 1985).

51. It is difficult to be confident about mortality rates in the United States before 1900, when the death registration areas began regular reporting. The evidence suggests that mortality rates between 1850 and 1880 remained relatively constant, with wide annual variations depending on the presence of epidemics. In the 1880s the mortality rates began to decline, and continued this decline, with minor fluctuations, throughout the period from 1890 to 1915. The major component of the decline was in infant mortality, especially mortality rates from the infectious diseases and infant diarrhea. This pattern is consistent with the thesis that the extension of municipal water systems and the filtration of water supplies played a major role in the decline in mortality. The pasteurization of milk was probably also an important contributing factor. On the estimation of mortality rates for the period, see Edward Meeker, "The Improving Health of the United States, 1850–1915," *Explorations in Economic History* 9 (1972): 353–73; Michael R. Haines, "The Use of Model Life Tables to Estimate Mortality for the United States in the Late Nineteenth Century," *Demography* 16 (1979): 289–312; Frederick L. Hoffman, "The General Death Rate of Large American Cities, 1871–1904," *Publications of the American Statistical Association* 10 (1906–1907): 1–75. For a general discussion of the social impact of infectious diseases, see John Duffy, "Social Impact of Disease in

the Late Nineteenth Century," *Bulletin of the New York Academy of Medicine* 47 (1971): 797–811.

52. Nelson M. Blake, *Water for the Cities* (Syracuse: Syracuse University Press, 1956).

53. Ellis Sylvester Chesbrough, who had learned his skills from army and railroad engineers, created the first comprehensive sewerage system for Chicago in the 1860s; Colonel George E. Waring, an energetic engineer-publicist, created a sewerage system for Memphis in the 1880s and then became consultant to sewerage construction projects all over the United States. See Louis P. Cain, "Raising and Watering a City: Ellis Sylvester Chesbrough and Chicago's First Sanitation System," *Technology and Culture* 13 (1972): 353–72; James H. Cassedy, "The Flamboyant Colonel Waring: An Anticontagionist Holds the American Stage in the Age of Pasteur and Koch," *Bulletin of the History of Medicine* 36 (1962): 163–76.

54. Joel A. Tarr, Terry Yosie, and James McCurley, "Disputes over Water Quality Policy: Professional Cultures in Conflict, 1900–1917," *American Journal of Public Health* 70 (1980): 427–35. In Baltimore, the resistance of the oyster fishermen, who saw their livelihood threatened by municipal and industrial wastes, eventually forced the City Council to install the most advanced sewage treatment system then available. See John Capper, Garrett Power, and Frank Shivers, Jr., *Chesapeake Waters: Pollution, Public Health, and Public Opinion, 1607–1972* (Centreville, Md.: Tidewater Publishers, 1983), pp. 85–105.

55. Joel A. Tarr, "The Separate vs. Combined Sewer Problem: A Case Study in Urban Technology Design Choice," *Journal of Urban History* 5 (1979): 308–99.

56. Morris Knowles, "Public Health Service Not a Medical Monopoly," *American Journal of Public Health* 3 (1913): 111–22.

57. Chester H. Wells, "A Plea for More General Recognition of the Qualifications of the Sanitary Engineer for Administrative Public Health Work," *American Journal of Public Health* 3 (1913): 123–25; Knowles, "Public Health Service Not a Medical Monopoly," pp. 119–22; H. P. Eddy, C.-E. A. Winslow, W. H. Sanders, "Discussion," *American Journal of Public Health* 3 (1913): 126–30.

58. William T. Sedgwick, Cincinnati address, as cited in *A Pioneer of Public Health*, pp. 76–77.

Chapter 2   Competition for the First School of Hygiene and Public Health

1. The story of the planning of public health education in the offices of the General Education Board and in the leading American medical schools has been partially told; Greer Williams has written the most complete account to date, which, though perceptive, is also a defense of Harvard as having been ill treated in the competition for the first endowed school of public health. See Greer Williams, "Schools of Public Health: Their Doing and Undoing," *Milbank Memorial Fund Quarterly* 54 (1976): 489–527. Though much that Williams says is true, the main point of uncovering this history is not to trade punches in the old academic battle between Harvard and Hopkins, but to understand better how these decisions have influenced the subsequent shape of public health education.

2. Abraham Flexner, *I Remember: An Autobiography* (New York: Simon & Schuster, 1960), p. 134.

3. Raymond Fosdick, *Chronicle of a Generation: An Autobiography* (New York: Harper & Brothers, 1958), p. 255.

4. John A. Ferrell, "Public Health Work as a Career," address delivered at the commencement exercises of the Medical College of Virginia, Richmond, June 2, 1914, pp. 1–2, Record Group (RG) 1.1, Ser. 200, RFA.

5. George Rosen, "The Efficiency Criterion of Medical Care, 1900–1920," *Bulletin of the History of Medicine* 50 (1976): 28–44.

6. For the efficiency argument applied to public health, see, for example, Max von Pettenkofer, *The Value of Health to a City: Two Popular Lectures,* translated, with an introduction, by Henry E. Sigerist (Baltimore: Johns Hopkins Press, 1941), pp. 15–52; Hibbert Winslow Hill, *The New Public Health* (New York: Macmillan Co., 1920); Alice Hamilton and Gertrude Seymour, "The New Public Health," *Survey* 37 (1916): 166–69, and *Survey* 38 (1916): 59–62.

7. Abraham Flexner, *Medical Education in the United States and Canada* (New York: Carnegie Foundation for the Advancement of Teaching, Bulletin no. 4, 1910); for Flexner's interest in preventive medicine, see Gert H. Brieger, "The Flexner Report: Revised or Revisited?" *Medical Heritage* (1985): 25–34.

8. Executive Committee of the International Health Commission, Minutes, 12/19/13, RG 1.1, Ser. 200, RFA.

9. Much of the credit for the Rockefeller involvement in public health and medicine must go to Frederick Gates, the original architect of the Rockefeller philanthropies. For Gates's role, see esp. E. Richard Brown, *Rockefeller Medicine Men* (Berkeley and Los Angeles: University of California Press, 1979) and John Ettling, *The Germ of Laziness: Rockefeller Philanthropy and Public Health in the New South* (Cambridge: Harvard University Press, 1981).

10. The relationships among the Rockefeller trusts are fully explained in Raymond B. Fosdick, *The Story of the Rockefeller Foundation* (New York: Harper & Brothers, 1952).

11. On Biggs's efforts in reorganizing the New York State Department of Health, see C.-E. A. Winslow, *The Life of Hermann M. Biggs: Physician and Statesman of the Public Health* (Philadelphia: Lea & Febiger, 1929), pp. 251–88.

12. Charles-Edward A. Winslow, "The Place of Public Health in a University" *Science* 62 (October 16, 1925): 335.

13. *University of Pennsylvania: Courses in Public Health, 1909–1910* (Philadelphia: University of Pennsylvania, 1909). This catalog gives a complete listing of courses leading to the diploma in public health.

14. A. C. Abbott to A. Flexner, 1/20/14, RG 1.1, Ser. 200, RFA.

15. E. P. Lyon to A. Flexner, 1/12/14, RG 1.1, Ser. 200, RFA.

16. William W. Ford to A. Flexner, 1/16/14, RG 1.1, Ser. 200, RFA.

17. Milton J. Rosenau, "Courses and Degrees in Public Health Work," *Journal of the American Medical Association* 64 (1915): 794–96. See also "Catalogue and Announcement," *Circular of the School for Health Officers* 1 (1913): 1–41.

18. Jean Curran, *Founders of the Harvard School of Public Health, with Biographical Notes, 1909–1946* (New York: Josiah Macy, Jr., Foundation, 1970), p. 7.

19. Milton J. Rosenau, *Preventive Medicine and Hygiene* (New York: D. Appleton & Co., 1913).

20. Milton J. Rosenau, "Memorandum" and letter to Abraham Flexner, 1/9/14, RG 1.1, Ser. 200, RFA.

21. J. D. Greene to A. Flexner, 2/20/14, RG 1.1, Ser. 200, RFA.

22. Wickliffe Rose, "First Report to the General Education Board: Training for Public Health Service," 5/28/14, RG 1.1, Ser. 200, RFA.

23. Ibid., p. 3.

24. E. Seligman to A. Flexner, 10/10/14, RG 1.1, Ser. 200, RFA.

25. Ibid., p. 2.

26. W. Rose to A. Flexner, 10/7/14, RG 1.1, Ser. 200, RFA.

27. Daniel Fox, "Abraham Flexner's Unpublished Report: Foundations and Medical Education, 1909–1928" *Bulletin of the History of Medicine* 54 (1980): 475–96.

28. H. Biggs to A. Flexner, 10/15/14, RG 1.1, Ser. 200, RFA.

29. Transcript of General Education Board meeting, 10/16/14, p. 21, RG 1.1, Ser. 200, RFA.

30. William H. Welch, transcript of General Education Board meeting, 10/16/14, p. 30.

31. Frederick T. Gates, transcript of General Education Board meeting, 10/16/14, p. 47.

32. William H. Welch, transcript of General Education Board meeting, 10/16/14, p. 47.

33. Williams, "Schools of Public Health," pp. 489–527.

34. Hermann Biggs, transcript of General Education Board meeting, 10/16/14, p. 48, RG 1.1, Ser. 200, RFA.

35. Theobald Smith, transcript of General Education Board meeting, 10/16/14, p. 85.

36. A. C. Abbott to A. Flexner, 10/10/14, RG 1.1, Ser. 200, RFA.

37. John Duffy, "The American Medical Profession and Public Health: From Support to Ambivalence," *Bulletin of the History of Medicine* 53 (1979): 1–22.

38. Ibid., p. 21.

39. Transcript of General Education Board Meeting, 10/16/14, pp. 67–68, RG 1.1, Ser. 200, RFA.

40. Wickliffe Rose, transcript of General Education Board meeting, 10/16/14, pp. 71–80.

41. Abraham Flexner, transcript of General Education Board meeting, 10/16/14, p. 110.

42. G. Whipple to A. Flexner, 10/22/14, RG 1.1, Ser. 200, RFA.

43. G. Blumer to A. Flexner, 10/28/14, 11/2/14, RG 1.1, Ser. 200, RFA.

44. E. Seligman to A. Flexner, 12/23/14, RG 1.1, Ser. 200, RFA.

45. E. H. Lewinski-Corwin to E. Seligman, 9/15/14, RG 1.1, Ser. 200, RFA.

46. W. Rose to A. Flexner, 10/27/14, RG 1.1, Ser. 200, RFA.

47. W. Rose to A. Flexner, 3/17/15, RG 1.1, Ser. 200, RFA.

48. Wickliffe Rose, "School of Public Health," May 1915, p. 10, RG 1.1, Ser. 200, RFA.

49. Ibid., p. 11.

Notes to Pages 32–40 / 243

50. For a description of these programs, see Raymond B. Fosdick, *Adventure in Giving: The Story of the General Education Board* (New York: Harper & Row, 1962); and Abraham Flexner, *The General Education Board, 1902–1914* (New York: General Education Board, 1915), pp. 18–70.

51. W. Rose, "School of Public Health," May 1915, p. 8, Archives, RG 1.1, Ser. 200, RFA.

52. Welch based this summary on a report prepared for him by William W. Ford of Johns Hopkins Medical School, "The Present Status and the Future of Hygiene or Public Health in America," March 1915, Box 118, William Henry Welch Papers, AMCMA.

53. William H. Welch, "Institute of Hygiene," 5/27/15, p. 11, RG 1.1, Ser. 200, RFA.

54. Ibid., p. 8.

55. Rose, "School of Public Health," May 1915, p. 12, RG 1.1, Ser. 200, RFA.

56. Welch, "Institute of Hygiene," 5/27/15, p. 8, RG 1.1, Ser. 200, RFA.

57. Curran, *Founders of the Harvard School of Public Health*, pp. 9–12.

58. G. Whipple to A. Flexner, 6/12/15, RG 1.1, Ser. 200, RFA.

59. C.-E. A. Winslow to A. Flexner, 6/14/15, RG 1.1, Ser. 200, RFA.

60. W. Park to A. Flexner, 7/3/15, RG 1.1, Ser. 200, RFA.

61. F. A. Cleveland to A. Flexner, 6/11/15, RG 1.1, Ser. 200, RFA.

62. E. Seligman to A. Flexner, 8/10/15, p. 4, RG 1.1, Ser. 200, RFA.

63. A. Flexner to E. Seligman, 9/13/15, RG 1.1, Ser. 200, RFA.

64. A. Flexner to W. Rose, 9/13/15, RG 1.1, Ser. 200, RFA.

65. W. Rose to A. Flexner, 9/16/15, RG 1.1, Ser. 200, RFA.

66. A. Flexner, "Memorandum on the Subject of Public Health," 6/13/15, RG 1.1, Ser. 200, RFA.

67. J. D. Greene to A. Flexner, 6/29/15, RG 1.1, Ser. 200, RFA.

68. A. Flexner to J. D. Greene, 7/1/15, RG 1.1, Ser. 200, RFA.

69. For the details of this story, see Curran, *Founders of the Harvard School of Public Health*, pp. 12–14.

70. W. Buttrick, A. Flexner, J. D. Greene, and W. Rose, "Memorandum Regarding Request to Endow School for Tropical Medicine at Harvard University," 6/29/15, RG 1.1, Ser. 200, RFA.

71. A. L. Lowell to the Trustees of the Rockefeller Foundation, 6/30/15, RG 1.1, Ser. 200, RFA.

72. W. Rose to A. Flexner, 9/16/15, RG 1.1, Ser. 200, RFA.

73. For the historical context of the struggle for control of hospital appointments, see Charles E. Rosenberg, "Inward Vision and Outward Glance: The Shaping of the American Hospital, 1880–1914," *Bulletin of the History of Medicine* 53 (1979): 346–91.

74. "Conference on Public Health: Harvard University, Cambridge, Massachusetts, November 3–5, 1915," p. 54, RG 1.1, Ser. 200, RFA.

75. Ibid., p. 1.

76. A. Flexner to W. T. Sedgwick, 11/6/15, RG 1.1, Ser. 200, RFA.

77. W. T. Sedgwick to A. Flexner, 11/8/15, RG 1.1, Ser. 200, RFA.

78. W. T. Sedgwick to A. Flexner, 11/26/15, p. 4, RG 1.1, Ser. 200, RFA.

79. Ibid., p. 3.

80. "Conference held at the University of Pennsylvania, November 8, 1915," p. 19, RG 1.1, Ser. 200, RFA.

81. "Conference at Columbia University, November 13 and 15, 1915," pp. 4–6, RG 1.1, Ser. 200, RFA.

82. N. M. Butler to E. Seligman, 11/22/15, RG 1.1, Ser. 200, RFA.

83. "Conference at Columbia University, November 13 and 15, 1915," pp. 44–46, RG 1.1, Ser. 200, RFA.

84. "Meeting at Johns Hopkins Hospital to Consider the Establishment of a School of Hygiene in Connection with the Johns Hopkins University," January 18, 1916, p. 23, RG 1.1, Ser. 200, RFA.

85. Ibid., p. 32.

86. Ibid., pp. 62, 63, 71.

87. Ibid., p. 84.

88. Ibid., p. 98.

89. Ibid., p. 141.

90. Ibid., p. 152.

91. William Howard later became the author of *Public Health Administration and the Natural History of Disease in Baltimore, Maryland* (Washington, D.C.: Carnegie Institution, 1924).

92. "Meeting at Johns Hopkins Hospital to Consider the Establishment of a School of Hygiene in Connection with the Johns Hopkins University," January 18, 1916, p. 158, RG 1.1, Ser. 200, RFA.

93. Ibid., p. 179.

94. Ibid., p. 184.

95. "Institute of Public Health: Final Report of the General Education Board," 1/26/16, pp. 9, 10, RG 1.1, Ser. 200, RFA.

96. Williams, "Schools of Public Health," pp. 489–527.

97. C. W. Eliot to A. Flexner, 2/1/16, RG 1.1, Ser. 200, RFA.

98. A. Flexner to C. W. Eliot, 2/11/16, RG 1.1, Ser. 200, RFA.

99. C. W. Eliot to A. Flexner, 2/18/16, RG 1.1, Ser. 200, RFA.

100. C. W. Eliot to J. D. Greene, 3/29/16, RG 1.1, Ser. 200, RFA.

101. J. D. Greene to C. W. Eliot, 3/30/16, RG 1.1, Ser. 200, RFA.

102. Abraham Flexner, *I Remember*, p. 197.

103. "Conference at Columbia University, November 13 and 15, 1915," p. 77, RG 1.1, Ser. 200, RFA.

104. Ibid., p. 45.

105. Johns Hopkins was the first medical school to move toward the full-time system for both clinical and preclinical departments. By 1916, the full-time system had been instituted for three of the major clinical departments: medicine, surgery, and pediatrics. See Thomas B. Turner, *Heritage of Excellence: The Johns Hopkins Medical Institutions, 1914–1947*, esp. pp. 3–22 (Baltimore: Johns Hopkins University Press, 1974); Alan M. Chesney, *The Johns Hopkins Hospital and the Johns Hopkins University School of Medicine*, vol. 3 (Baltimore: Johns Hopkins Press, 1963).

106. Jerome D. Greene, "Institute of Hygiene: Report of the Sub-Committee," 5/24/16, RG 1.1, Ser. 200, RFA.

107. F. Goodnow to J. D. Greene, 5/1/15, RG 1.1, Ser. 200, RFA.

108. W. W. Ford, "Plan of Organization of a School of Hygiene," May 1916, pp. 1–2, Box 118, William Henry Welch Papers, AMCMA.'

109. W. H. Welch and W. H. Howell, "Suggestions Regarding Organization of an Institute or School of Hygiene," Box 118, William Henry Welch Papers, AMCMA.

110. Ford, "Plan of Organization of a School of Hygiene: Schedule," Box 118, William Henry Welch Papers, AMCMA.

111. Ibid., pp. 12–13.

112. W. H. Welch and W. H. Howell, "Suggestions Regarding Organization of an Institute or School of Hygiene," p. 1, Box 118, William Henry Welch Papers, AMCMA.

113. W. H. Welch to S. Flexner, 5/21/16, RG 1.1, Ser. 200, RFA.

114. W. H. Welch, "The School of Hygiene and Public Health at the Johns Hopkins University. Report made at the Commencement Exercises of the Johns Hopkins University, June 13, 1916," Box 118, William Henry Welch Papers, AMCMA.

115. J. H. Preston to W. H. Welch, 6/13/16, RG 1.1, Ser. 200, RFA.

116. W. H. Welch to J. D. Greene, 6/13/16, RG 1.1, Ser. 200, RFA.

117. J. D. Greene to W. H. Welch, 6/14/16, RG 1.1, Ser. 200, RFA.

Chapter 3 Working It Out: William Henry Welch and the Art of Negotiation

1. William H. Welch to Daniel C. Gilman, 12/18/16, pp. 3–4, Daniel C. Gilman Papers, Special Collections, Milton S. Eisenhower Library, Johns Hopkins University, Baltimore, Maryland.

2. F. P. Mall to A. Flexner, 1/13/17; A. Flexner to F. P. Mall, 1/20/17; A. Flexner to J. W. Williams, 2/19/17; RG 1.1, Ser. 200, RFA. Howell was reluctant to leave his professorship in the School of Medicine, but was persuaded to accept the new position in part by an increase in his salary from $5,000 to $7,500. On the establishment of faculty salaries at the new school, see William H. Welch to Simon Flexner, 6/12/16, RG 1.1, Ser. 200, RFA; Jerome D. Greene to William H. Welch, 6/13/16, RG 1.1, Ser. 200, RFA. J. Whitridge Williams, professor of obstetrics and gynecology at the Medical School, urged setting salaries higher than originally anticipated; he wrote to Abraham Flexner: "It would be unwise to give ordinary university salaries, and that much better work will be obtained were really living salaries paid. I would suggest $7,500 as the minimum." J. W. Williams to A. Flexner, 6/28/16, RG 1.1, Ser. 200, RFA.

3. S. Flexner to A. Flexner, 6/21/16, RG 1.1, Ser. 200, RFA.

4. William H. Welch, "Memorandum on the Establishment of a School of Hygiene and Public Health by the Rockefeller Foundation," 6/14/16, RG 1.1, Ser. 200, RFA.

5. For more details on Welch's activities during this period, see Simon Flexner and James Thomas Flexner, *William Henry Welch and the Heroic Age of American Medicine* (New York: Viking Press, 1941), pp. 365–83. See also, W. H. Welch to G. E. Vincent, 12/16/17, RG 1.1, Ser. 200, RFA.

6. Abraham Flexner to President Goodnow, 2/15/17, RG 1.1, Ser. 200, RFA.

7. Advisory Board Minutes of the School of Hygiene and Public Health, vol. 1, note signed by Louise Durham, 2/23/17, p. 1, AMCMA.

8. George E. Vincent had been president of the University of Minnesota before becoming president of the Rockefeller Foundation in 1917. Alan Gregg (of the Rockefeller Foundation) described him as "a genial and alert eagle, attentive, spirited and eager." Raymond B. Fosdick, *The Story of the Rockefeller Foundation, 1913–1950* (New York: Harper & Brothers, 1952), p. 29.

9. G. E. Vincent to S. Flexner, 3/14/17, RG 1.1, Ser. 200, RFA.
10. Ibid., p. 1.
11. G. E. Vincent to W. H. Welch, 3/14/17, RG 1.1, Ser. 200, RFA.
12. See Harry J. Prebluda, "The Newer Knowledge of Animal Nutrition: The Road Ahead," in *Agricultural and Food Chemistry, Past, Present, and Future,* edited by Roy Tetaniski, (Westport, Conn.: USDA, AVI Publishing Company, 1978), pp. 352–66. Prebluda notes that administrators at the University of Wisconsin did not at first publicize McCollum's experiments for fear of criticism; the Wisconsin legislature was not expected to look kindly on the expenditure of taxpayers' money to provide room and board for farmers' pests.
13. Elmer V. McCollum, *From Kansas Farm Boy to Scientist: The Autobiography of Elmer Verner McCollum* (Lawrence: University of Kansas Press, 1964), p. 157.
14. Ibid., p. 140.
15. E. V. McCollum to W. H. Howell, 3/8/17, 5/23/17, Office of the Dean's Correspondence, RG 3, Ser. A, Box 4, AMCMA; F. Goodnow to G. E. Vincent, 5/14/17, RG 1.1, Ser. 200, RFA.
16. W. H. Welch to G. E. Vincent, 11/4/17, RG 1.1, Ser. 200, RFA.
17. R. Pearl to W. H. Howell, 12/31/17, Office of the Dean's Correspondence, RG 3, Ser. A, Box 5, AMCMA.
18. Robert Hegner, *An Introduction to Zoology* (New York: Macmillan Co., 1910); *College Zoology* (New York: Macmillan Co., 1912). The latter text went through seven editions from 1912 to 1959.
19. G. E. Vincent, "Memorandum of Suggestions: School of Hygiene and Public Health," 11/1/17; see also W. H. Welch to G. E. Vincent, 10/30/18, RG 1.1, Ser. 200, RFA.
20. G. E. Vincent to W. H. Welch, 6/4/18, RG 1.1, Ser. 200, RFA.
21. W. H. Welch, "Memorandum: School of Hygiene and Public Health," 11/8/17, p. 2, RG 1.1, Ser. 200, RFA.
22. Charles-Edward A. Winslow, *The Evolution and Significance of the Modern Public Health Campaign* (New Haven: Yale University Press, 1923), pp. 53, 55. See also, C. E. A. Winslow, "Public Health at the Crossroads," *American Journal of Public Health,* 16 (1926): 1075–85.
23. William Henry Welch, *Public Health in Theory and Practice: An Historical Review* (New Haven: Yale University Press, 1925), pp. 42–43, 47. Yale University Press published this version of Welch's Sedgwick Memorial Lecture, delivered at MIT in January 1924, in the same series as Winslow's book. Both accounts of the history of public health clearly display their authors' different biases and Welch's account reads as though it were a direct response to Winslow.
24. Sir Arthur Newsholme, *The Last Thirty Years in Public Health: Recollections and Reflections on My Official and Post-Official Life* (London: George Allen & Unwin, 1936), p. 403.
25. As cited in C. E. A. Winslow, *The Life of Hermann M. Biggs* (Philadelphia: Lea & Febiger, 1929), p. 202.
26. Allen Weir Freeman, *Five Million Patients: The Professional Life of a Health Officer* (New York: Scribner, 1946).
27. H. S. Cumming to W. H. Frost, 7/12/22; W. H. Frost to H. S. Cumming, 7/16/22; H. S. Cumming to W. H. Frost, 6/20/29; letters from the personal files of Susan Frost Parrish, Washington, D.C.

28. For details of Simon's life and career, see A. McGehee Harvey, "Pioneer American Virologist: Charles E. Simon," *Johns Hopkins Medical Journal* 142 (1978): 161–86.

29. Charles E. Simon, *An Introduction to the Study of Infection and Immunity* (Philadelphia: Lea & Febiger, 1912); *Human Infection Carriers: Their Significance, Recognition, and Management* (Philadelphia: Lea & Febiger, 1919).

30. Freeman, *Five Million Patients*, pp. 240–41.

31. "Memorandum on a System of Foreign Scholarships and Fellowships in connection with the Proposed School of Public Health," 1/24/16, pp. 2–3, RG 1.1, Ser. 200, RFA.

32. Wickliffe Rose, "Conference with Dr. W. H. Howell at Baltimore, January 5, 1918," RG 1.1, Ser. 200, RFA.

33. For degree requirements, see Advisory Board Minutes of the School of Hygiene and Public Health, 12/21/17, AMCMA.

34. Ibid., 1/30/19.

35. Ibid., 3/13/19.

36. A. Flexner to W. H. Howell, 4/23/17, RG 1.1, Ser. 200, RFA.

37. George Huntington Williams, personal interview, 10/29/80.

38. Marie L. Koch, personal interview, 3/11/80.

39. In March 1922, the Public Health Service held a major conference in Washington on "The Future of Public Health in the United States and the Education of Sanitarians." The conference speakers included a long list of distinguished names such as Hugh Cumming, the surgeon general, George Vincent, president of the Rockefeller Foundation, and Welch, Winslow, Ferrell, Whipple, Rosenau, and Biggs. The issues were the familiar ones: What kinds of public health workers were needed? How could more and better health officers be recruited? How should they be trained? Conference speakers emphasized the need to persuade more medical students to enter the field and to improve the salaries and job security of public health officers to make the career more attractive. Existing training for health officers was said to be deficient in some of the newer areas of public health concern (and this criticism was presumably directed largely at the Hopkins school), specifically mental hygiene, child hygiene, economic and social aspects of public health, physical education, industrial hygiene, and public health education. Equal attention was given to the problem of how to improve the training of public health officers already employed. Most agreed that the best method was the short intensive postgraduate course lasting about six weeks in connection with a school of public health. Other suggestions included summer schools, special institutes, bulletins and periodicals, and consultant services to local health departments from the Public Health Service. Most conference members felt that the training of existing health officers had been sadly neglected and should receive much more attention; they were also concerned that the grand schemes for training future sanitarians would create "impractical idealists." "In our zeal for training the super-sanitarian of the future," said C. E. Turner, "we must not forget to train practical useful health officers" (p. 7). Said W. F. Draper: "There is a danger of an over-production of sanitary supermen" (p. 7). Several emphasized the need for a grounding in political and practical realities and suggested that students should be taught more about history, politics, and local government rather than simply scientific theory. In regard to the specialties that ought to be recognized within public health, the highest number of votes (in order) went to

sanitary engineering, administration, epidemiology, child hygiene, laboratory work, vital statistics, industrial hygiene, public health education, and public health nursing. Fields mentioned but considered less important included mental hygiene, social hygiene, school hygiene, nutrition, and physical education. "The Opinions of Conference Members on Certain Unanswered Questions Arising from the Conference, March 14 and 15, on the Future of Public Health in the United States and the Education of Sanitarians," Box 10, William Henry Welch Papers, AMCMA.

40. John A. Ferrell, "Measures for Increasing the Supply of Competent Health Officers," *Journal of the American Medical Association* 77 (1921): 513–16. This calculation referred only to medical directors; it did not include the public health nurses, sanitary inspectors, technical and clerical employees also needed by health departments.

41. George Whipple, "The Education of Health Officers," *Public Health Reports* (1921): Reprint no. 703, p. 4.

42. C.-E. A. Winslow, "The Untilled Fields of Public Health," *Modern Medicine* 2 (1920): 8.

43. As reported by Lee K. Frankel in "The Plans and Purposes of the American Public Health Association," *Modern Medicine* 1 (1919): 329.

44. Advisory Board Minutes of the School of Hygiene and Public Health, 4/28/21, vol. 1, p. 117, AMCMA.

45. Report on the School of Hygiene and Public Health, 1920–21, 11/9/21, pp. 3–4, RG 1.1, Ser. 200, RFA.

46. W. H. Howell to G. E. Vincent, 10/30/18; G. E. Vincent to W. H. Welch, 1/20/19; F. F. Russell to W. H. Welch, 5/23/21; W. H. Welch to F. F. Russell, 5/27/21; R. W. Hegner to J. A. Ferrell, 10/19/21; J. A. Ferrell to R. W. Hegner, 11/5/21; all letters in RG 1.1, Ser. 200, RFA.

47. B. M. Rhetta to W. H. Welch, 2/12/22, Box 11, Office of the Dean's Correspondence, 1922–23, AMCMA.

48. W. H. Howell to B. M. Rhetta, 3/3/22, Box 11, Office of the Dean's Correspondence, 1922–23, AMCMA.

49. F. F. Russell to W. H. Welch, 5/23/21; W. H. Welch to F. F. Russell, 5/27/21; RG 1.1, Ser. 200, RFA.

50. E. V. McCollum to W. H. Welch, 3/13/20; W. H. Welch to E. V. McCollum, 3/15/20; Box 4, Office of the Dean's Correspondence, AMCMA; Report of the School of Hygiene and Public Health, 1920–21, pp. 12–13, RG 1.1, Ser. 200, RFA; see also E. V. McCollum to G. E. Vincent, 12/23/19, RG 1.1, Ser. 200, RFA.

51. William Howell, "Preliminary Announcement of the School of Hygiene and Public Health of the Johns Hopkins University," n.d., Box 117, William Henry Welch Papers, AMCMA.

52. Advisory Board Minutes of the School of Hygiene and Public Health, 2/12/18, vol. 1, AMCMA.

53. E. Harris to W. H. Howell, 8/25/21; W. H. Howell to E. Harris, 8/27/21; Box 7, Office of the Dean's Correspondence, 1922–23, AMCMA.

54. G. E. Vincent, "Memorandum of Suggestions: School of Hygiene and Public Health," 11/1/17, RG 1.1, Ser. 200, RFA.

55. This lecture series was funded by a portion of a bequest left to the Johns Hopkins Medical Institutions by Captain Joseph De Lamar. The De Lamar Fund also supported the *American Journal of Hygiene*.

56. Advisory Board Minutes of the School of Hygiene and Public Health, Special Meeting, 10/20/19, vol. 1, p. 56, AMCMA.

57. Ibid., pp. 56–57.

58. G. E. Vincent to W. H. Welch, 1/24/19, RG 1.1, Ser. 200, RFA.

59. Advisory Board Minutes of the School of Hygiene and Public Health, 10/20/19, vol. 1, p. 57, AMCMA.

60. Ibid., p. 57.

61. Raymond Pearl, "Report of Committee on Plans for the Development of the School of Hygiene," 11/4/19, p. 2, Box 117, William Henry Welch Papers, AMCMA.

62. William Welch, "School of Hygiene and Public Health, Johns Hopkins University: Plans of Organization and Development," 11/15/19, p. 4, RG 1.1, Ser. 200, RFA.

63. Ibid., p. 10.

64. Committee for the Study of Nursing Education, *Nursing and Nursing Education in the United States* (New York: Macmillan Co., 1923).

65. Raymond Pearl, "Plans for the Development of the Department of Biometry and Vital Statistics," November 1919, Box 117, William Henry Welch Papers, AMCMA.

66. Ibid., p. 1.

67. See, for example, Sir Arthur Newsholme, *Fifty Years in Public Health: A Personal Narrative with Comments* (London: George Allen & Unwin, 1935).

68. William Cort and Robert Hegner, "Plans for the Expansion of the Department of Protozoology and Medical Zoology," November 1919, p. 4, RG 1.1, Ser. 200, RFA.

69. Minutes of the Executive Board of the Rockefeller Foundation, 2/25/20, RG 1.1, Ser. 200, RFA.

70. W. H. Welch to E. R. Embree, 11/20/19, RG 1.1, Ser. 200, RFA.

71. Simon Flexner, "Notes Regarding Budget, School of Hygiene and Public Health, Johns Hopkins, January 1 to July 1, 1920," p. 4, RG 1.1, Ser. 200, RFA.

72. Minutes of the Executive Board of the Rockefeller Foundation, 2/25/20, RG 1.1, Ser. 200, RFA.

73. "Memorandum Regarding an Additional Building near the Medical School," 5/15/16, p. 2, RG 1.1, Ser. 200, RFA.

74. J. D. Greene to F. Goodnow, 6/13/16, RG 1.1, Ser. 200, RFA.

75. R. B. Keyser to J. D. Greene, 7/6/17, RG 1.1, Ser. 200, RFA.

76. J. D. Greene to R. B. Keyser, 7/12/17, RG 1.1, Ser. 200, RFA.

77. F. Goodnow to G. E. Vincent, 10/10/17, RG 1.1, Ser. 200, RFA.

78. G. E. Vincent to F. Goodnow, 7/15/18, RG 1.1, Ser. 200, RFA.

79. Ibid., p. 2.

80. G. E. Vincent to F. Goodnow, 8/6/18, 8/26/18, 8/28/18, 9/10/18; F. Goodnow to G. E. Vincent, 9/18/18; RG 1.1, Ser. 200, RFA.

81. Telegram, R. Pearl to G. E. Vincent, 11/28/19, RG 1.1, Ser. 200, RFA.

82. "Special Memorandum: Conference on Proposed New Building for School of Hygiene and Public Health at Johns Hopkins," 1/26/22, RG 1.1, Ser. 200, RFA.

83. "Special Memorandum: Baltimore, Maryland Club, February 1, 1922: Memorandum of Conference Concerning Proposed New Building for School of Hygiene, Johns Hopkins," RG 1.1, Ser. 200, RFA.

84. Minutes of the Executive Board of the Rockefeller Foundation, 2/24/22, p.4, RG 1.1, Ser. 200, RFA.
85. *Baltimore Sun*, March 1, 1922.
86. Ibid., p. 1.
87. William H. Welch, "The Endowment of the School of Hygiene and Public Health by the Rockefeller Foundation," March 1922, p. 3, Box 118, William Henry Welch Papers, AMCMA.
88. *British Medical Journal*, November 20 and 27, 1926; as cited in *Annual Reports to the President of the University*, 1926–1927, p. 2, RG 1.1, Ser. 200, RFA.
89. "New Johns Hopkins Building Will Be Dedicated Tomorrow," *Baltimore Sun*, October 21, 1926.
90. Andrew Balfour, "Hygiene as a World Force," *Science* 54 (November 12, 1926): 439–66.

Chapter 4   Creating New Disciplines, I: The Pathology of Disease

1. Wickliffe Rose, Record of Interviews, 12/1/26, RG 1.1, Ser. 200, RFA.
2. Calista Causey, personal interview, 12/14/84.
3. Johns Hopkins University School of Hygiene and Public Health, *Catalogue and Announcement for 1924–25* (Baltimore: Johns Hopkins Press, 1924), p. 43.
4. Robert W. Hegner, *Big Fleas Have Little Fleas, or, Who's Who among the Protozoa* (Baltimore: Williams & Wilkins, 1938), p. 85.
5. Ibid., pp. 87–98, 149–57.
6. For an informative and detailed account of Hegner's views and the research program in medical zoology, see Lloyd E. Rozeboom, "Medical Zoology at the Johns Hopkins University School of Hygiene and Public Health: A History (Somewhat Anecdotal)," manuscript, 1986.
7. Gerald Winfield, personal interview, 9/10/82.
8. For the range of student research, see issues of *American Journal of Hygiene* for the 1920s.
9. Robert W. Hegner and William Cort, *Diagnosis of Protozoa and Worms Parasitic in Man* (Baltimore: Johns Hopkins University School of Hygiene and Public Health, 1921); Robert W. Hegner, William Cort, and Francis Root, *Outlines of Medical Zoology: With Special Reference to Laboratory and Field Diagnosis* (New York: Macmillan Co., 1923); Robert Hegner, *College Zoology* (New York: Macmillan Co., 1926–1949), 5 editions; Hegner, *Big Fleas Have Little Fleas.*
10. Hegner, *Big Fleas Have Little Fleas*, p. 29.
11. Ibid.
12. Robert Hegner, "The Relation of Medical Zoology to Public Health Problems," *Journal of the American Medical Association* 75 (1920): 1607–10.
13. Wickliffe Rose to R. Hegner, 1/10/21, RG 1, Ser. 100, RFA.
14. R. Hegner to F. F. Russell, 4/7/23, RG 1, Ser. 100, RFA.
15. Robert Hegner, "Medical Research in Malaria," *Southern Medical Journal* 18 (1925): 438–40.
16. R. Hegner to F. F. Russell, 10/22/25; F. F. Russell to R. Hegner, 10/29/25; RG 1, Ser. 100, RFA.
17. Most of these studies were published in the *American Journal of Hygiene*; a

summary of some of the research is given in Robert W. Hegner, "Studies on Bird Malaria," *Southern Medical Journal* 19 (1926): 377–81.

18. Robert Hegner, "Parasite Reactions to Host Modifications," *Journal of Parasitology* 23 (1937): 1–12.

19. Hegner, *Big Fleas Have Little Fleas*, pp. 257–65.

20. William Cort, "Autobiography," manuscript, distributed on the occasion of his eightieth birthday, April 28, 1967, p. 5.

21. Norman R. Stoll, "Remarks at the Dedication of the Cort Library, School of Hygiene and Public Health, The Johns Hopkins University, 21 May, 1954," address, pp. 1–2, RG 1.1, Ser. 200, RFA.

22. W. W. Cort to W. H. Welch, 6/30/21, RG 1, Ser. 100, RFA.

23. W. Rose to W. W. Cort, 11/29/21, RG 1, Ser. 100, RFA.

24. See William W. Cort, "Investigations on the Control of Hookworm Disease: 1. General Introduction," *American Journal of Hygiene* 1 (1921): 557–68. This was the first of a series of forty-five papers on hookworm investigations at Johns Hopkins and contains an outline of the possible problems of field research. For an account of field studies, see note 26 below, and William Cort, *Studies on Hookworm, Ascaris, and Trichuris in Panama, Embodying the Results of the Researches of an Expedition to the Republic of Panama* (Baltimore: American Journal of Hygiene, Monographic Ser. no. 9, 1929).

25. W. W. Cort to G. Williams, interview, n.d., RG 3, Ser. 908, RFA.

26. William Cort, *Researches on Hookworm in China, Embodying the Results of the Work of the China Hookworm Commission* (Baltimore: American Journal of Hygiene, Monographic Ser. no. 7, 1926).

27. Cort, "Autobiography," p. 6.

28. W. W. Cort to F. F. Russell, 3/31/31, RG 1, Ser. 100, RFA.

29. C. W. Stiles to W. W. Cort, 5/18/31, p. 1, RG 1, Ser. 100, RFA.

30. "Brought Parasites from China in Own Stomach for Study," *Baltimore Sun*, November 20, 1925.

31. Ibid.

32. See, for example, correspondence between Francis Root, H. H. Howard, and George Bevier about Colombian mosquitoes, G. Bevier to H. H. Howard, 5/12/34; F. M. Root to H. H. Howard, 5/18/34, 6/8/34; RG 1.1, Ser. 311, RFA.

33. W. H. Welch to F. F. Russell, 3/12/24, RG 5, Ser. 1, RFA.

34. Francis Root, "Dragon Flies Collected at Point Pelee and Pelee Island Ontario, in the Summers of 1910 and 1911," *Canadian Entomologist* (1912): 208–9.

35. Robert Hegner, "Francis Metcalf Root," *Journal of Parasitology* 21 (1935): 67–69.

36. Advisory Board Minutes of the School of Hygiene and Public Health, 10/25/34, AMCMA.

37. Lloyd Rozeboom, personal interview, 11/12/82.

38. William H. Howell, "Charles E. Simon," *American Journal of Hygiene* 8 (1928): i–vi.

39. For a contemporary description of the field, see Charles E. Simon, "The Filterable Viruses," *Physiological Reviews* 2 (1923): 483–508.

40. Charles E. Simon, "Report of the Work of the Division of Filterable Viruses of the Department of Medical Zoology, 1922–23," Box 52, William Henry Welch Papers, AMCMA.

41. Charles E. Simon to William H. Welch, 3/21/23, Box 52, William Henry Welch Papers, AMCMA.

42. "An Appreciation," n.d., Box 117, William Henry Welch Papers, AMCMA.

43. Howard Andervont, as cited in A. McGehee Harvey, "Pioneer American Virologist: Charles E. Simon," Johns Hopkins Medical Journal 142 (1978): 175. Harvey's article provides an excellent summary of Simon's work.

44. Ibid., p. 176.

45. William W. Ford, Bacteriology (New York: Harper & Brothers, 1939). For a sketch of Ford's career, see Alan Chesney, The Johns Hopkins Hospital and the Johns Hopkins School of Medicine, vol. 2, (Baltimore: Johns Hopkins Press, 1958), pp. 360–61.

46. For a brief description of this research, see W. W. Ford to W. H. Howell, 3/24/24; "Report to Committee raising new endowment fund for University," March 1924, Box 16, Office of the Dean's Correspondence, AMCMA.

47. See catalogs of the School of Hygiene and Public Health, 1918–30, for the listing and content of courses, Interdepartmental Library, School of Hygiene and Public Health, Baltimore, Maryland.

48. Samuel Damon, Food Infections and Food Intoxifications (Baltimore: Williams & Wilkins, 1928).

49. For a brief description of the research cited, see annual reports to the president of the university, 1922–28, RG 1.1, Ser. 200, RFA.

50. Simon Flexner and James Flexner, William Henry Welch and the Heroic Age of American Medicine (New York: Viking Press, 1941), pp. 207–10.

51. Carroll Gideon Bull, "How Bacteria Are Destroyed in the Living Organism," Half-Century Fund Reports, March 1924, RG 3, Series A, Box 16, Office of the Dean's Correspondence, AMCMA.

52. Ibid., p. 2.

53. See Noel R. Rose, Felix Milgrom, and Carrel J. Van Oss, "Scope and Background of Immunity," in Principles of Immunity, edited by Rose, Milgrom, and Van Oss (New York: Macmillan Co., 1973), pp. 3–13.

54. Roscoe Hyde, "Complement-deficient Guinea Pig Serum," Journal of Immunology 8 (1924): 267–86; "The Activation of Complement-deficient Guinea Pig Serum with Heated Sera," American Journal of Hygiene 4 (1924): 62–64; "Complement-deficient Guinea Pig Serum and Supersensitized Corpuscles," American Journal of Hygiene 4 (1924): 65–66; "Corpuscle Counts on Normal and Complement-deficient Guinea Pigs," American Journal of Hygiene 4 (1924): 169–87; "The Activation of Yeast-absorbed Complement with Heated Sera," American Journal of Hygiene 5 (1925): 145–48; R. R. Hyde and Elizabeth Parsons, "Quantitative Interdependence of Sensitizer and Complement in Hemolysis," American Journal of Hygiene 7 (1927): 11–21; R. R. Hyde, "The Complement Deficient Guinea Pig: A Study of an Inherited Biochemical Structure in Relation to a Toxic Immune Body," American Journal of Hygiene 7 (1927): 619–28; "The Complementing Properties of Blood Plasma," American Journal of Hygiene 8 (1928): 859–69.

55. See Sidney Raffel, "Fifty Years of Immunology," Annual Review of Microbiology 36 (1982): 1–26.

56. The School of Hygiene and Public Health of the Johns Hopkins University (Baltimore: American Journal of Hygiene, Monographic Ser. no. 6, 1926), p. 39.

57. Marie L. Koch, personal interview, 11/3/81.

1. W. H. Howell, "The Relations of Public Health and Medicine," Trimble lecture, given at 129th annual session, April 26–28, 1927, Baltimore, *Transactions of the Medical and Chirurgical Faculty of the State of Maryland* (1925–29), p. 220.

2. W. H. Howell, "Scientific Research and Public Health," *Transactions of the Royal Canadian Institute* 13 (1921): 7–8.

3. W. H. Howell, "Hurry and Health," *Baltimore Health News* 12 (1934): 148–50.

4. W. H. Howell, "Scientific Research and Public Health," p. 8.

5. W. H. Howell to G. W. McCoy, 2/7/21, Box 5, Office of the Dean's Correspondence, 1917–21, AMCMA.

6. R. A. Spaeth, "The Prevention of Fatigue in Manufacturing Industries," *Journal of Industrial Hygiene* 1 (1919): 435.

7. An authority on radiation and lighting, Clark acted as consultant to several corporations, including the Baltimore Gas and Electric Company. See Janet Howell Clark, *Lighting in Relation to Public Health* (Baltimore: Williams & Wilkins, 1924); Elizabeth Fee and Anne Clark Rodman, "Janet Howell Clark: Physiologist and Biophysicist (1889–1969)," *The Physiologist* 28 (1985): 397–400.

8. W. H. Howell, "Department of Physiological Hygiene," *American Journal of Hygiene* 6 (1926): 40.

9. W. H. Howell, *Textbook of Physiology for Medical Students and Physicians* (Philadelphia: W. B. Saunders Co., fourteen editions, 1905 to 1940).

10. Janet H. Clark, "Biography: William Henry Howell," manuscript, n.d., p. 23, written by Howell's daughter, private collection of Anne C. Rodman, Aberdeen, Maryland. For a warm appreciation of Howell by his well-known student A. M. Baetjer, see "An Anniversary Tribute to the Memory of the Late William Henry Howell, Faculty of Hygiene and Public Health," *Bulletin of the Johns Hopkins Hospital* 109 (1961): 16.

11. "Will Test Effects of Climate on Body: Hopkins Scientists Plan Experiments with New Apparatus," *Baltimore Sun*, April 14, 1926.

12. W. H. Howell, "Humidity and Comfort," *Science* 73 (1931): 453–55.

13. For more details on Howell's work and ideas, see Elizabeth Fee, "William Henry Howell: Physiologist and Philosopher of Health," *American Journal of Epidemiology* 119 (1984): 293–300. Howell's physiological contributions are more fully described in J. Erlanger, "William Henry Howell," *Biographical Memoirs of the National Academy of Sciences* 26 (Washington, D.C.: National Academy of Sciences, 1951): 153–80. Howell continued his physiological research long after his formal retirement from the School of Hygiene.

14. "Elmer Verner McCollum: Dr. Vitamin," *Time* 58 (September 24, 1951): 93–94.

15. E. Neige Todhunter, "Rats in Nutrition Research," *Chemistry* 52 (1979): 8–11.

16. Ernestine McCollum, personal interview, 5/25/82.

17. E. V. McCollum, Nina Simmonds, H. T. Parsons, P. G. Shipley, and E. A. Park, "Studies on Experimental Rickets: I. The Production of Rachitis and Similar Diseases in the Rat by Deficient Diets," *Journal of Biological Chemistry* 45 (1921): 333–34; "Studies on Experimental Rickets: 2. The Effect

of Cod Liver Oil Administered to Rats with Experimental Rickets," *Journal of Biological Chemistry* 45 (1921): 343–48.

18. P. G. Shipley, E. A. Park, E. V. McCollum, and Nina Simmonds, "The Function of the Organic Factor as Exemplified by Cod Liver Oil," *Transactions of the American Pediatric Society* 33 (1921): 131–39.

19. P. G. Shipley, E. A. Park, G. F. Powers, E. V. McCollum, and Nina Simmonds, "The Prevention of the Development of Rickets in Rats by Sun-light," *Proceedings of the Society for Experimental Biology and Medicine* 19 (1921): 43–47.

20. E. V. McCollum, Nina Simmonds, J. Ernestine Becker, and P. G. Shipley, "Studies on Experimental Rickets: 21. An Experimental Demon-stration of the Existence of a Vitamin Which Promotes Calcium Deposition," *Journal of Biological Chemistry* 53 (1922): 304.

21. The stages of this research are described in twenty-three papers on "Studies on Experimental Rickets," published in the *Journal of Biological Chemistry* in 1921 and 1922. See also Harry G. Day, "Elmer Verner McCollum: A Biographical Memoir," *Biographical Memoirs* 45 (1974): 263–335, National Academy of Sciences, Washington, D.C.

22. "Magnesium for Philanthropists," *New York Times* (October 30, 1934): 18. See also Harry G. Day, "E. V. McCollum and Magnesium in Nutrition," *Trends in Biochemical Sciences* 7 (1982): 112–13.

23. Harry G. Day, "On Making Stannous Fluoride Useful," *The Review* 17 (Indiana University, 1975): 1–17.

24. Harry G. Day, "Nutrition and Dental Health," *Chemistry* 52 (1979): 12–15.

25. Harry J. Prebluda, personal communication, 10/3/86; see also Donald K. Tressler, *The Memoirs of Donald K. Tressler* (Westport, Conn.: Avi Publishing Co., 1976).

26. Elmer V. McCollum, *From Kansas Farm Boy to Scientist* (Lawrence: University of Kansas Press, 1964), p. 177. See also Agatha Rider, "Elmer Verner McCollum, 1879–1967," *Journal of Nutrition* 100 (1970): 3–10.

27. Johns Hopkins University Circular, School of Hygiene and Public Health, *Catalogue and Announcement for 1925–26* (Baltimore: Johns Hopkins Press, 1925), p. 38.

28. E. V. McCollum and Nina Simmonds, *Food, Nutrition, and Health* (Baltimore: Lord Baltimore Press, 1925); E. V. McCollum, *The Newer Knowl-edge of Nutrition* (New York: Macmillan Co., 1918).

29. *McCall's* magazine, September 1925, June 1928, July 1932, September 1937, and May 1946.

30. Franklin C. Bing and Harry J. Prebluda, "E. V. McCollum: Pathfinder in Nutrition Investigations and World Agriculture," *Agricultural History* 54 (1980): 157–66.

31. E. V. McCollum, *A History of Nutrition: The Sequence of Ideas in Nutrition Investigations* (Boston: Houghton Mifflin, 1957), p. 421.

32. For a more extensive account of early epidemiological methods, see C.-E. A. Winslow, Wilson G. Smillie, James A. Doull, and John E. Gordon, *The History of American Epidemiology* (St. Louis: C. V. Mosby, 1952).

33. Abraham Lilienfeld, "Wade Hampton Frost: Contributions to Epi-demiology and Public Health," *American Journal of Epidemiology* 117 (1983): 380.

34. W. H. Frost, "The Importance of Epidemiology as a Function of Health Departments," *Medical Officer* 29 (1923): 113–14.

35. W. H. Frost, "Epidemiology," *Papers of Wade Hampton Frost, M.D.: A Contribution to Epidemiological Method* (New York: Commonwealth Fund, 1941), p. 497.

36. Editorial, "Public Health Balloons," *American Journal of Public Health* 31 (1941): 990.

37. W. H. Frost, "Report to the Committee on Organization and Activities," November 8, 1919, p. 2, Box 118, William Henry Welch Papers, AMCMA.

38. W. H. Frost, "Epidemiology," *Nelson Loose Leaf System, Public Health—Preventive Medicine*, vol. 2 (New York: Nelson & Sons, 1927), p. 163. Reprinted in Kenneth F. Maxcy, ed., *Papers of Wade Hampton Frost, M.D.*, pp. 493–542.

39. W. H. Frost, "What Every Health Officer Should Know: Epidemiology," paper prepared for the American Public Health Association meeting, New York City, October 1937, pp. 1–2, manuscript in personal collection of Susan Frost Parrish, Washington, D.C.

40. Ibid., p. 5.

41. W. H. Frost, "Infection, Immunity, and Disease in the Epidemiology of Diphtheria, with Special Reference to Some Studies in Baltimore," *Journal of Preventive Medicine* 2 (1928): 325–43.

42. V. A. Van Volkenburgh and W. H. Frost, "Acute Minor Respiratory Diseases Prevailing in a Group of Families Residing in Baltimore, Maryland, 1928–1930; Prevalence, Distribution, and Clinical Description of Observed Cases," *American Journal of Hygiene* 17 (1933): 122–53.

43. W. H. Frost, "The Age Selection of Mortality from Tuberculosis in Successive Decades," *American Journal of Hygiene* 30 (1939): 91–96; Philip E. Sartwell, "The Contributions of Wade Hampton Frost," *American Journal of Epidemiology*, 104 (1976): 388; Lowell Reed also worked closely with Frost in developing the statistical methods used for analyzing epidemiological data. The two developed a mathematical model for simulating the progress of disease epidemics known as the "Reed-Frost epidemic theory." Although neither published the theory, it was widely discussed and became a strong influence on students and later model builders. See Philip E. Sartwell, "Memoir on the Reed-Frost Epidemic Theory," *American Journal of Epidemiology* 103 (1976): 138–40.

44. W. H. Frost, "Report to the Committee on Organization and Activities," November 8, 1919, p. 1, AMCMA.

45. For a description of this teaching method, see *American Journal of Hygiene* 6 (1926): 17–19.

46. Margaret Merrell, "The Reed-Frost Collaboration," *American Journal of Epidemiology* 104 (1976): 365.

47. Ernest Stebbins, personal interview, 10/12/81.

48. John A. Ferrell to W. H. Frost, 3/2/27, RG 1.1, Ser. 200, RFA.

49. John A. Ferrell, "Epidemiology in North America in the Past Twenty Years," *Supplement to the American Journal of Public Health* 32 (1942): 143–47.

50. Six months after his appointment at the school, for example, Pearl wrote: "The economic situation is becoming daily more impossible. I simply cannot live in decency and comfort on the salary I get. My wife must spend the

greater portion of her time in household drudgery because we cannot afford even the modestly necessary service. We would like to have more children, and I feel we would be doing some slight service at least to the nation if we did. But again the economic situation sternly forbids." (R. Pearl to W. H. Welch, 8/14/19, Box 45, Welch Correspondence, AMCMA). In the same letter, Pearl wrote that he had been offered a position as "head of the department of a large and developing oil company" and also "membership in one of the largest and wealthiest industrial companies in this country," both paying much more than his university salary.

51. Morton Kramer, personal interview, 6/23/82.

52. Merrell, "The Reed-Frost Collaboration," p. 369.

53. Ibid., p. 366.

54. John B. Grant, oral history, vol. 1, p. 104, RG 13, RFA.

55. The School of Hygiene and Public Health of the Johns Hopkins University, *American Journal of Hygiene* monographic ser. no. 6 (1926): 19–24.

56. Johns Hopkins University Circular, School of Hygiene and Public Health, *Catalogue and Announcement for 1922–23*, p. 60.

57. See chart in *American Journal of Hygiene* 6 (1926): 24.

58. Raymond Pearl and Lowell Reed, "On the Rate of Growth of the Population of the United States Since 1790 and Its Mathematical Representation," *Proceedings of the National Academy of Sciences* 6 (1920): 275–88. See also Lowell J. Reed, "Evolutionary Changes in the Seasonal Curve of the Birth Rates," *American Journal of Public Health* 15 (1925): 948–50.

59. Raymond Pearl, *Studies in Human Biology* (Baltimore: Williams & Wilkins, 1924), p. 585.

60. For a more complete history and analysis of the logistic curve, see Sharon Kingsland, "The Refractory Model: The Logistic Curve and the History of Population Ecology," *Quarterly Review of Biology* 57 (1982): 29–52.

61. Raymond Pearl, "A Plan for Research on the Biology of Life Duration and Extension," 3/25/24, p. 1, RG 1.1, Ser. 200, RFA.

62. Ibid., p. 2.

63. Raymond Pearl, "A Note on the Inheritance of the Duration of Life in Man," *American Journal of Hygiene* 2 (1922): 229–33.

64. Raymond Pearl, "Differential Fertility," *Quarterly Review of Biology* 2 (1927): 102–18.

65. Raymond Pearl, "Preliminary Account of an Investigation of Factors Influencing Longevity," *Journal of the American Medical Association* 82 (1924): 259–64.

66. See, for example, Raymond Pearl and Agnes Bacon, "Biometrical Studies in Pathology: I. The Quantitative Relations of Certain Viscera in Tuberculosis," *Johns Hopkins Hospital Reports* 21 (1922): 157–230.

67. Raymond Pearl, *The Biology of Death* (Philadelphia: J. B. Lippincott Co., 1922), p. 225.

68. Ibid., p. 226.

69. Raymond Pearl to Edwin Embree, 12/21/25, p. 2, RG 1.1, Ser. 200, RFA.

70. Ibid., p. 5.

71. Raymond Pearl, *Alcohol and Longevity* (New York: Knopf, 1926).

72. Thomas B. Turner, personal communication, 10/17/86.

73. The establishment of the Bureau of Contraceptive Advice and the

Baltimore Birth Control Clinic are described in the chapter on "The Community as Public Health Laboratory."

74. Raymond Pearl, "Foreword," *Human Biology* 1 (1929): 1.

75. Raymond Pearl, "Foreword," *Quarterly Review of Biology* 1 (1926): 1–3.

76. Raymond Pearl to George Vincent, 12/11/28, RG 1.1, Ser. 200, RFA; Raymond Pearl, A. C. Sutton, and W. T. Howard, "Experimental Treatment of Cancer with Tuberculin," *Lancet* 216 (1929): 1078–80.

77. Joseph Ames to Max Mason, 4/3/30, RG 1.1, Ser. 200, RFA.

78. Merrell, "The Reed-Frost Collaboration," pp. 364–69.

79. Ibid., p. 367.

80. Ibid., p. 365.

81. Morton Kramer, personal interview, 6/23/82. For more on Reed's views of the profession, see Lowell Reed, "Some Aspects of Multidisciplinary Professions," *American Journal of Public Health* 48 (1958): 3.

82. Margaret Merrell, personal interview, 11/16/81. Roger M. Herriott noted that one of Reed's papers was helpful to virologists in improving estimates of virus titration, and was universally adopted by them and others. See Lowell J. Reed and Hugo Muench, "A Simple Method of Estimating Fifty Per Cent Endpoints," *American Journal of Hygiene* 27 (1938): 493–97.

83. Allen Freeman, *Five Million Patients: The Professional Life of a Health Officer* (New York: Scribner, 1946), p. 238.

84. Ibid., pp. 237–38.

85. Ibid., p. 245.

86. The School of Hygiene and Public Health of the Johns Hopkins University, *American Journal of Hygiene* monographic ser. no. 6 (1926): 14.

87. Freeman, *Five Million Patients*, p. 259.

88. Ibid., pp. 275–76.

89. *Report of the Committee on Municipal Health Department Practice of the American Public Health Association*, Public Health Bulletin no. 136 (Washington, D.C.: Government Printing Office, 1923).

90. Freeman, *Five Million Patients*, p. 250.

91. Charles J. Tilden, "The Course in Civil Engineering," *Johns Hopkins Alumni Magazine* 2 (1914): 234–301, quote on p. 301.

92. Annual reports of the president of the Johns Hopkins University, 1920s, Hamburger Archives, Johns Hopkins University, Baltimore, Maryland.

93. "Urged Purified Water When Idea Seemed Over-Fastidious," *Baltimore Evening Sun*, November 21, 1933.

94. Abel Wolman, "Recent Trends in Public Health Engineering Practice," *American Journal of Public Health* 27 (1937): 44. For other statements of Wolman's views in the 1930s, see Abel Wolman, "The Public Health Engineer's Work," *American Journal of Public Health* 23 (1933): 329–32; Abel Wolman, "Changing Public Health Practices and Problems," *American Journal of Public Health* 27 (1937): 1029–35. For a brief review of Wolman's career, see Gina Maranto, "If You Want to Know about Water, Ask Abel Wolman," *Johns Hopkins Magazine* 33 (April 1982): 11–16.

95. *Abel Wolman: His Life and Philosophy*, an oral history by Walter Hollander, Jr. (Chapel Hill: Universal Printing and Publishing Co., 1981), p. 663; Abel Wolman, personal interview, 9/7/83; Maranto, "If You Want to Know about Water, Ask Abel Wolman," p. 13.

96. William Thompson Sedgwick, *Principles of Sanitary Science and the*

Public Health with Special Reference to the Causation and Prevention of Infectious Diseases (New York: Macmillan Co., 1902).

97. *Abel Wolman*, an oral history by Walter Hollander, Jr., p. 885.

98. Ibid., p. 673.

99. Ibid., p. 667.

100. For an eloquent statement of the continuing need on a global scale for environmental improvement, including safe water and sanitation, see Abel Wolman, "Give Health a Chance—with Healthy Surroundings," and "Discussion," *World Health Forum* 7 (1986): 107–13, 113–30.

Chapter 6   Surviving the Thirties

1. W. H. Welch to W. H. Howell, 3/25/25, Box 19, Office of the Dean's Correspondence, AMCMA.

2. Robert S. Morison, "The Foundation Interest," talk given at the fiftieth anniversary of the Institute of the History of Medicine, Johns Hopkins University, October 18, 1979.

3. Handwritten menu of Maryland dinner in honor of Dr. W. H. Welch, 12/20/26, AMCMA.

4. "Dr. Welch Declares Average Life Could Be Extended to 100 Years; Urges as Much Care of Human Bodies as of Autos," *Baltimore Sun*, January 20, 1927.

5. W. H. Welch to Hugh Young, as cited in Donald Fleming, *William H. Welch and the Rise of Modern Medicine* (Boston: Little, Brown & Co., 1954), p. 159.

6. See, for example, letter to Andrew Balfour, 6/14/27, Box 20, Office of the Dean's Correspondence, 1926–27, AMCMA.

7. Minutes of the Board of Trustees, 3/4/19, Hamburger Archives, Johns Hopkins University, Baltimore, Maryland.

8. School of Hygiene and Public Health, *Catalogue and Announcement*, 1920–21, Interdepartmental Library, School of Hygiene and Public Health, Baltimore, Maryland.

9. William H. Howell, "Explanatory Note," January 1929, Minutes of the Executive Committee, School of Hygiene, AMCMA.

10. G. Nuttall to W. H. Welch, 7/12/20, Box 43, William Henry Welch Papers, AMCMA.

11. W. H. Welch to C. E. Simon, 6/31/20, RG 3, Ser. A, Box 1, Office of the Dean's Correspondence, 1920–21, AMCMA.

12. A. W. Hedrich to W. H. Welch, 1/13/21, Box 26, William Henry Welch Papers, AMCMA.

13. Report to the president of the university, School of Hygiene and Public Health, 1926–27, p. 22, RG 1.1, Ser. 200, RFA. See also William J. Curtis, "Joseph De Lamar," *Johns Hopkins Hospital Bulletin* 34 (April 1923): 135–37.

14. William H. Welch, "Introduction," *American Journal of Hygiene* 1 (1921): iv.

15. McCollum's papers also appeared in a variety of other publications: *American Journal of Physiology, American Journal of Public Health, Proceedings of the American Philosophical Society, Journal of Agricultural Research, Journal of the American Medical Society, Bulletin of the Johns Hopkins Hospital,* and the *American Food Journal.* Howell also published fairly frequently in *Science* and the

Journal of the American Medical Association, among others. Pearl published with some regularity in *Science, The American Naturalist*, and the *Journal of the National Academy of Sciences*.

16. The few papers outside the dominant pattern of laboratory research on pathogenic organisms covered diverse topics: Raymond Pearl, "A Note on the Inheritance of Duration of Life in Man," *American Journal of Hygiene* 2 (1922): 229–33; G. H. Robinson, "Some Observations on a Case of Rat-Bite Fever," *American Journal of Hygiene* 2 (1922): 324; Robert Woodbury, "The Relation between Breast and Artificial Feeding and Infant Mortality," *American Journal of Hygiene* 2 (1922): 668–87.

17. Editorial, "Change in Name," *American Journal of Epidemiology* 81 (1965): 1.

18. Report to the president of the university for the School of Hygiene and Public Health, 1927–28, p. 32, RG 1.1, Ser. 200, RFA.

19. Report of the director of the School of Hygiene and Public Health, 1929–30, pp. 17–18, RG 1.1, Ser. 200, RFA.

20. W. H. Howell, "Report upon the Work of the School of Hygiene and Public Health during the Session of 1926–27," RG 1.1, Ser. 200, RFA.

21. Conversation with Wade Hampton Frost as cited in "Memorandum by Dr. Heiser re General Impressions, obtained from members of the Hopkins School's staff, on lack of interest of doctors in public health instruction," 2/1/27, p. 2, RG 1.1, Ser. 200, RFA.

22. Kenneth F. Maxcy to W. H. Howell, 2/11/27, RG 1.1, Ser. 200, RFA.

23. "Memorandum by Dr. Heiser," 2/1/27, p. 1.

24. "Memorandum: Summer Training of Undergraduate Medical Students," 12/10/35, RG 1.1, Ser. 200, RFA.

25. W. H. Howell, "Report to the president for School of Hygiene and Public Health, 1927–28," p. 36, RG 1.1, Ser. 200, RFA.

26. Ayodhya N. Das personal communication, 8/18/82.

27. "Memorandum, School of Hygiene and Public Health, Baltimore, June 14, 1922," p. 1, RG 1.1, Ser. 200, RFA.

28. Ibid., p. 2.

29. L. E. Burney, "Life of the School in 1931–32 from Perspective of a Student and Reflections on the Nature of My Education," 1983, School of Hygiene and Public Health.

30. Margaret Merrell, personal interview, 11/16/81.

31. Minutes of the Executive Board, 3/27/30, 3/24/33, AMCMA.

32. The remainder of the school's operating costs came from tuition fees, the De Lamar Fund, and various short-term fellowships and special grants.

33. The other members of the committee on physiology were Elmer McCollum, Robert Hegner, and William Ford; members of the committee on organization were Lowell Reed, Hegner, and Ford. See Advisory Board Minutes of the School of Hygiene and Public Health, 10/30/30, vol. 2, p. 365, AMCMA.

34. "Committee on Organization of the School," 12/2/30, Box 1, RG 2, Ser. C, AMCMA.

35. William H. Howell, Revision of Welch-Rose Report, "Institute of Hygiene," June 1918, p. 17, Subject Reference Files, AMCMA.

36. "Final Report, Committee on Organization of the School," 10/29/31, p. 2, Box 1, RG 2, Ser. C, AMCMA.

37. Ibid.

38. Ibid., p. 3.
39. "Duties of the Committee Designated to Survey Space," 11/9/31, Box 135, RG 3, Ser. A, Office of the Dean's Correspondence, AMCMA.
40. Committee on Organization, 3/10/31.
41. Ibid., 12/9/30.
42. Ibid.
43. Committee on Organization, First Progress Report, 2/16/31.
44. Ibid., 2/16/31.
45. Ibid., 3/3/31.
46. Ibid., Second Progress Report, 4/30/31.
47. Ibid., Final Report, 10/29/31, p. 5.
48. Committee on the Animal Farm, 2/25/32, Box 135, RG 3, Ser. A, Office of the Dean's Correspondence, AMCMA.
49. Minutes of the Advisory Board, 3/26/31, vol. 2, p. 381; Minutes of the Executive Board, 3/26/31, AMCMA.
50. "Report of the Committee on the Department of Physiology," 10/1/31, Box 135, RG 3, Ser. A, Office the Dean's Correspondence, AMCMA.
51. Ibid., p. 1.
52. Janet Clark was the author of the book *Lighting in Relation to Public Health* (Baltimore: Williams & Wilkins, 1924), and numerous research papers (currently on file at the American Physiological Society). Anna Baetjer's early research concerned the physiological effects of high temperature and humidity, the relationship of potassium and calcium salts to blood flow and heart rhythm, and the effects of blood plasma salts on muscle contraction.
53. Committee on Policy, 11/3/31, Box 135, RG 3, Ser. A, Office of the Dean's Correspondence, AMCMA.
54. Report of Committee on Policy, 5/26/32, Box 135, RG 3, Ser. A, Office of the Dean's Correspondence, AMCMA.
55. Ibid., p. 1.
56. Advisory Board Minutes of the School of Hygiene and Public Health, 10/29/31, 12/17/31, AMCMA.
57. Report of Committee on Policy, 1/18/33, Box 135, RG 3, Ser. A, Office of the Dean's Correspondence, AMCMA.
58. Advisory Board Minutes of the School of Hygiene and Public Health, 1/31/35; 2/28/35; 12/17/36, AMCMA.
59. For a more complete account of Janet Clark's life and work see Elizabeth Fee and Anne Clark Rodman, "Janet Howell Clark: Physiologist and Biophysicist (1899–1969)," *The Physiologist* 28 (1985): 397–400.
60. Anna Baetjer, personal interview, 2/11/81.
61. William H. Howell, Addendum to Report of the Department of Physiological Hygiene, 1939, pp. 3–4, Box 136, Office of the Dean's Correspondence, AMCMA.
62. Anna Baetjer, personal interview, 2/11/81.
63. Anna Baetjer, *Women in Industry: Their Health and Efficiency*, published under the auspices of the National Research Council (New York: W. B. Saunders Co., 1946); Anna Baetjer, "Pulmonary Carcinoma in Chromate Workers: 1. A Review of the Literature and Report of Cases," *Archives of Industrial Hygiene and Occupational Medicine* 2 (1950): 487–504; "Pulmonary Carcinoma in Chromate Workers: 2. Incidence on the Basis of Hospital Records," ibid., pp. 505–16.

64. Anna Baetjer, personal interview, 2/11/81.

65. If one uses a sliding scale, faculty earning over $3,500 lost 10 percent of their salaries; those earning between $1,000 and $3,500 lost 5 percent. Staff salaries over $1,000 were cut by 10 percent; no cuts were made for those making less than $1,000.

66. W. H. Frost, "To Members of the Advisory Board of the School of Hygiene and Public Health," 2/16/34, Box 135, RG 3, Ser. A, Office of the Dean's Correspondence, AMCMA.

67. Committee on External Relations, Report to President Ames, 4/18/33, p. 1, Box 135, RG 3, Ser. A, Office of the Dean's Correspondence, AMCMA.

68. W. H. Frost, "Memorandum to Members of the Faculty," 9/25/33, Box 135, RG 3, Ser. A, Office of the Dean's Correspondence, AMCMA.

69. Committee on External Relations, 4/18/33, p. 2.

70. Ibid., p. 3.

71. Advisory Board Minutes of the School of Hygiene and Public Health, 6/5/33, 10/5/33, AMCMA.

72. Ibid., 3/26/25, 5/27/26, 3/31/27.

73. Ibid., 3/29/28, 2/27/30, 3/28/29.

74. Ibid., 12/17/25, 3/21/27, 9/20/26, 3/29/28, 10/5/33.

75. Ibid., 5/26/32, 4/26/34.

76. Ibid., 5/29/30, 10/2/30, 3/31/32.

77. Ibid., 10/4/28, 3/28/29, 9/29/32, 1/25/34.

78. Ibid., 11/18/26, 3/28/29, 4/25/29, 5/29/30.

79. Ibid., 3/26/31, 6/5/33, 10/5/33.

80. Ibid., 2/26/30, 11/20/30, 12/18/30, 4/30/31, 5/26/32.

81. Ibid., 10/2/30, 3/26/31, 2/25/32, 10/4/34.

82. See resolutions on overhead administrative charges, ibid., 3/28/29.

83. Preliminary Report of the Policy Committee, 10/22/34, AMCMA.

84. Advisory Board Minutes of the School of Hygiene and Public Health, vol. 3, 5/31/34, AMCMA.

85. Report of the Policy Committee, 1/21/37.

86. For a useful outline of the history of federal and state funding for public health, see Harry S. Mustard, *Government in Public Health* (New York: Commonwealth Fund, 1945). The broader context of scientific funding is discussed in A. Hunter Dupree, *Science in the Federal Government* (Cambridge: Harvard University Press, 1957).

Chapter 7   The Community as Public Health Laboratory

1. Dean's report to the president of the university, 1929–30, Box 137, RG 3, Ser. A, Archive of the School of Hygiene, AMCMA.

2. Report of the School of Hygiene and Public Health, 1920–21, 11/9/21, RG 1.1, Ser. 200, RFA.

3. Ibid., p. 7.

4. Memorandum to the General Director of the International Health Board, 1921, RFA as cited by George Comstock, "Hagerstown Health and Morbidity Studies," De Lamar lecture, School of Hygiene and Public Health, April 26, 1983, p. 3.

5. John S. Fulton, "Report of the Washington County Demonstration

Unit," 7/18/23, Box 14, Office of the Dean's Correspondence, 1924–25, AMCMA.

6. Comstock, "Hagerstown Health and Morbidity Studies," pp. 7–8.

7. For Sydenstricker's work, see Edgar Sydenstricker, "A Study of Illness in a General Population Group. Hagerstown Morbidity Studies No. 1: The Method of Study and General Results," *Public Health Reports* 41 (1926): 2069–88, and the papers in Richard V. Kasius, ed., *The Challenge of Facts: Selected Public Health Papers of Edgar Sydenstricker* (New York: Prodist, 1974).

8. W. H. Frost to F. F. Russell, 6/29/23, RG 1.1, Ser. 200, RFA.

9. Wade Hampton Frost, "Proposed Training Area for School of Hygiene and Public Health, Baltimore," June 1923, p. 4, Box 14, Office of the Dean's Correspondence, AMCMA.

10. Ibid., p. 6.

11. Ibid., p. 8.

12. W. H. Frost to F. F. Russell, 6/29/23, RG 1.1, Ser. 200, RFA.

13. F. F. Russell to W. H. Frost, 7/12/23, RG 1.1, Ser. 200, RFA.

14. W. H. Frost to F. F. Russell, 7/23/23, RG 1.1, Ser. 200, RFA.

15. Report of the director of the School of Hygiene and Public Health, 1929–30, p. 2, RG 1.1, Ser. 200, RFA.

16. Simon Flexner and James Thomas Flexner, *William Henry Welch and the Heroic Age of American Medicine* (New York: Viking Press, 1941), p. 133.

17. "Mayor Picks Man for New Health Post," *Baltimore Sun*, July 15, 1931.

18. Huntington Williams, personal interview, 10/29/80.

19. Ibid.

20. W. H. Frost to F. F. Russell, 11/21/31; F. F. Russell to W. H. Frost, 12/28/31; W. H. Frost to F. F. Russell, 1/4/32, 1/5/32; RG 1.1, Ser. 200, RFA.

21. "Confidential Proposal for Establishing a Public Health Training Area for Baltimore," 4/1/32; Joseph Ames to F. F. Russell, 5/31/32, RG 1.1, Ser. 200, RFA.

22. "Proposal for the Establishment of a Public Health Training Area in Baltimore," 5/31/32, RG 1.1, Ser. 200, RFA.

23. Huntington Williams to F. F. Russell, 6/9/32, RG 1.1, Ser. 200, RFA.

24. Huntington Williams, personal interview, 10/29/79; Huntington Williams, *Huntington Williams, M.D., Commissioner of Health, 1931–1962*, published for family and friends (Baltimore, 1983), pp. 49–51.

25. Joseph W. Mountin, *A Study of Health and Hospital Service in Baltimore, Maryland: Summary and Major Recommendations* (Washington, D.C.: United States Public Health Service, June 9, 1932), p. 10.

26. Ibid., p. 32.

27. Executive Committee Minutes, 6/13/32, RG 1.1, Ser. 200, RFA.

28. W. H. Frost to F. F. Russell, 6/17/32, RG 1.1, Ser. 200, RFA.

29. Huntington Williams, personal interview, 10/29/79.

30. "New Health Area Begins Functions: Dr. Mustard Takes Over His Duties in Sixth and Seventh Wards," *Baltimore Sun*, September 22, 1932.

31. "Proposed New Health Agency Near Reality," *Baltimore Sun*, August 15, 1932; "New Health Area Begins Functions," *Baltimore Sun*, September 22, 1932.

32. C. Howe Eller, "Door-to-Door Health Control," *Johns Hopkins Alumni Magazine* 28 (November 1939): 14.

33. W. H. Frost to F. F. Russell, 9/11/34, RG 1.1, Ser. 200, RFA.

34. W. G. Smillie to D. L. Edsall, 11/27/33, RG 1.1, Ser. 200, RFA.

35. "Where Doorbells Are Always Ringing," *Evening Sun,* September 13, 1939.

36. Lowell J. Reed and Huntington Williams, "The Unique Nature of the Eastern Health District: The District Census Surveys," *Baltimore Health News* 25 (September 1948): 60–61.

37. "Where Doorbells Are Always Ringing," *Evening Sun,* September 13, 1939.

38. Ibid., p. 2.

39. See, for example, R. E. Wheeler, "A Study of Mortality and Morbidity in Children Exposed to Household Contact with Pulmonary Tuberculosis in Adults" (Dr.P.H. diss., School of Hygiene and Public Health, Johns Hopkins University, 1932); James Perkins, "A Study of the Care of Cases of Tuberculosis Occurring in Residents of the Eastern Health District" (Dr.P.H. diss., School of Hygiene and Public Health, Johns Hopkins University, 1933); C. Howe Eller, "A Study of the Cases of Tuberculosis Reported in the Eastern Health District, 1923–32" (Dr.P.H. diss., School of Hygiene and Public Health, Johns Hopkins University, 1934); Floyd Feldman, "Tuberculosis Service in the Eastern Health District" (Dr.P.H. diss., School of Hygiene and Public Health, Johns Hopkins University, 1934); Ross Gauld, "A Study of Reported Cases of Tuberculosis and Their Family Contacts" (Dr.P.H. diss., School of Hygiene and Public Health, Johns Hopkins University, 1935).

40. Wade Hampton Frost, "How Much Control of Tuberculosis?" in Kenneth Maxcy, ed., *Papers of Wade Hampton Frost: A Contribution to Epidemiological Method* (New York: Commonwealth Fund, 1941), p. 607.

41. Martin Frobisher, "Some Recent Advances in Diphtheriology," *American Journal of the Medical Sciences* 195 (1938): 417–25; Martin Frobisher, "Types of *Corynebacterium diphtheriae* in Baltimore, Maryland," *American Journal of Hygiene* 28 (1938): 13–35; C. Howe Eller and John J. Phair, "Diphtheria Immunization, Natural and Artificial in the Eastern Health District of Baltimore, 1922–1940," *American Journal of Hygiene* 34 (1941): 28–37; J. J. Phair and Mary R. Smith, "Diphtheria in Baltimore: The Carrier Rate in Twelve Surveys, 1921–1939," *American Journal of Hygiene* 35 (1942): 47–54.

42. Eller and Phair, "Diphtheria Immunization," pp. 28–37.

43. C. Howe Eller, "Door-to-Door Health Control," *Johns Hopkins Alumni Magazine* 28 (1939): 11–16.

44. Jean Gregoire, "A Study in Infant Hygiene" (Dr.P.H. diss., School of Hygiene and Public Health, Johns Hopkins University, 1935). See also Mehmet Olcar, "Births in the Eastern Health District in 1935: The Characteristics of the Families in Which the Births Occurred" (Dr.P.H. diss., School of Hygiene and Public Health, Johns Hopkins University, 1938).

45. "Baltimore Experiment in Public Health Work," *Baltimore Sun,* October 23, 1938.

46. Jean Downes and Selwyn Collins, "A Study of Illness among Families in the Eastern Health District in Baltimore," *Milbank Memorial Fund Quarterly* 18 (1940): 5–26; Jean Downes, "Chronic Disease among Middle and Old-Age Persons," *Milbank Memorial Fund Quarterly* 19 (1941): 5–24.

47. Downes, "Chronic Disease among Middle and Old-Age Persons," p. 5; Sally Preas and Ruth Phillips, "The Severity of Illness among Males and

Females," *Milbank Memorial Fund Quarterly* 20 (1942): 221–44.

48. Preas and Phillips, "The Severity of Illness among Males and Females," p. 224.

49. Edgar Sydenstricker, *Health and Environment* (New York: McGraw-Hill, 1933), as cited in Jean Downes, "Illness in the Chronic Disease Family," *American Journal of Public Health* 32 (1942): 598.

50. Clifford W. Beers, *A Mind That Found Itself* (New York: Longmans, Green & Co., 1908).

51. Paul Lemkau, "Notes on the Development of Mental Hygiene in the Johns Hopkins School of Hygiene and Public Health," *Bulletin of the History of Medicine* 35 (1961): 169–74.

52. Barbara A. Dreyer, "Adolph Meyer and Mental Hygiene: An Ideal for Public Health," *American Journal of Public Health* 66 (1976): 998–1003.

53. Raymond Fosdick, *Adventure in Giving: The Story of the General Education Board* (New York: Harper & Row, 1962), p. 259.

54. J. A. Ferrell to W. H. Frost, 1/29/34, RG 1.1, Ser. 200, RFA.

55. W. H. Frost to J. A. Ferrell, 3/2/34, RG 1.1, Ser. 200, RFA.

56. J. A. Ferrell, "Memorandum to Doctor Russell," 5/28/34, RG 1.1, Ser. 200, RFA.

57. W. H. Frost to J. A. Ferrell, 6/8/34, RG 1.1, Ser. 200, RFA.

58. J. A. Ferrell to W. H. Frost, 6/18/34, RG 1.1, Ser. 200, RFA.

59. W. H. Frost to J. A. Ferrell, 6/19/34, RG 1.1, Ser. 200, RFA.

60. A. W. Freeman to F. F. Russell, 8/27/34, 9/25/34, RG 1.1, Ser. 200, RFA.

61. A. W. Freeman to J. A. Ferrell, 8/26/38, RG 1.1, Ser. 200, RFA.

62. Ibid., p. 1.

63. A. W. Freeman and Bernard M. Cohen, "Preliminary Observations on the Epidemiology of Mental Disease," *American Journal of Public Health* 29 (1939): 633–35.

64. "Two Field Studies in Mental Hygiene," *International Health Department Newsletter*, April 1938, RG 1.1, Ser. 200, RFA.

65. Bernard M. Cohen and Ruth E. Fairbank, "Statistical Contributions from the Mental Hygiene Study of the Eastern Health District of Baltimore: 1. General Account of the 1933 Mental Hygiene Survey of the Eastern Health District," *American Journal of Psychiatry* 94 (1937–38): 1153–61.

66. Ibid., 2. "Psychosis in the Eastern Health District," *American Journal of Psychiatry* 94 (1937–38): 1377–95.

67. For an extended critique, see Gerald N. Grob, "The Origins of Psychiatric Epidemiology," *American Journal of Public Health* 75 (1985): 229–36.

68. Ibid., p. 233.

69. Bernard Cohen, Ruth Fairbank, and Elizabeth Greene, "Statistical Contributions from the Mental Hygiene Study of the Eastern Health District: 3. Personality Disorder in the Eastern Health District in 1933," *Human Biology* 2 (1939): 112–29.

70. Bernard Cohen, Christopher Tietze, and Elizabeth Greene, "Statistical Contributions from the Mental Hygiene Study of the Eastern Health District of Baltimore: 4. Further Studies on Personality Disorder in the Eastern Health District in 1933," *Human Biology* 2 (1939): 485–512.

71. Ruth Fairbank, "Mental Hygiene from the Epidemiological View-

point," *Contributions Dedicated to Dr. Adolf Meyer by His Colleagues, Friends, and Pupils*, edited by S. Katzenelbogen (Baltimore: Johns Hopkins Press, 1938), pp. 89–94.

72. Ibid., p. 90.

73. "Louis Azrael Says—," *Baltimore News Post*, March 5, 1938.

74. Elizabeth Adamson, "A Community Program for Prevention of Mental Disease," *American Journal of Public Health* 26 (1936): 480.

75. Ruth Fairbank, "Mental Hygiene Component of a City Health District," *American Journal of Public Health* 27 (1937): 250, 252.

76. Douglas A. Thom, *Everyday Problems of the Everyday Child* (New York: D. Appleton & Co., 1927); William Emet Blatz, Dorothy Millichamp, and Margaret Fletcher, *Nursery Education, Theory and Practice* (New York: Morrow, 1935); Esther L. Richards, *Behavior Aspects of Child Conduct* (New York: Macmillan Co., 1934).

77. Fairbank, "Mental Hygiene Component of a City Health District," p. 250.

78. Arnold Gesell, *Infancy and Human Growth* (New York: Macmillan Co., 1928); Charlotte Bühler, *The First Year of Life* (New York: John Day Co., 1930).

79. For more details, see Marcia Cooper, *Evaluation of the Mothers' Advisory Service. Monographs of the Society for Research in Child Development*, vol. 12, 1947 (Washington, D.C.: Society for Research in Child Development, National Research Council, 1948).

80. Marcia Cooper, "Evaluation of the Mothers' Advisory Service" (Dr.P.H. diss., School of Hygiene and Public Health, Johns Hopkins University, 1947), p. 19.

81. Ibid.

82. Fairbank, "Mental Hygiene Component of a City Health District," p. 250.

83. Paul Lemkau, personal interview, 6/4/82.

84. Allen Freeman, "Mental Hygiene and the Health Department," *American Journal of Public Health* 28 (1938): 242.

85. P. Lemkau, C. Tietze, and M. Cooper, "Mental Hygiene Problems in an Urban District: 1. Description of the Study," *Mental Hygiene* 25 (1941): 624–46; "2. Psychotics, the Neurotics," *Mental Hygiene* 26 (1942): 100–19; "3. The Epileptics and Mental Deficients," *Mental Hygiene* 26 (1942): 275–88; "4. Mental Hygiene Problems in Children Seven to Sixteen Years of Age," *Mental Hygiene* 27 (1943): 279–95; P. Lemkau, C. Tietze, and M. Cooper, "Complaint of Nervousness and the Psychoneuroses," *American Journal of Orthopsychiatry* 12 (1942): 214–23; P. Lemkau, C. Tietze, and M. Cooper, "Report of Progress in Developing a Mental Hygiene Component of a City Health District," *American Journal of Psychiatry* 97 (1940–41): 805–11.

86. Paul Lemkau, *Mental Hygiene in Public Health* (New York: McGraw-Hill, 1949).

87. Paul Lemkau, "What Can the Public Health Nurse Do in Mental Hygiene?" *Public Health Nursing* 40 (1948): 299–303.

88. First Report of the Bureau for Contraceptive Advice, Baltimore, Maryland, 1929, Baltimore Birth Control Clinic, III/62/3, Adolph Meyer Archive, AMCMA.

89. Organization Meeting of Committee on Contraceptive Information,

March 22, 1926, Baltimore Birth Control Clinic, III/62/1, Adolph Meyer Archive, AMCMA.

90. Second Meeting of Committee on Contraceptive Information, May 5, 1926, Baltimore Birth Control Clinic, III/62/1, Adolph Meyer Archive, AMCMA.

91. Third Meeting of Committee on Contraceptive Information, October 18, 1926, Baltimore Birth Control Clinic, III/62/1, Adolph Meyer Archive, AMCMA.

92. Committee on Contraceptive Information, May 5, 1927; Report of the Finance Committee, December 9, 1927; Baltimore Birth Control Clinic, III/62/2, Adolph Meyer Archive, AMCMA.

93. "To the Physicians of Maryland," October 17, 1927, Baltimore Birth Control Clinic, III/62/3, Adolph Meyer Archive, AMCMA.

94. Bureau for Contraceptive Advice Incorporated, Minutes of First Meeting of Board of Directors, May 24, 1926. Baltimore Birth Control Clinic, III/62/3, Adolph Meyer Archive, AMCMA.

95. Bessie Moses, Contraception as a Therapeutic Measure (Baltimore: Williams & Wilkins, 1936), pp. 1–2.

96. First Report of the Bureau for Contraceptive Advice, Baltimore, Maryland, 1929, p. 6, Baltimore Birth Control Clinic, III/62/3, Adolph Meyer Archive, AMCMA.

97. Moses, Contraception as a Therapeutic Measure, pp. 24–25.

98. First Report of the Bureau for Contraceptive Advice, Baltimore, Maryland, 1929, pp. 7–10, Baltimore Birth Control Clinic, III/62/3, Adolph Meyer Archive, AMCMA.

99. Ibid., p. 8.

100. Ibid., p. 6.

101. Moses, Contraception as a Therapeutic Measure, p. 58.

102. Ibid., p. 60.

103. Ibid., p. 61.

104. Ninth Meeting of Board of Directors. Bureau for Contraceptive Advice, November 5, 1931, Baltimore Birth Control Clinic, III/62/4, Adolph Meyer Archive, AMCMA.

105. Jean H. Keyser to Adolph Meyer, April 28, 1933, Baltimore Birth Control Clinic, III/62/4, Adolph Meyer Archive, AMCMA.

106. Baltimore Birth Control Clinic, Inc., 1937, "Purpose and Program," Baltimore Birth Control Clinic, Adolph Meyer Archive, AMCMA.

107. Ibid., "What We Are Doing."

108. Ibid., "Some Letters from Mothers."

109. Thomas Parran, Shadow on the Land: Syphilis (New York: Reynal & Hitchcock, 1937); Thomas Parran and R. A. Vonderlehr, Plain Words about Venereal Disease (New York: Reynal & Hitchcock, 1941).

110. W. A. McIntosh to A. Freeman, 8/28/36, RG 1.1, Ser. 200, RFA.

111. Turner later became dean of the Johns Hopkins Medical School. See his lively autobiographical account: Thomas B. Turner, Part of Medicine, Part of Me: Musings of a Johns Hopkins Dean (Baltimore: Waverly Press, 1981).

112. Baltimore City Health Department Annual Report, 1933, p. 93, Maryland Room, Enoch Pratt Public Library, Baltimore, Maryland.

113. Thomas B. Turner et al., "Studies on Syphilis in the Eastern Health District of Baltimore City: 1. Principles Concerned in Measuring the Frequency

of the Disease," *American Journal of Hygiene* 37 (1943): 259–72; 2. "Discovery Rates as an Index of Trend," *American Journal of Hygiene* 37 (1943): 273–88.

114. Thomas B. Turner, "Memorandum to Dr. Ferrell," 7/19/38, RG 1.1, Ser. 200, RFA.

115. See note 113; also, E. Gurney Clark and Thomas B. Turner, "Studies on Syphilis in the Eastern Health District of Baltimore City. 3. Study of the Prevalence of Syphilis based on Specific Age Groups of an Enumerated Population," *American Journal of Public Health* 32 (1942): 307–13; George M. Leiby, Thomas B. Turner, E. Gurney Clark, Robert Dyar, Fred C. Kluth, "Studies of Syphilis in the Eastern Health District of Baltimore City: 4. Syphilis among Parturient Women as an Index of the Trend of Syphilis in the Community," *American Journal of Hygiene* 46 (1947): 260–67; E. Gurney Clark, "Studies on Syphilis in the Eastern Health District of Baltimore City. 6. Prevalence in 1939, by Race, Sex, Age, and Socioeconomic Status," *American Journal of Syphilis, Gonorrhea, and Venereal Diseases* 29 (1945): 455–73.

116. Turner, *Part of Medicine, Part of Me*, pp. 74–77.

117. Excerpt from Trustees Confidential Report, November, 1950, "The Fitness of the Environment," RG 1.1, Ser. 200, RFA.

118. For the development of district health organizations in several cities, see Christie W. Gordon, "Administration of Health Department Functions through District Health Organizations in Urban Communities of 500,000–1,000,000 Population in the United States" (Dr.P.H. diss., School of Hygiene and Public Health, Johns Hopkins University, 1947).

119. Ernest Stebbins, personal interview, 10/15/79.

120. Some of the general problems of district health administration are discussed in a paper by George Silver and Abraham Lilienfeld, "Observations on Current Practices in Municipal District Health Administration," *American Journal of Public Health* 41 (1951): 1263–67.

121. Huntington Williams, personal interview, 10/29/80.

122. Ibid.

123. Ibid.

124. Ernest Stebbins, personal interview, 10/15/79; Huntington Williams, personal interview, 10/29/80.

125. Executive Committee Minutes of the International Health Division, 11/18/38, RG 1.1, Ser. 200, RFA.

Chapter 8   Extending the Hopkins Model

1. Jean Alonzo Curran, *Founders of the Harvard School of Public Health, with Biographical Notes, 1909–1946* (New York: Josiah Macy, Jr., Foundation, 1970), p. 17.

2. Ibid., pp. 19–20.

3. E. O. Jordan, J. C. Whipple, C.-E. A. Winslow, *A Pioneer of Public Health: William Thompson Sedgwick* (New Haven: Yale University Press, 1924).

4. Curran, *Founders of the Harvard School of Public Health*, pp. 28–31. See also D. L. Edsall to W. Rose, 1/25/21, RG 1.1, Ser. 200, RFA.

5. Curran, *Founders of the Harvard School of Public Health*, pp. 87–91.

6. See note 1 for full citation.

7. W. S. Leathers et al., Committee on Professional Education of the American Public Health Association, "Public Health Degrees and Certificates

Granted in 1936," *American Journal of Public Health* 27 (1937): 1267–72.

8. Thomas Parran and Livingston Farrand, "Report to the Rockefeller Foundation on the Education of Public Health Personnel," 10/28/39, RG 1.1, Ser. 200, RFA.

9. Ibid.

10. Alan Gregg's diary, Baltimore, 3/24/38, RG 1.1, Ser. 200, RFA.

11. Leathers et al., "Public Health Degrees," pp. 1270 -72; Arthur P. Miller, "Undergraduate Engineering Training in Public Health and Related Activities in Engineering Colleges of the United States," *Public Health Reports* 54 (1939): 29–35.

12. *The Rockefeller Foundation Annual Report, 1913–14* (New York: Rockefeller Foundation, 1915), p. 40.

13. George Vincent, *The Rockefeller Foundation: A Review for 1921* (New York: Rockefeller Foundation, 1922), p. 36.

14. *The Rockefeller Foundation Annual Report, 1926* (New York: Rockefeller Foundation, 1927), pp. 27–28.

15. Donald Fisher, "Rockefeller Philanthropy and the British Empire: The Creation of the London School of Hygiene and Tropical Medicine," *History of Education* 7 (1978): 120–43. See also Sir Philip Manson-Bahr, *History of the School of Tropical Medicine in London, 1899–1949* (London: H. K. Lewis, 1956), esp. pp. 64–67; Catherine A. Clark and James Mackintosh, *The School and the Site: A Historical Memoir to Celebrate the Twenty-fifth Anniversary of the School* (London: H. K. Lewis, 1954), esp. pp. 55–61.

16. R. D. Defries, "Postgraduate Teaching in Public Health in the University of Toronto, 1913–1955," *Canadian Journal of Public Health* 48 (1957): 285–94; R. D. Defries, *The First Forty Years: Connaught Medical Research Laboratories, University of Toronto* (Toronto: University of Toronto Press, 1969).

17. Raymond B. Fosdick, *The Story of the Rockefeller Foundation, 1913–1950* (New York: Harper & Brothers, 1952), pp. 42–43.

18. J. A. Ferrell to T. Parran, 5/12/38, RG 1.1, Ser. 200, RFA.

19. J. A. Ferrell to M. Eliot, 5/13/38; T. Parran to J. A. Ferrell, 5/31/38; M. Eliot to J. A. Ferrell, 6/24/38; J. A. Ferrell to W. S. Leathers, 9/1/38; RG 1.1, Ser. 200, RFA.

20. J. A. Ferrell, "University Facilities in the United States for Training Public Health Personnel," 9/26/38, RG 1.1, Ser. 200, RFA.

21. Ibid., p. 11.

22. Livingston Farrand had previously worked for the International Health Board as director of the tuberculosis program in France during World War I; he had been chairman of the Central Committee of the American Red Cross, treasurer of the American Public Health Association, and also president of the University of Colorado. He was president of Cornell University from 1921 to 1937.

23. A. J. Warren, "Confidential Report on Institutes of Hygiene and Schools of Public Health in Europe," 10/31/39, p. 10, RG 1, Ser. 100, RFA. All these institutes and schools were studied in 1937 by a committee of the Health Section of the League of Nations, composed of Sir Wilson Jameson of the London school, Dr. Andrija Stampar of Yugoslavia, and Dr. Pittaluga of Spain. Their report was published in the *Bulletin of the Health Organization of the League* 7, no. 2 (April 1938). For later development of the European schools, see

F. Grundy and J. M. Mackintosh, *The Teaching of Hygiene and Public Health in Europe* (Geneva: World Health Organization, 1957); J. D. Cottrell, *The Teaching of Public Health in Europe* (Geneva: World Health Organization, 1969); *Travelling Seminar on Organization and Administration of Schools of Public Health* (Washington, D.C.: Pan American Health Organization, Scientific Publication no. 94, 1964).

24. Thomas Parran and Livingston Farrand, "Report to the Rockefeller Foundation on the Education of Public Health Personnel," 10/28/39, p. 21, RG 1.1, Ser. 200, RFA. Page references for subsequent quotations appear in the text.

25. For useful discussion of the contributions of the social sciences to public health, see George Rosen, "Social Science and Health in the United States in the Twentieth Century," *Clio Medica* 11 (1976): 245–68; George Rosen, "The Evolution of Social Medicine," in *Handbook of Medical Sociology*, edited by Howard E. Freeman, Sol Levine, and Leo G. Reeder (Englewood Cliffs, N.J.: Prentice Hall, 1972), pp. 17–61.

26. Thomas Parran and Livingston Farrand, "Report to the Rockefeller Foundation on the Education of Public Health Personnel," 10/28/39, p. 64, RG 1.1, Ser. 200, RFA. Page references for subsequent quotations appear in the text.

27. George E. Vincent, *The Rockefeller Foundation: A Review for 1920* (New York: Rockefeller Foundation, 1921), p. 4.

28. Ibid., *The Rockefeller Foundation: A Review for 1924* (New York: Rockefeller Foundation, 1925), pp. 22–23.

29. W. S. Leathers, "Undergraduate Instruction in Hygiene and Preventive Medicine to Medical Students," 7/8/31, p. 4, RG 1, Ser. 100, RFA.

30. "Proposed Future Program," Rockefeller Foundation Agenda for Special Meeting at the Westchester Country Club, April 11, 1933, p. 73, RG 3, Ser. 906, RFA.

31. Alan Gregg to W. G. Smillie, 10/16/34, 1/7/35, 1/8/34; RG 1, Ser. 100, RFA.

32. Alan Gregg to Charles Smith, 12/21/35, RG 1, Ser. 100, RFA.

33. Russell A. Nelson, "Organizational Relationships of Schools of Public Health with Schools of Medicine," in *Schools of Public Health: Present and Future*, edited by John Z. Bowers and Elizabeth Purcell (New York: Josiah Macy, Jr., Foundation, 1974), pp. 11–14.

34. Ibid., p. 12.

35. John C. Hume, "Relationship of Schools of Public Health and Schools of Medicine," in *Schools of Public Health in Latin America* (New York: Josiah Macy, Jr., Foundation, 1974), pp. 167–68.

36. Luis Fernando Duque, "The Future of Schools of Public Health in Latin America," in *Schools of Public Health in Latin America* (New York: Josiah Macy, Jr., Foundation, 1974), p. 3, report of a Macy Conference, Medellin, Colombia, November 17–19, 1974.

37. Guillermo Arbona, "Future Role of Schools of Public Health," in *The Past, Present, and Future of Schools of Public Health* (Chapel Hill: University of North Carolina, 1963), pp. 81–89.

38. Conrad Seipp, ed., *Health Care for the Community: Selected Papers of Dr. John B. Grant* (Baltimore: Johns Hopkins Press, 1963).

39. John B. Grant, "Mutatis Mutandis," in *Health Care for the Community*, p. 182.

40. Milton I. Roemer, "More Schools of Public Health: A Worldwide Need," *International Journal of Health Services* 14 (1984): 493–94.

41. Charles-Edward A. Winslow, "Public Health at the Crossroads," *American Journal of Public Health* 16 (1926): 1075–85.

42. See especially the Committee on the Costs of Medical Care's final report, *Medical Care for the American People* (1932; reprinted, Washington, D.C.: U.S. Department of Health, Education, and Welfare, 1970).

43. Henry Sigerist, "The Medical Student and the Social Problems Confronting Medicine Today," *Bulletin of the History of Medicine* 4 (1936): 411–22; see also Milton I. Roemer, ed., *Henry E. Sigerist on the Sociology of Medicine* (New York: M.D. Publications, 1960). For an overview of Sigerist's influence, see Milton Terris, "The Contributions of Henry E. Sigerist to Health Service Organization," *Milbank Memorial Fund Quarterly* 53 (1975): 489–530.

44. Edgar Sydenstricker, "The Changing Concept of Public Health," *Milbank Memorial Fund Quarterly* 13 (1935): 301–10. See also E. Sydenstricker, "Health in the New Deal," *Annals of the American Academy of Political and Social Science* 176 (1934): 131–37 and E. Sydenstricker, *Health and Environment* (New York: McGraw-Hill, 1933).

45. See especially Arthur J. Viseltear, *Emergence of the Medical Care Section of the American Public Health Association, 1926–1948: A Chapter in the History of Medical Care in the United States* (Washington, D.C.: American Public Health Association, 1972); Milton I. Roemer, "The American Public Health Association as a Force for Change in Medical Care," *Medical Care* 11 (1973): 338–51; Milton Terris, "Evolution of Public Health and Preventive Medicine in the United States," *American Journal of Public Health* 65 (1975): 161–69.

46. For details of this debate, see Viseltear, *Emergence of the Medical Care Section of the American Public Health Association*, esp. pp. 7–10.

47. W. G. Smillie, *Proceedings of the Conference on Preventive Medicine and Health Economics, September 30–October 4, 1946* (Ann Arbor: School of Public Health, University of Michigan, 1946), p. 146. See George Rosen, *Preventive Medicine in the United States, 1900–1975: Trends and Interpretations* (New York: Science History Publications, 1975), esp. pp. 60–61.

48. See Milton Terris, "The World Need for Schools of Public Health," *Journal of Public Health Policy* 3 (1982): 111–16.

49. For a variety of perspectives on public health education, see *Higher Education for Public Health: A Report of the Milbank Memorial Fund Commission* (New York: Prodist, 1976); and the essays in *Schools of Public Health*, edited by Bowers and Purcell; *The Past, Present, and Future of Schools of Public Health*; *Schools of Public Health in Latin America* (cited in notes 36 and 37).

50. L. E. Burney, "The Future Role of Schools of Public Health," in *The Past, Present, and Future of Schools of Public Health*, pp. 139–40.

51. Milton I. Roemer, "More Schools of Public Health: A Worldwide Need," *International Journal of Health Services* 14 (1984): 493.

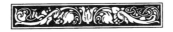

Index

Committee on Maternal Health, 205
Commonwealth Fund, 179
Community, as public health laboratory,
182–215
Community-based studies, in mental
hygiene, 199–204; Winslow on, 230
Complement, study of effect of,
118–119
Contraception: forms of, 207; as medical
problem, 207. *See also* Birth Control
Cooper, Marcia: and Hopkins Mental
Hygiene Study, 204; on Mothers'
Advisory Service, 202–203
Cort, William: conducts short courses,
79–80; as editor, 160, 162; on first
faculty, 64, 65; 1919 plan of, 88; re-
search of, 104–108, 178, 179
Cottage cheese, as treatment, 100
Cox, Herald R., 120
C.P.H., demand for, 75. *See* table, 77
Crewe, Lord, 221
Cumming, Hugh S. (Surgeon General),
70, 83
Curran, Jean Alonzo, on Harvard
School of Public Health, 217–218

Damon, Samuel Reed, 116
Das, Ayodhya, on student experience,
166–167
Davis, Harry L., 68
Day, Harry G., and fluoride, 130
De Lamar, Joseph, endowment of, 161
De Lamar Endowment: funds journal,
161; and lectures, 163
De Lamar Institute of Public Health,
218
De Lamar Lectures, success of, 83
Demography, role of, in new school, 54,
55
Duration of life, research on, 141
Diarrhea, flagellate, 100
Diphtheria, research on, 117–118, 134,
194
Disease(s): causes of, 10; concept of, 9;
Eastern Health District, study of
chronic, 194–197; Howell, on study
of chronic, 125; decline in infectious,
23; endemic, 10–11; epidemic,
10–11, 12 and public health, 21; and

sanitary engineering, 22–24; scientific
concept of, 20–22
Disease control: Chapin on, 20; and
epidemiological research, 136; Frost's
contribution to, 136; requirements
for, 122–123
Dogs, hookworm research on, 107, 108
Dr.P.H. degree: candidates for, 74–76;
demand for, 78; recruiting candidates
for, 84. *See* table, 77
Drinker, Cecil and Philip, 217
Duffy, John, 37
Duque, Luis Fernando, 229
Durham, Louise, 61, 158

Eastern Health District: and Bureau of
Contraceptive Advice, 204–210;
establishment of, 184–192; as example of cooperation, 235; future of,
212–214; mental hygiene studies in,
197–204; photos, 191, 195, 202;
studies in, 192–197; syphilis study in,
210–212
Edsall, David L., 217
Efficiency, as criterion, 29
Eli Lilly Company, 178
Eliot, Calista P., work of, 116
Eliot, Charles W.: and Harvard's efforts
in public health education, 216; on
selection of site, 50
Eliot, Martha, 222–223
Eller, Howe, 213
Embree, Edwin: at budget meetings, 89;
and new building, 92
Emergency Committee in Aid of Dis-
placed Foreign Physicians, 179
Emerson, Haven, 47, 83; and Columbia
University's department of public
health, 226; opposed national health
plan, 231
Entomology, medical: as discipline, 97,
98, 109; research in, 65
Environmental factors, course on, 125
Environmental health: Howell's defini-
tion of, 124; research in, 126. *See also*
Physiological hygiene
Epidemiology: "armchair," 133; defini-
tion of, 132, 134; Frost's work in department, 132–136; as fundamental

Epidemiology (contd.)
discipline, 68–70; increase in research in, 162; laboratory method of teaching, 135; "shoe leather," 133
Everyday Problems of the Everyday Child (Thom), 201
Executive Committee: and budget deficit, 172; responsibility of, 159

Faculty: first, 59–73; profile of, 181
Faculty-student relationships, 167
Fairbank, Ruth, pin charts of, 200–201
Farrand, Livingston, 83: background of, 269n.22; and evaluation of schools of public health, 223–226. See also Parran-Farrand report
Fatigue, Spaeth on, 125
Feirer, William, 178
Ferrell, John H.: on demand for public health officers, 78; and evaluation of schools of public health, 222–223; as first candidate for Dr.P.H., 75–76; on growth of epidemiological services, 136; on mental hygiene program funding, 198; on public health officer, 29
Fertility control, success rate of, 208–209
Field work: in Eastern Health District, 192–214; need for, 41; with U.S. Public Health Service, 188–189; in Washington County; 183–184
Filterable viruses. See Viruses
Filtration, definition of, 111
Fisher, Irving, 18
Fitzgerald, John, survey of, on teaching of preventive medicine, 228
Five Million Patients (Freeman), 68, 71, 73
Flexner, Abraham: admiration of, for Welch, 51; and Eliot, 50; and founding of new school, 26; and General Education Board, 29–35; and medical model of public health, 43–44; on Rose, 27; on Seligman, 43; and site visits, 44–49; urges opening of school, 61
Flexner, Simon, 51; and beginnings of new school, 52–55; on budget control, 89; as De Lamar lecturer, 83; as editor, 160; photo, 53

Flexner Report, and medical education, 29–30
Fluorides, research on, 130
Food, Nutrition, and Health (McCollum), 131
Food Infections and Food Intoxifications (Damon), 116
Ford, William: as editor, 160, 162; on first faculty, 60; 1919 report of, 87; photo, 115, 118; and plans for new school, 54; research of, 114–115, 178; on training facilities, 31
Forssman antigen, 119
Founders of the Harvard School of Public Health (Curran), 217
Fowl plague. See Hühner
Fox, Daniel, 34
Freeman, Allen Weir: as dean, 179; on early faculty, 68, 71–73; and health center, 186; and mental hygiene program, 198; on Mothers' Advisory Service, 203–204; and physiology committee, 168, 172–175; as teacher, 147; work of, in public health administration, 146–149
Frobisher, Martin, Jr., 78; Eastern Health District, work of, 190, 195; work of, 116
Frost, Wade Hampton: on attracting physicians to public health, 164; as chair of organization committee, 168; collaboration of, with Reed, 143; as dean, 171; and Eastern Health District, 184–189; as editor, 160, 162; on first faculty, 68, 70; as head of public health administration, 67; and mental hygiene program, 197–198; photo, 69; 1919 plans of, 87; as teacher, 135; work of, in epidemiology, 132–136

Gates, Frederick, on attractions of medical practice, 36
General Education Board (of Rockefeller Foundation): and first school of hygiene and public health, 29–56; and hookworm research, 17
Giardia. See Diarrhea
Gilman, Daniel C., 57

Goldberger, Joseph, pellagra studies of, 22

Goldmark Report, 85

Goodnow, Frank: on first faculty, 60; and new building, 91–93; and plans for new school, 53–54

Gorgas, William (Surgeon Major, later Surgeon General), 17, 61

Gorgas Memorial Laboratory, 178

Grant, John B., 79; on integrated health services, 229–230; on Reed as teacher, 139

Greene, Jerome D.: and first school of hygiene and public health, 27, 32; on Rose, 50–51; and site visits, 44–49

Gregory, John H., career of, 88, 150–151, 152

Gunn, Selskar, recommended for faculty, 66, 82

Hackett, Lewis, as Rockefeller Fellow, 79

Hagerstown Morbidity Studies, 184

Hamilton, Alice: on Howell as teacher, 125–126; and industrial hygiene, 21–22

Harcourt, Lewis, 221

Harlan, Henry D. (Judge), 48

Harvard Medical School, relationship of, to Harvard School of Public Health, 217

Harvard-MIT School for Health Officers, 31–32, 38; restructuring of, 216–217. See also Harvard School of Public Health

Harvard School of Public Health, 216–217; compared with Hopkins School of Hygiene and Public Health, 217–218; Parran-Farrand report on, 225–226

Harvard University, proposal of, for School of Tropical Medicine, 44; site visit to, 44–46

Health: beginnings of physiology of, 126; study of, reviewed, 234

Health education, popular, McCollum's work in, 131, 132. See also Public health education

Health systems, provision for integrated, 229–230

Hedrich, W. W., and Welch, 160

Hegner, Robert: bibliography of, 101; conducts short courses, 79–80; as editor, 160; on first faculty, 64–65; on medical zoology, 99; photo, 100, 102; 1919 plan of, 88; poetry of, 101–102; research of, on parasitology, 99–104, 178–179

Heiser, Victor C.: on appeal of public health to medical school graduates, 163, 164; as De Lamar lecturer, 83

Helmholtz, Henry F., 163

Helminthology: research in, 65; research and teaching, 104–109; as separate discipline, 97, 98

Heparin, Howell isolates, 126

Heredity, Pearl on importance of, 141

Hexylresorcinol, research in, 116

Hill, Hibbert Winslow, on modern scientific methods, 20–21

History of Nutrition (McCollum), 132

Hooker, Donald, and contraceptive bureau, 205, 206

Hookworm: campaign against, 27–29; Cort's research on, 104–108; early research on, 17–18; international programs for control of, 219

Hospital, teaching, seen as essential to public health education, 42

Howard, William T.: as assistant health commissioner, 49; courses of, 139

Howell, William H.: appendix of, to Welch-Rose Report, 168–169; and black physicians, 81; and contraceptive bureau, 204–205, 209; dual commitment of, 96, 122, 124; as editor, 160; as executive manager, 53–55; on first faculty, 59–60; and first school of hygiene and public health, 26–27; on need for field work, 182–183; photo, 59, 77; 1919 report of, 86; on public health employment, 164; retirement of, 168; as school administrator, 158; on school as research institute, 81, 82; site committee visits, 49; on training public health nurses, 81; vision of public health of, 124

Howland, John, 48; research of, on rickets, 129

Lederle Laboratories, 178
Lemkau, Paul: and mental hygiene, 203–204; on role of public health nurses, 204
Leonard, Veader, 178; research of, 116
Lewinski-Corwin, E. H., on public health issues, 39
Liver fluke, Barlow's research on, 108–109
London School of Hygiene and Tropical Medicine, 220–221; as central school, 222
Lowell, A. L., on Flexner, 45
Lusk, Graham, as editor, 160
Lynch, Ruth Stocking, 65
Lyon, E. P., on training for health officials, 31

McCall's, articles on nutrition in, 131
McCleary, George F., 163
McCollum, Elmer Verner: as advocate of special training, 81–82; commitment to popular health education, 131–132; contributions of, 126–132; as director of physiological hygiene department, 174, 175; as editor, 160, 162; on first faculty, 62–63; first use of rats as experimental animals, 62–63, 127–129; photo, 128; 1919 report of, 86–87; philosophy of teaching of, 130; and student grants, 178
McCollum, Ernestine, on nutrition experiments, 127–128
McCoy Hall, fire destroys, 92
MacNutt, J. Scott, 21
Macy, Josiah, Jr., Foundation, 179
Magnesium, 130
Malaria: Hegner's research on, 103–104; photo, 103
Malaria control programs, Root's work with, 110–111
Manganese, 130
Manual for Health Officers (MacNutt), 21
Marine Hospital Service, 11
Markle, John and Mary, Foundation, 179
Marshall, G.A.K., 83
Masters of Public Health, as recommended degree, 170

Maxcy, Kenneth F., 116; awarded fellowship, 79; and European survey, 223; on medical graduates' interest in public health, 164
Meader, Percy D., as faculty member, 116
Mead Johnson Company, 178
Medical education: relationship of, to public health, 37; Y plan of, 25
Medical practitioners, opposition of, to profession of public health, 52. See also Physicians
Medical schools: and emphasis on research, 232; importance of, to schools of public health in Welch-Rose report, 42–43; relationship to public health, 37
Medical zoology, department of, 98–103; 1922 faculty photo, 80
Medicine, relation of, to public health, 2, 6, 164–165, 227–236. See also Tensions
Mencken, H. L., 138
Mental Hygiene in Public Health (Lemkau), 204
Mental hygiene studies, of Eastern Health District, 197–204
Merrell, Margaret: and recollection of student days, 167; on Reed, 139; on Reed-Frost collaboration, 143
Meyer, Dr. Adolf: and contraceptive bureau, 205; and Eastern Health District, 197, 198, 199; mental hygiene activities of, 197
Meyer, Arthur: appointment not renewed, 172; course of, on environmental factors, 125; as faculty member, 86
Milbank Memorial Fund, 179; financing of contraceptive study by, 208–209
Milk and milk products, research on bacteriology of, 114–115, 178
Mind That Found Itself, A (Beers), 197
Miner, John R., courses of, 139
Mortality rates, U.S., 240n.51
Moses, Dr. Bessie: and contraceptive bureau, 205–209; and Planned Parenthood, 210
Moses, Jacob (Judge), 205

Mosquitoes, as cause of yellow fever, 17
Mothers' Advisory Service, 201–204; appraisal of, 203; photo, 202
Mountin, Joseph W., Public Health Service report of, 188–189
Muench, Hugo, 78
Municipal housekeeping, 14
Murphy, Starr J., at budget meeting, 89
Museum, hygienic: opening exhibit, 94–95; Welch's plans for, 83
Mustard, Harry Stoll, as Eastern Health District officer, 189–192, 212

National Cancer Institute, 179
National Committee on Federal Legislation, 206
National Committee on Maternal Health, 82, 179
National Committee for Mental Hygiene, 197
National Dental Association, 178
National Health Conference, recommends national health program, 231
National health program, controversy over, 230–232
National Research Council, grants of, 178
Negroes, exclusion of, from School of Hygiene, 81; infectious diseases of, 48, 49
Nelson, Russell, on cooperative efforts of medical and public health schools, 229
Nelson, S. Page, as business manager, 158
New Deal: and failure to create national health program, 231–232; impact of public funding of, 180, 181; influence of, on public health service, 236
Newer Knowledge of Nutrition, The (McCollum), 131
New Public Health, The (Hill), 20–21
Newsholme, Sir Arthur: conducts short course for health officers, 79; first departmental plan of, 88; philosophy of, 67
Noguchi, Hideyo, 83
Norris, Ethel, 158
Nosology, attempts to provide psychiatric, 199–200

Nursery Education (Blatz, Millichamp, and Fletcher), 201
Nursing: in Eastern Health District, 190; excluded from School of Hygiene, 81; photos, 12, 191, 195; in schools of public health, 233
Nutrition: McCollum's work in, 86–87, 126–132, 234–235; research in, 62–63, 130–131; scientific study of, 132. See also Chemical hygiene
Nuttall, George, 160
Nutting, Mary Adelaide, 33, 47
Nydegger, James, 75

Occupational health, emergence of department of, 176. See also Baetjer, Anna
Oppenheimer, Ella Hutzler, 78
Organization of School of Hygiene, committee on, 168–172
Otto, Gilbert, 65; hookworm research of, 107
Oyster fishermen, and Baltimore sewerage system, 241n.54

Parasitology, research on, 99–104
Park, Edward A., work of, on rickets, 129
Park, William H.: as De Lamar lecturer, 83; as editor, 161; and first school of hygiene and public health, 33, 35; on Welch-Rose Report, 43
Parker, Sylvia, 65
Parran, Thomas: and evaluation of schools of public health, 222, 223–226; and syphilis study, 210
Parran-Farrand report, 224–226
Parsons, Helen, 65, 86
Patents, control of, 177
Pathological disciplines, as dominant, 159–160
Pathological Division, of new school, 55
Pathological hygiene, 5; disciplines of, 97–121
Paton, Stewart, 163
Paula, Geraldo de Souza, 76
Pearce, Richard, and new building, 92
Pearl, Raymond: character of, 138; and contraceptive bureau, 204–209; contributions of, 136–146; as editor, 160; on first faculty, 63–64; heads organi-

zational committee, 85, 87; outline of research of, 139–140; photo, 137; research activities of, 142–143; research grants for, 178, 179

Pearson, Karl, 63, 64

Peirce, Katherine, work of, in Eastern Health District, 190

Peking Union Medical College, 220

Pellagra, research on cause of, 22

Personal hygiene: course on, 125–126; Howell, on importance of, 124

Personality disorders: and low economic status, 199–200; rates of, 200

Pettenkofer, Max von: concept of, 54, 57; on economics of public health, 29; Institute of Hygiene of, as model, 122; on value of sanitary reform, 14

Phillips, Amy, 65

Phipps Clinic, 197–199

Physicians: attraction to public health in 1930s, 181; encouragement of, by Rockefeller Foundation, 165; as first students, 73–75; less exclusive role in public health, 233; need for, in public health, 78; not attracted to public health, 163–165; and professional struggle with sanitary engineers, 22–25, 150. See also Medicine; Tension

Physiological Division, of new school, 54–55

Physiological hygiene, 5; changes in department of, 174–176; disciplines of, 123–124; research and teaching, 124–126; survival of, 180

Physiology, committee on, 168, 172–176

Pin charts, and social problems, 200–201

Plague, 10

Planned Parenthood, 210

Plasmodium, Hegner's research on, 103

Plotz, Ella Sachs, Foundation, 178

Pneumonia, research on immunity to, 117

Policy, committee on, 171

Political patronage, impact of, on public health officers, 1–2; decrease in influence of, 16; relationship of political interests to public health, 2–3

Population dynamics, as discipline, 143

Porter, William, on hookworm research, 107

Poverty, concept of, 9

Powdermaker, Florence, 65; on faculty, 79; wins fellowship, 79

Preston, James H. (Mayor of Baltimore), and naming of school, 56

Preventive medicine: focus on, 227; teaching of, 228

Preventive Medicine and Hygiene (Rosenau), 32

Pritchett, Ida, 65; on faculty, 79; wins fellowship, 79

Privacy, individual's right to, 199

Promotion, criteria for, 170

Protozoology: as discipline in new school, 55, 97, 98; research in, 65, 99–104; staff photo, 102

Prudden, T. Mitchell, and laboratory method, 19

Public funding, impact of, on school, 180–181. See also New Deal; Social Security

Public health: aims and goals of, 18–19; attraction of medical graduates to, 181; broad approach to, 122; disease-oriented approach to, 20–22; dominance of, by medical men, 22–23; influence of bacteriology on, 19–20; medical schools' lack of interest in, 217; the "new," 96–97, 114–116; practice of, on local level, 235; process of professionalization of, 1–5, 14–15; relationship of, to medicine, 2, 6, 164–165, 227–236; relationship of, to other disciplines, 5–6; social conception of, 39

Public health administration: department of, 146–149; faculty appointments in, 66–68

Public health education: contrasting views on, 66; debates about, 6–7; early concepts of, 215; English method of, 6; federal funding for, 181, 218; German method of, 6–7; Hopkins model of, 235–236; main tasks of, 3–6; medical model for, 232; social orientation to, 234

Public health employment, structure of, 164–165

Public health nursing: neglect of, 233; reluctance to train in, 169; role of in mental hygiene programs, 204; training in considered by school, 185; training in denied, 81

Public health officers: before twentieth century, 9–16; demand for, 78–79; federal funds for training, 181, 218; Ferrell on, 29; qualifications for, 24–25; relationship of, to medicine, 37

Public health policy, McCollum's work in, 131–132

Public health practice, Freeman's work in, 148

Public health schools. *See* Schools of public health

Public health services: delivery of, 182–214; as expanding, 224; funding for, 181; impact of Welch-Rose Report on, 236

Quarantine regulations, and disease control, 10–11

Quarterly Review of Biology, 142

Rabbits: "Dutchbelt," 119; as experimental animals, 117, 119

Radiation, Clark's course on physiological effects of, 125

Raffel, Sidney, research of, 119

Rask, Olaf, courses of, 131

Rat, as experimental animal, 62–63, 127

Reagents, preparation of, 119–120

Records, patients': in Bureau of Contraceptive Advice, 209; statistical analysis of, 208

Reed, Lowell: personality of, 138–139; contributions of, 138–146; as dean, 181; on demand for public health training, 218–219; on editorial board, 162; on first faculty, 64; photo, 144–145; as teacher, 139; work of, in biostatistics, 143–146

Reed, Walter, cause of yellow fever diagnosed by, 17

Reed-Frost epidemic curve, 143

"Reed-Frost epidemic theory," 256n.43

Reform, public health, 13–16

Regionalization of health services, concept of, 229–230

Research: emphasis on shared, 233; as focus of Welch report, 41; new emphasis on applied, 180–181; primary role of, 215–216

Research Corporation, 179

Research grants, handling of, 177–179

Rhetta, Dr. B. M., and segregation, 81

Richards, Esther, courses of, 181

Rickets, McCollum's research on, 128–129

Ricksettia, research on, 120

Riley, Robert, 78

Robinson, George H., on faculty, 116

Rockefeller, John D., begins public health investment, 17

Rockefeller Foundation: awards for new building, 92–93; and budget for school, 88–89; fellowships of, in international public health, 219–220; fellowship program of, 79; funds mental hygiene program, 197–198; goal of, in public health education, 220; intervention of, in professionalization of public health, 26–56; on medical education–public health relationship, 227; and public health as profession, 3, 4, 7, 17, 25; reputation of, 30; summer public health fellowships of, 165; on teaching of preventive medicine, 228; on tripartite mission of the school, 84–85, 89

Rockefeller philanthropies, description of, 30

Rockefeller Sanitary Commission, 30; campaign of against hookworm, 27–29. *See also* International Health Board

Rockefeller Sanitary Commission for the Eradication of Hookworm Disease, 17, 105; photo, 28

Rodent ecology project, 212

Roemer, Milton, on medical vs. public health education, 230

Root, Francis, 98; conducts short courses, 79–80; on first faculty, 64, 65; research of, 109–111

Rose, Wickliffe, 3, 26; and conception

Shipley, Paul, work of, on rickets, 129
Sigerist, Henry, promotes national
  health program, 230
Silver, George, and Eastern Health District, 213
Simmonds, Nina, 65, 86; courses of,
  131; photo, 128
Simon, Charles E.: first course on
  viruses, 71; as managing editor of
  American Journal of Hygiene, 160–162;
  research of, 111–113
Sinai Hospital, and Eastern Health Dis-
  trict, 187
Smillie, Wilson G.: on administrative
  problems of Eastern Health District,
  190; on changes needed to effect
  national health program, 232
Smith, Charles, survey of, on teaching
  of preventive medicine, 228
Smith, Homer, 78
Smith, Theobald: as editor, 161; and
  first school of hygiene and public
  health, 33, 35, 36, 38; on Welch-
  Rose Report, 42
Smith-Lever Act of 1914, 40
Socialized medicine: Freeman on, 148;
  Newsholme on, 67; preventive medi-
  cine as, 228
Social problems, transformed into emo-
  tional problems, 201–203
Social sciences, Parran-Farrand report
  on neglect of, 225
Social Security Act, impact of, 181. *See
  also* New Deal
Society of Hygiene, 162–163
Soper, Fred, as Rockefeller fellow, 79
Sources and Modes of Infection, The
  (Chapin), 20
Spaeth, Reynold: on fatigue, 125; report
  of, 86
"Species sanitation," principle of, 109
Squibb, E. R., and Sons, 178
Stebbins, Ernest: and Eastern Health
  District, 212–213; on Frost as
  teacher, 135
Sternberg, George, 19
Stiles, Charles Wardell, 17, 83; on
  hookworm research, 107–108
Stitt, E. R., as editor, 161

Stoll, Norman, 78; and hookworm research, 106
Stuart, Harold, work of, in child health,
  217
Students: career track of, 163–165; first,
  73–85; high proportion of international, 222; mix of, 165–167; "special," 74, 80
Sunshine, as treatment for rickets, 129
Sydenstricker, Edgar, 78; and expanded
  view of public health, 230–231; morbidity study of, 184; and pellagra
  studies, 22; research of, 70
Syphilis study, by Eastern Health District, 210–212. *See also* Venereal disease control

Taliaferro, William H., 65
Teaching, problems of, 167
Tensions: between laboratory and field
  research, 155; between medicine and
  public health, 164–165; between
  pathology and physiology, 155; be-
  tween physicians and sanitary en-
  gineers, 150; between pure and applied sciences, 155
Textbook of Physiology (Howell), 125
Thies, Elizabeth, 158
Tietze, Christopher, and mental hygiene
  study, 204
Tilden, Charles: on curriculum, 150; on
  first faculty, 60
Toronto. *See* University of Toronto
  School of Hygiene
Trace elements, studies on, 129–130
Training, separate for nurses, doctors,
  and sanitary engineers, 219; criticism
  of, 223
Tressler, Donald K., 130
Tropical medicine: development in, 86;
  foundation interest in, 84; Harvard
  proposal for school of, 44: interest in,
  44, 64; London School of, 220–221
Tuberculosis, research on, 135, 193–194
Turner, Thomas B., "Tommy": and
  syphilis control program, 211–212;
  work of, 116
Typhoid fever, transmission of, 19

Ubiquiteers, formation of, 166
United States Bureau of Fisheries, 178
United States Public Health Service: conference of, 248–249n.39; expansion of, 18; Frost's work with, 135–136; research grants of, 179; supports Eastern Health District, 188; and syphilis study, 210–212; and Washington County Health Unit, 183–184
University of California, public health funding for, 226
University of Maryland Hospital and Training School for Nurses, 187
University of Michigan: creates division for public health, 218; as regional, 224; short courses at, 226
University of Minnesota, public health funding for, 226
University of North Carolina, public health funding for, 226
University of Pennsylvania first public health graduates, 31; site visit to, 46
University of Toronto School of Hygiene, 220, 221–222; evaluation of, 225; Parran-Farrand report on, 225

Vanderbilt University: funding of, for short courses, 226; as regional, 224
Vaughn, Victor C., 19; as editor, 161
Venereal disease control, 116; federal funding for, 218; and syphilis study, 210–212
Vincent, George: on British system of public health service, 221; and emphasis on popular health education, 82; Gregg on, 246n.8; on new building, 89, 91–96; as Rockefeller Foundation president, 61
Virology, 113. See also Viruses
Viruses, filterable: Simon's work with, 111–113; study of, 97, 98
Viseltear, Arthur, on APHA and scope of public health, 231
Vital statistics, 54, 55; study of, in public health, 63–64. See also Biometry
Vitamin A, discovery of, 62, 127
Vitamin B, discovery of, 62
Vitamin D, discovery of, 129

Wagner Bill, and national health program, 231
Wander Company, research grants of, 179
Waring, George E. (Colonel), sewerage system of, 241n.53
Warren, Andrew J., evaluation of, 223
Washington, Booker T., 18
Washington County Health Unit, 183–184; objectives of, 183
Water supply, improvements in public, 23–24
Watson, Bob, as Rockefeller fellow, 79
Welch, William Henry, 3, 18, 26, 33; active in mental hygiene movement, 197; and art of negotiation, 57–95; and conception of students, 73; death of, 180; defines public health education, 215; dual commitment of, 122; and first school of hygiene and public health, 35, 38–39; introduces laboratory for teaching public health, 19; lack of interest in public health administration, 66; on longevity, 157–158; mail system of, 158; management philosophy of, 96; meets with site committee, 48; network of, 186–187; and organization plan, 85–89; photo, 53, 58, 77; reputation of, as gastronome, 157; retirement of, 156–158; on sanitary reform, 14; on school as research institute, 81, 82; selected as director, 53–56; serves in WWI, 61; as "statesman," 56; on training for public health, 36
Welch bacillus, research on, 117
Welch Medical Library, 157
Welch-Rose Report, 40–44; continuing influence of, 236; emphasis of, 42; Howell appendix to, 168–169; reactions to, 42–43; Rose version of, 40–41, 42; Welch version of, 41, 42
Wells, H. Gideon, 163
Western Maryland–Fairfield Farms Dairy, 178
"West Points of Public Health," 220
Whipple, George C.: as De Lamar lecturer, 83; on demand for public health officers, 78; and first school of

Whipple, George C. (contd.)
hygiene and public health, 26, 33,
35; on Welch-Rose Report, 42
White, Joseph, and world public health,
219
Willcox, W. F., 83
Williams, Greer: on schools of public
health, 241n.1; on Welch, 36
Williams, George Huntington: 76; as
Baltimore's commissioner of health,
186–192; and Eastern Health District,
212–214
Williams, J. Whitridge: on advantages
of Baltimore, 49; and contraceptive
bureau, 204–208; offers lecture
course, 82
Wilson, Edwin B., 143
Wilson Laboratories, 178
Winfield, Gerald, and experimental
animals, 100–101
Winslow, Charles-Edward A.: on community medical services, 230; and
concept of public health, 21; as De
Lamar lecturer, 83; as editor, 161;
and first school of hygiene and public

health, 26, 32, 33, 35; on lack of personnel, 78–79; on Welch-Rose Report, 42–43; at Yale Medical School,
226; at Yale's Department of Public
Health, 218
Wolfe Street, as divided, 232
Wolman, Abel: on Birth Control
Clinic, 209; career of, 151–154; chal-
lenges medical bias, 233; on first
faculty, 70–71; and national health
program, 231; as teacher, 152–154
Women: discrimination against,
173–176; and public health reforms,
13–14
World Health Organization, 154

Yale University: appraisal of, 226; public
health education in, 34, 39, 218
Yellow fever, research on, 10, 17
Y plan, for medical education, 25

Zinsser, Hans, 33, 60; as editor, 161
Zoology, medical: definition of, 99; as
department, 97; research in, 98